Taking SIDES

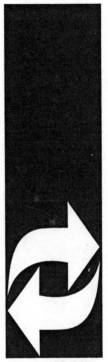

Clashing Views on Controversial Issues in Health and Society

Second Edition

Taking SIDES

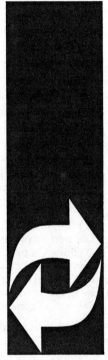

Clashing Views on Controversial Issues in Health and Society

Second Edition

Edited, Selected, and with Introductions by

Eileen L. Daniel
State University of New York College at Brockport

Dushkin Publishing Group/Brown & Benchmark Publishers
A Times Mirror Higher Education Group Company

To Mom and Dad with thanks

Photo Acknowledgments

Part 1   Capitol Building/Congressional News Photos
Part 2   State of Minnesota Department of Economic Development
Part 3   Drug Enforcement Agency
Part 4   American Cancer Society
Part 5   Digital Stock
Part 6   General Electric Company
Part 7   Pam Carley/DPG

Cover Art Acknowledgment

Charles Vitelli

Library of Congress Cataloging-in-Publication Data

Main entry under title:
    Taking sides: clashing views on controversial issues in health and society/edited, selected, and with introductions by Eileen L. Daniel.—2nd ed.
    Includes bibliographical references and index.
    1. Health. 2. Medical care—United States. 3. Medical ethics. 4. Social medicine—United States. I. Daniel, Eileen L., *comp.*

362.1

1-56134-444-3   95-74673

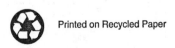

Printed on Recycled Paper

PREFACE

This book contains 40 articles arranged in 20 *pro* and *con* pairs. Each pair addresses a controversial issue in health and society, expressed in terms of a question in order to draw the lines of debate more clearly.

The questions that are included here relate to health topics of current concern, such as AIDS, abortion, environmental health, and drug use and abuse. The authors of these articles take strong stands on specific issues and provide support for their positions. Although we may not agree with a particular point of view, each author clearly defines his or her stand on the issues.

This book is divided into seven parts, each containing related issues. Each issue is preceded by an *introduction*, which sets the stage for the debate, gives historical background on the subject, and provides a context for the controversy. Each issue concludes with a *postscript*, which offers a summary of the debate, some concluding observations, and suggestions for further reading on the subject. The postscript also raises further points because all issues have more than two sides. At the back of the book is a listing of all the *contributors to this volume*, which gives information on the physicians, professors, journalists, theologians, and scientists whose views are debated here.

Taking Sides: Clashing Views on Controversial Issues in Health and Society is a tool to encourage critical thought on important health issues. Readers should not feel confined to the views expressed in the selections. Some readers may see important points on both sides of an issue and may construct for themselves a new and creative approach, which may incorporate the best of both sides or provide an entirely new vantage point for understanding.

Changes to this edition   This second edition of *Taking Sides: Clashing Views on Controversial Issues in Health and Society* includes some significant changes from the first edition. Eight completely new issues have been added: *Is There a Health Care Crisis in the United States?* (Issue 1); *Should the Government Require U.S. Medical Schools to Produce More Primary Care Doctors?* (Issue 2); *Is Gun Control a Public Health Issue?* (Issue 5); *Does Health Care Delivery and Research Benefit Men at the Expense of Women?* (Issue 12); *Is AIDS a Major Threat to the Heterosexual, Non-Drug-Abusing Population?* (Issue 13); *Is Yo-Yo Dieting Dangerous?* (Issue 14); *Is the Gulf War Syndrome Real?* (Issue 16); and *Does Exposure to Electromagnetic Fields Cause Cancer?* (Issue 18). For four of the issues retained from the previous edition, the issue question has been significantly modified and both selections have been replaced in order to focus the debate more sharply and to bring it up to date: Issue 6 on healthy behavior; Issue 8 on secondhand smoke; Issue 9 on the disease model of addiction; and Issue 15 on vitamin C. For the issues on physician-assisted suicide (Issue 3), health care

i

for the elderly (Issue 4), positive mental attitude (Issue 7), drug legalization (Issue 10), and chiropractors (Issue 20), one or both of the selections have been replaced to provide new points of view. In all, 31 of the 40 selections are new.

A word to the instructor   An *Instructor's Manual With Test Questions* (multiple-choice and essay) is available through the publisher for instructors using *Taking Sides* in the classroom. Also available is a general guidebook, *Using Taking Sides in the Classroom*, which discusses teaching techniques and methods for integrating the pro-con approach of *Taking Sides* into any classroom setting.

Acknowledgments   Special thanks to John, Diana, and Jordan. Also, thanks to my colleagues at the State University of New York College at Brockport for all their helpful contributions. I was also assisted in preparing this edition by the valuable suggestions from the adopters of *Taking Sides* who filled out comment cards or returned questionnaires:

Barry Brock
Barry University

Gary L. Chandler
Gardner-Webb University

David B. Claxton
Western Carolina University

Barbara Cole
Texas Tech University

Gina Giovinco
University of Central Florida

Barney R. Groves
Virginia Commonwealth
   University

MaryAnn Janosik
Lake Erie College

Kim Lim
SUNY College at Cortland

Marge A. O'Leary
College of Saint Francis

Linda Peterson
North Seattle Community
   College

Cheryl Rainey
Clemson University

Nancy Schlapman
Indiana University at
   Kokomo

Richard C. Vallone
University of North Florida

Many of your recommendations were incorporated into this edition. Finally, I appreciate the assistance of Mimi Egan, publisher for the Taking Sides series, David Dean, administrative assistant, and David Brackley, copy editor, of Dushkin Publishing Group/Brown and Benchmark Publishers.

Eileen L. Daniel
State University of New York College at Brockport

CONTENTS IN BRIEF

CONTENTS

Nancy F. McKenzie, executive director of Health/PAC, maintains that health
care in America has gone well beyond the crisis point. Irwin M. Stelzer,
director of Regulatory Policy Studies at the American Enterprise Institute,
argues that although there is some need for reform, overall, the health care
system in the United States is based on reasonable costs and the provision of
high-quality care.

James Nolan, physician and chair of the Department of Medicine at the State
University of New York at Buffalo, argues that government regulation of med-
ical schools would help meet the need for primary care physicians. Richard A.
Cooper, dean of the Medical College of Wisconsin and director of its Health
Policy Institute, strongly objects to government regulation of the educational
process.

Timothy E. Quill, M.D., describes a physician-assisted suicide and asserts that
doctors have roles other than healing and fighting against death. Physicians
Herbert Hendin and Gerald Klerman argue that there is a great potential for
abuse if physician-assisted suicide is legalized.

Hastings Center director Daniel Callahan believes that medical care for elderly people should not involve expensive health care services that serve
only to forestall death. Physicians Ezekiel J. Emanuel and Linda L. Emanuel
argue that cost savings due to limitations in medical care at the end of life are
not likely to be substantial.

Physician Jerome P. Kassirer argues that guns, particularly guns in the household, are a major public health threat. Journalist J. Neil Schulman argues that
the issue of gun control is not an epidemiological concern but a criminological
one.

Michael F. Jacobson, the director of the Center for Science in the Public Interest, claims that federal policies emphasizing healthy behavior would reduce health care spending. Physician Faith T. Fitzgerald argues that there is a need to reassess the role of preventive medicine, which she feels should not try to control people's behavior for their own good.

Author Marc Barasch asserts that some people can cure themselves of disease by maintaining an optimistic, upbeat attitude. Freelance writer Ellen Switzer argues that state of mind does not significantly affect the outcome of an illness.

The editors of *Consumer Reports* argue that there is sound scientific data proving that secondhand smoke causes lung cancer and other illnesses. Editor and journalist Jacob Sullum argues that there is no evidence that secondhand smoking carries the dangers associated with actually smoking.

Physician George E. Vaillant maintains that alcoholism should be treated as a disease and not as a behavioral problem or character flaw. Journalist Joann Ellison Rodgers argues that the theory that alcoholism and drug addiction are diseases is outdated.

Theologian Joseph P. Kane asserts that legalizing drugs will help prevent crime and violence. Gerald W. Lynch, president of the John Jay College of Criminal Justice, and Roberta Blotner, director of the City University of New York's substance abuse prevention programs, claim that legalizing drugs would increase drug usage and addiction.

Author Mary Gordon believes that abortion is an acceptable means to end an unwanted pregnancy. Editor Jason DeParle argues that the 3 out of 10 pregnancies that currently end in abortion raise many moral questions.

Health and medical reporters Leslie Laurence and Beth Weinhouse claim that women have been excluded from most research on new drugs and medical treatments. Physician Andrew G. Kadar argues that women actually receive more medical care and benefit more from medical research than do men.

William B. Johnston, the vice president of the Hudson Institute, and Kevin R. Hopkins, an adjunct senior fellow of the Hudson Institute, warn that unless people make a serious attempt to alter behaviors that put them at risk for AIDS, the heterosexual population will be facing an AIDS epidemic. Michael Fumento, a former AIDS analyst, claims that AIDS will not devastate white, middle-class heterosexuals.

Nutritionist Frances M. Berg contends that yo-yo dieting, or weight cycling, is associated with an elevated risk of physical and mental health problems. The National Task Force on the Prevention and Treatment of Obesity maintains that there is no convincing evidence that weight cycling has any major effects on health or the effectiveness of future diets.

Patricia Long, a journalist who specializes in health issues, suggests that people would benefit from higher levels of vitamin C than those currently recommended by the government. Physician and attorney Victor Herbert maintains that megadoses of vitamin C may harm more people than they help.

Journalists Dennis Bernstein and Thea Kelley claim that disabling, sometimes life-threatening medical problems related to environmental and chemical exposure are currently affecting thousands of soldiers who fought in the Persian Gulf War. Michael Fumento, a science and economics reporter, argues that medical experts have not found any evidence to support the existence of a syndrome related to the war.

Pesticide researchers Lawrie Mott and Karen Snyder maintain that fruits and vegetables sold to consumers are contaminated with harmful pesticide residues. Professor of biochemistry and molecular biology Bruce Ames argues that any risks from pesticides in foods are minimal.

Journalist Paul Brodeur argues that exposure to electromagnetic fields (EMFs) emitted from high-voltage power lines can cause cancer. Reporter Gary Taubes contends that selective reporting of scientific evidence has generated unnecessary public anxiety about electromagnetic fields.

Health writer Royce Flippin argues that all children should be immunized against potentially dangerous childhood diseases. Health journalist Richard Leviton maintains that many vaccines are neither safe nor effective.

Rick Weiss, a staff writer for *Health* magazine, contends that patients with back pain who are treated by chiropractors are generally more satisfied with their treatment than those treated by medical doctors. The editors of the *Harvard Medical School Health Letter* argue that many chiropractors adhere to a philosophy that is unproven at best and harmful at worst.

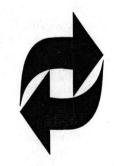

INTRODUCTION

Dimensions and Approaches to the Study of Health and Society

Eileen L. Daniel

WHAT IS HEALTH?

Traditionally, being healthy meant being absent of illness. If someone did not have a disease, then he or she was considered to be healthy. The overall health of a nation or specific population was determined by numbers measuring illness, disease, and death rates. Today, this rather negative view of assessing individual health and health in general is changing. A healthy person is one who is not only free from disease but also fully well.

Being well, or wellness, involves the interrelationship of many dimensions of health: physical, emotional, social, mental, and spiritual. This multifaceted view of health reflects a holistic approach, which includes individuals' taking responsibility for their own well-being.

Our health and longevity are affected by the many choices we make every day: Medical reports tell us that if we abstain from smoking, taking drugs, excessive alcohol consumption, and eating foods that contain too much fat and cholesterol, and if we exercise regularly, our rate of disease and disability will significantly decrease. These reports, while not totally conclusive, have encouraged many people to make positive lifestyle changes. Millions of people have quit smoking; alcohol consumption is down; and more and more individuals are exercising regularly and eating low-fat diets. While these changes are encouraging, many people who have been unable or unwilling to make these changes are left feeling worried or guilty over continuing their negative health behaviors.

But disagreement exists among the experts about the exact nature of positive health behaviors, which causes confusion. For example, some scientists claim that overweight people should make efforts to lose weight, even if it takes many tries. Other researchers claim that dieting itself can be more dangerous than being overweight. Who do you believe? Experts disagree on a wide variety of topics, including the health risks of being exposed to electromagnetic fields from power lines or appliances, whether or not chiropractors are legitimate health providers, and the role of vitamin C in preventing cancer and heart disease.

Health status is also affected by society and government. Societal pressures have helped pass smoking restrictions in public places, mandatory safety belt legislation, and laws permitting condom distribution in public schools. The government plays a role in the health of individuals as well, although it has failed to provide even minimal health care for many low-income Americans.

Unfortunately, there are no absolute answers to many questions regarding health and wellness issues. Moral questions, controversial concerns, and individual perceptions of health matters all can create opposing views. As you evaluate the issues in this book, you should keep an open mind toward both sides. You may not change your mind regarding the morality of abortion or the limitation of health care for the elderly, but you will still be able to learn from the opposing viewpoints.

WELLNESS, BEHAVIOR, AND SOCIETY

The issues in this book are divided into seven parts. The first deals with health and society. Issue 1 debates whether or not there is a health care crisis in the United States. The importance of this issue is clear: approximately 35 to 40 million Americans have no health insurance; there has been a nationwide resurgence in infectious diseases, such as tuberculosis; antibiotic-resistant strains of bacterial infections threaten thousands of Americans; and those enrolled in government programs such as Medicaid often have difficulty finding physicians who will accept them as patients because reimbursements are so low and the paperwork is so cumbersome. On the other hand, Americans continue to live longer and longer, and for the majority of the population, the health care available in the United States is among the best in the world. Issue 2 deals with a related topic: whether or not the disproportionate number of medical specialists as compared to primary care physicians has caused a crisis in health care costs and a high demand for general practitioners. Issue 3 deals with whether or not physicians should participate in the deaths of hopelessly ill patients. Although many people agree that doctors should not prolong the lives of terminally ill patients, particularly if doing so goes against the patients' wishes, do elderly people who want to live as long as possible deserve special consideration? In Issue 4, Daniel Callahan, the director of the Hastings Center, argues that the increasing proportion of health care dollars that is going to the elderly should be curbed because it is a major contributor to the high cost of health care. Physicians Ezekiel J. Emanuel and Linda L. Emanuel disagree with Callahan, claiming that there would not be a significant saving if health care for the elderly were rationed. The fifth controversy in this section is about the epidemic of gun-related deaths and the potential benefits of more stringent gun control. Many doctors and public health officials claim that homicide involving guns is increasing in the United States and that this trend is escalating health care costs and diminishing quality of life. They feel that gun control would help reduce the number of shootings and deaths. Opponents argue that under gun control, only criminals would have access to guns, not law-abiding citizens. They also contend that doctors should leave the gun control issue to criminologists.

MIND/BODY RELATIONSHIP

Part 2 discusses two important issues related to the relationship between mind and body: Should Healthy Behavior Be Mandated? and, Can a Positive Mental Attitude Overcome Disease? Over the past 10 years, both laypeople and the medical profession have placed an emphasis on the prevention of illness as a way to improve health. Not smoking, for instance, certainly reduces the risk of developing lung cancer. However, the current U.S. health care system places an emphasis on treatment rather than prevention, even though prevention is less expensive, less painful, and more humane. In Issue 6, microbiologist Michael F. Jacobson claims that the emphasis on treatment has neglected prevention. Physician Faith T. Fitzgerald argues that overpromotion of prevention and blaming the sick for causing their own illnesses by smoking or overeating is not productive. Not everyone, she adds, is capable of making positive lifestyle changes.

As Jacobson claims, we can be responsible for much of our own well-being by practicing positive health behaviors. Marc Barasch, in Issue 7, argues that we can also control our health by maintaining a positive mental attitude. He claims that the mind can influence the body by affecting the immune system. A positive mental attitude can boost the immune system, which, in turn, can help fight disease. Ellen Switzer counters that there is no concrete proof that people can prevent or slow a disease's progress by maintaining a positive mental state. Blaming people for causing their own diseases through negative states of mind, she argues, ignores the real causes of disease.

SUBSTANCE USE AND ABUSE

Part 3 introduces current issues related to drug use and abuse. Millions of Americans use and abuse drugs that alter their minds and affect their bodies. These drugs range from illegal substances, such as crack cocaine and opiates, to the widely used legal drugs alcohol and tobacco. Use of these substances can lead to physical and psychological addiction and the related problems of family dysfunction, reduced worker productivity, and crime. Particularly because of crime involving illegal drugs, many experts have argued for the legalization of drugs, particularly marijuana. The logic is that if drugs were legalized, the enormous profits from illegal drug sales would not exist, drug dealers would be out of business, and law enforcement officials could therefore focus on other areas of crime.

The drug crisis in America is often related to changes in or a breakdown of traditional values. The collapse of strong family and religious influences may affect drug usage, especially among young people. It has been argued, however, that some people, regardless of societal or familial influences, will use drugs based on some inherent need or inherited factor. This is particularly true in relation to alcoholism. For some time, experts have maintained that addiction to drugs and alcohol is an inherited disease because it appears to run in families. Other experts disregard the disease model of addiction and argue that drug abuse and excessive drinking are voluntary behaviors that are within an individual's control.

Also in this section is a debate on secondhand smoke. Some studies have shown that nonsmokers who are forced to breathe tobacco smoke run a higher risk of developing lung cancer and other diseases that are primarily related to smoking. The tobacco industry and some journalists respond that the Environmental Protection Agency has altered the data on the relationship between passive smoking and health and that secondhand smoke is not nearly as dangerous as actually smoking.

SEXUALITY AND GENDER ISSUES

The issues in Part 4 debate topics related to gender and sexuality. A particularly divisive topic is the use of abortion to end an unwanted pregnancy. Mary Gordon believes that abortion is acceptable and argues in Issue 11 that it is not an immoral choice for women. Jason DeParle, in opposition, discusses why liberals and feminists do not like to talk about the morality of abortion. The abortion issue continues to cause major controversy. More restrictions have been placed on the right to abortion as a result of the political power wielded by the pro-life faction. Pro-choice followers, however, argue that making abortion illegal again will force many women to obtain dangerous "back alley" abortions. Complicating the issue has been the recent killings and shootings of doctors and other personnel involved with abortion.

Issue 12 is a debate over whether or not our health care system favors men at the expense of women. Although women on average live longer than men, many women claim that they have been excluded from pharmaceutical tests and other medical research and that they receive inferior care when they see doctors. Reporters Leslie Laurence and Beth Weinhouse, arguing from this viewpoint, contend that women have been ignored in medical research, are not adequately treated for heart disease (a leading cause of death among women), and are not taken seriously by their doctors. Physician Andrew G. Kadar disagrees with this premise. He claims that women see their doctors more frequently than men, are hospitalized more often than men, and continue to outlive men by several years.

Issue 13 focuses on whether or not AIDS is a serious risk to the heterosexual, non-drug-abusing population. William B. Johnston and Kevin R. Hopkins feel that as heterosexuals become more sexually active, their risk of contracting AIDS increases. They argue that unless the heterosexual population drastically alters its sexual habits soon, a widespread AIDS epidemic is inevitable. Michael Fumento, on the other hand, believes that the AIDS epidemic has peaked and that heterosexual transmission has actually decreased. According to Fumento, the general population was *never* at a high risk for contracting the disease.

NUTRITION AND HEALTH

Is it healthier to remain overweight than to diet repeatedly? Will taking large doses of vitamins, particularly vitamin C, improve health? These questions are discussed in Part 5, which deals with nutrition and dieting. Millions of Americans are dieting, many going on one diet after another in an effort to achieve a lean figure. Does constant dieting increase one's risk of heart disease and other medical problems? And does it become harder to lose weight the more frequently one diets? These questions are explored in Issue 14.

Will taking megadoses of vitamins help prevent many serious diseases, such as cancer and heart disease? New research indicates that the current recommendations for many vitamins, including vitamin C, are inadequate for our changing lifestyles. People today are under considerable stress, are exposed to increasing amounts of environmental pollutants, often use drugs, and frequently eat away from home. These factors may make it impossible for individuals to meet their needs for vitamins via diet alone. While vitamins prevent deficiency diseases, it appears that specific vitamins may also be beneficial in the treatment and prevention of certain illnesses, such as cancer and heart disease, and may prolong life by several years. Experts warn, however, that the large doses often recommended to prevent disease can have side effects or be toxic and that it is still safest simply to eat a balanced diet that includes plenty of fruits and vegetables.

ENVIRONMENTAL ISSUES

Debate continues over fundamental issues surrounding the environment: human needs and the future of the environment. The debate becomes more heated as environmental issues move closer to human concerns, such as health, economic interests, and politics. In Issue 16, for example, the debate focuses on whether or not troops stationed overseas during the Persian Gulf War were exposed to harmful environmental or chemical substances during combat that caused the health problems many of the soldiers are currently suffering. Issue 17 discusses the safety of pesticide usage on fruits and vegetables. The Alar (a chemical growth regulator for apples) scare in the mid-1980s, in which it was widely reported that a by-product of Alar is a carcinogen, convinced many Americans that the apple supply was not safe and that an apple a day could cause cancer. At the same time, nutritionists as well as the Department of Agriculture were urging people to eat more fruits and vegetables to help *prevent* cancer. Another major issue is the alleged risk of exposure to electromagnetic fields (EMFs) given off by power lines and appliances that use electricity. Reports linking exposure to EMFs with leukemia and other cancers have made headlines. In Issue 18, Paul Brodeur argues that EMF exposure presents a genuine danger and that the power industry has gone to great lengths to cover it up. Gary Taubes maintains that there is no real proof that EMFs present a health risk.

MAKING CHOICES FOR THE HEALTH CARE CONSUMER

Part 7 introduces questions about particular issues related to choices about health care services. The questions here are, Should All Children Be Immunized Against Childhood Diseases? and, Are Chiropractors Legitimate Health Providers?

At the turn of the century, millions of American children developed childhood diseases such as tetanus, polio, measles, and pertussis (whooping cough). Many of these children died or became permanently disabled because of these illnesses. Today, vaccines exist to prevent all of these conditions; however, not all children receive their recommended immunizations. Some do not get vaccinated until the schools require them, and others are allowed exemptions. More and more, parents are requesting exemptions from some or all vaccinations based on fears over their safety and effectiveness. The pertussis vaccination seems to generate the biggest fears. Reports of serious injury to children following the pertussis vaccination (usually given in a combination of diphtheria, pertussis, and tetanus, or DPT) have convinced many parents to forgo immunization. As a result, the rates of measles and pertussis have been climbing after decades of decline. Is it safer to be vaccinated than to risk getting pertussis? Most medical societies and physicians believe so, but Richard Leviton, in Issue 19, argues that many vaccines are neither safe nor effective.

Current views of chiropractors and the practice of spinal manipulation are discussed in Issue 20. Due to demand by the public, chiropractors are achieving new legitimacy, despite the efforts of traditional medicine to discredit them. Traditionalists view chiropractors as a notch above quacks, but at the same time, more and more people are turning to spinal manipulation for relief from their backaches, headaches, and other conditions.

Will the many debates presented in this book ever be resolved? Some issues may resolve themselves because of the availability of resources. For instance, funding for health care for the elderly may become restricted in the United States, as it is in the United Kingdom, simply because there are increasingly limited resources to go around. An overhaul of the U.S. health care system to provide care for all while keeping costs down seems inevitable; most Americans agree that the system must be changed. Other controversies may require the test of time for resolution. Several more years may be required before it can be determined if electromagnetic field exposure is positively linked to cancer. The debates over the effectiveness of megadoses of vitamins may also require years of additional research.

Other controversies may never resolve themselves. There may never be a consensus over the issues of abortion, gun control, physician-assisted suicide, or the disease model of addiction. This book will introduce you to many ongoing controversies on a variety of sensitive and complex health-related topics. In order to have a good grasp of one's own viewpoint, it is necessary to be familiar with and understand the points made by the opposition.

PART 1

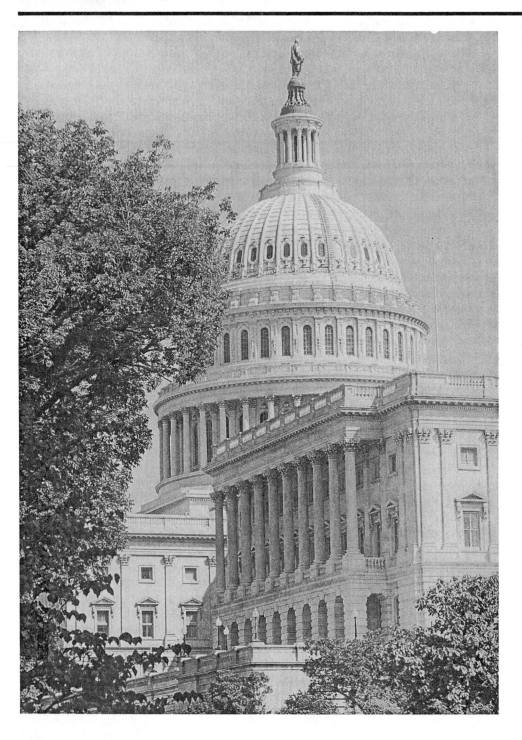

Health and Society

The United States currently faces many frightening health problems, including rising health care costs, an aging population, and a lack of health care insurance for millions of people. Society must confront the enormous financial burden of providing health care to a growing elderly population. At the same time, the government has not been able or willing to meet the health care needs of low-income Americans. Medical and financial resources remain limited for some, while demands increase. To further complicate the problem, public policy and medical ethics have not always kept pace with rapidly growing technology and scientific advances. This section discusses some of the major controversies concerning the role of society in health concerns.

- Is There a Health Care Crisis in the United States?

- Should the Government Require U.S. Medical Schools to Produce More Primary Care Doctors?

- Should Doctors Ever Help Terminally Ill Patients Commit Suicide?

- Should Health Care for the Elderly Be Limited?

- Is Gun Control a Public Health Issue?

ISSUE 1

Is There a Health Care Crisis in the United States?

YES: Nancy F. McKenzie, from "The Real Health Care Crisis," *The Nation* (February 28, 1994)

NO: Irwin M. Stelzer, from "What Health-Care Crisis?" *Commentary* (February 1994)

ISSUE SUMMARY

YES: Nancy F. McKenzie, executive director of Health/PAC, maintains that health care in America has gone well beyond the crisis point and that Americans are "currently suffering the effects of the skewed health financing policies of the past thirty years."

NO: Irwin M. Stelzer, director of Regulatory Policy Studies at the American Enterprise Institute, argues that although there is some need for reform, overall, the health care system in the United States is based on reasonable costs, the provision of high-quality care, and a private system that functions much more efficiently than publicly run programs.

In November 1992 Bill Clinton was elected president of the United States. In his inaugural address, referring to a campaign promise, Clinton claimed that he would "use what's right with American health care to fix what's wrong with American health care."

Many Americans have perceived serious wrongs with the current health care system. In general, people would like to see improvement in the following areas: (1) access to health care for the 35–40 million who are currently uninsured, (2) the ability to keep one's health insurance when one changes or loses a job, and (3) control over the escalating costs of health care.

Health care in the United States is handled by various unrelated agencies and organizations and through a number of programs, including private insurance, government-supported Medicaid for the needy, and Medicare for the elderly. Currently, about 16 percent of the population do not have any health insurance and do not qualify for government-sponsored programs. These people must often do without any medical care at all or suffer financial catastrophe if illness occurs. A *New York Times* article in 1992 claimed that 50 percent of personal bankruptcies in the United States have been attributed to medical costs.

U.S. health care is the most expensive in the world. The United States spends more on health care than any other nation, about $2,600 per capita. The share of the national output of wealth—the gross domestic product (GDP)—expended by the United States on health is 14 percent and rising. Yet the United States has a lower life expectancy, a higher infant mortality rate, and a higher percentage of low-birthweight infants than Canada, Japan, and most Western European nations. Considering the enormous amount of money spent on health care, it is ironic that the United States is the only industrialized nation other than South Africa that does not provide government-sponsored health care for all its citizens.

There are many explanations for why the American health care system costs so much. One argument is that malpractice lawsuits brought by patients against physicians have led to astronomical settlements. This, in turn, has led to rising premiums that doctors must pay for malpractice coverage and to physicians practicing "defensive medicine" by ordering excessive tests and procedures. Extra paperwork and administrative costs related to second-guessing of doctors' judgments by insurance companies have also driven up costs. Another argument involves the expense of advancing technology coupled with the often highly competitive medical market: if one hospital orders a million-dollar piece of equipment, competing hospitals in the same area often decide that they must have the same equipment for their patients.

Some argue that there is a health care crisis in America because medicine in the United States is run as a business that must generate profit rather than as a social service, as it is in other countries. Furthermore, the burden of social problems in the United States has significantly contributed to the demands on medicine. Homicides, assaults, drug abuse, escalating cases of infectious diseases such as tuberculosis, and the highest rate of acquired immunodeficiency syndrome (AIDS) cases in the industrialized world have all posed serious problems for the American health care system.

All of these issues have led much of the American public to believe that there is a major health care crisis in the United States. In the following selections, Nancy F. McKenzie, executive director of Health/PAC, argues that there is no health care system in the United States, just "a marketplace for the buying and selling of life and death." As a result, the poor and minorities receive substandard care and suffer more disability and premature death. Irwin M. Stelzer, director of Regulatory Policy Studies at the American Enterprise Institute, argues that the health care system in America is reasonably priced and that poor health and high mortality cannot be blamed solely on the system. He maintains that there is no crisis, only a few repairable concerns.

YES   Nancy F. McKenzie

THE REAL HEALTH CARE CRISIS

Lately, as the debate over health care reform has grown more heated, more scrambled and more overloaded by competing lobbies, a new approach has surfaced offering a respite to those overwhelmed by the mind-numbing details: Relax, there is no health care crisis. You can hear it from Clinton friend and foe alike. "Our country has health care problems, but no health care crisis," growled Senator Bob Dole in his televised response to the President's State of the Union Message. Days earlier, Democratic Senator Pat Moynihan said pretty much the same on *Meet the Press*. What nonsense!

In fact, health care in America is beyond crisis. We are currently suffering the effects of the skewed health financing policies of the past thirty years. The Reagan/Bush era saw the economic rout of everyone but the very rich, and in health care the dismantling of public programs, preventive care and basic physician education and training, as well as the failure to oversee private insurers. Cuts in safety-net programs between 1980 and 1992 were substantial: 23 percent in maternal health services, 28 percent in preventive health services, 40 percent in community clinics (after adjusting for the health care inflation rate), 63 percent in community development and housing assistance.

Today, only a small portion of doctors choose to provide primary care—family practice services, internal medicine, obstetrics/gynecology—and only a small percentage of those will treat poor patients. Public entitlements are so restrictive in their coverage and meager in their payments to physicians that many who do provide basic care are opting out of Medicaid altogether as well as parts of the Medicare program. The institutional exclusion of the sick poor also occurs in the private arena. A 1990 study in New York City found a total of just twenty-eight primary-care physicians for 1.6 million people in the city's nine lowest income communities. In New York State, only 15 percent of physicians regularly see Medicaid patients. And in major cities across the nation, 50 percent of all admissions to public hospitals are through the emergency room because so many individuals lack physicians. The result:

- The maternal mortality rate of women of color is three times that of white women. One-half to one-third of these deaths are unnecessary and could easily be avoided using preventive measures, given that they are primarily attributable to lack of prenatal care.

- Because they come so late to treatment, only 22 percent of women diagnosed with breast cancer at New York City's Harlem Hospital live five years, compared with 76 percent of white women and 64 percent of black women nationwide.

- A child in Chile or Malaysia is more likely to celebrate his first birthday than a black baby born in the Mississippi Delta.

- Black men in central Harlem are less likely to reach age 65 than men in Bangladesh.

- Estimates of HIV [human immunodeficiency virus] infection among homeless individuals go as high as 40 percent.

- After controlling for differences in age, sex, race and specific disease, the uninsured are as much as three times more likely to die during a hospital stay than the insured.

In the United States over the past twenty years, health care increasingly has been redefined to mean the provision of medical services alone. Broader threats to health, such as lead poisoning, stress and lack of housing, as well as rehabilitative strategies and long-term care, have all dropped out of health discourse. The predictable result is that the system is now besieged by public health crises it is unequipped to handle. For twelve years we have had an AIDS [acquired immunodeficiency syndrome] epidemic that, by international standards, is unnecessarily vast. In 1988 there was a syphilis scare. In 1989–90 there was a measles epidemic due to a national shrinking of childhood immunization programs. Now it is tuberculosis [TB].

In the past ten years, the United States has been ravaged by a tuberculosis epidemic of staggering proportions, largely among individuals between the ages of 25 and 44. Despite the preventability and curability of TB, cases in New York City, for example, have doubled since 1985, to 52 per 100,000 in 1992 (the national incidence was 10.5 cases per 100,000). New York City's black and Latino communities have five times the national average, and comprise 80 percent of cases in the state. Currently, 19 percent of TB cases in the city are multiple-drug resistant because of inconsistent treatment and individuals' lack of connection to health facilities. As a result, public health officials here and abroad are worried that America has created a new and essentially untreatable TB strain.

The response to the current TB epidemic reveals not only the inadequacy of the health care system but the limitations of the current debate on health care reform. The re-emergence and flourishing of this nineteenth-century disease is only the latest wave of health disasters to batter a population increasingly lacking in housing, employment and public and primary health care; that is, more and more people lack the basic human services essential for a community's well-being. The current debate ignores the fact that the public and primary health care infrastructure, which could be expected to treat TB patients, has been dismantled and abandoned, or increasingly replaced by managed-care cost containment programs.

* * *

To their credit, both Bill and Hillary Clinton have attacked the "no crisis" defense of the status quo. But for them, the crisis is centered not on the lack of care for the poorest and sickest among us but on the explosion in *costs*—burdening business and government alike—and on the insecurity of those millions lacking insurance coverage or in danger of losing it.

To address the cost and coverage problems, Clinton's health reform plan claims to establish a universal entitlement to health care for all Americans. But when the President talks about health security, he means health *insurance* security, immortalized in wallet-sized plastic. And this focus on private insurance has tremendous implications, as the past fifty years of employer-based coverage have shown us. The President tells us that under his plan, everyone—organized into large pools of consumers known as health alliances—will have access to insurance that does not discriminate by illness or past condition. But the plan also allows organizations with more than a certain number of employees (currently 5,000, though the Administration now says this is negotiable) to opt out of these alliances, pay a small payroll tax "penalty" and continue their own health plans. But if health alliances don't include the healthiest Americans—the relatively young, working middle-class individuals who tend to be employed by these companies—it will defeat the whole equitable "risk-sharing" rationale of community rating: that they mix individuals likely to be well with individuals likely to be ill.

State-controlled health alliances may attempt to regulate plans to insure that they are representative of the population's heterogeneity. But in fact, it will be difficult, if not impossible, to prevent plans from controlling their exposure to risk by carefully placing services in locations designed to filter out those considered to have undesirable racial and socioeconomic status, a longstanding practice. The same insurance industry that brought us "redlining" by disease and "cherry picking" of healthy people in order to increase profits, is now to be catapulted into the role of "caring" provider, expected to shed its lifelong exclusionary, actuarial habits! As one commentator put it, "Let the Buyer Be Well!"

This problem is easy to see when we look at New York City. The number of Medicaid recipients in New York is sizable. Any alliance that includes them will have a sicker, more vulnerable population. The fact that many people who work in New York City live elsewhere, and that any company with 5,000 employees will be able to have its own corporate alliance, will make New York's regional health alliance uncompetitive compared with those of its neighbors. The premiums city dwellers pay will be higher—they are already 40 percent higher than those of suburban areas. As it is, this two-tiered pattern will occur in all alliances, since the poor will be able to afford only the lowest-cost plan offered, and others will buy better services.

Perhaps that isn't alarming as long as everyone is covered. But the alliance approach doesn't produce any new infrastructure; it uses whatever institutions are already there. And in New York, as across the country, providers have been working very hard to avoid the poorest and sickest among us. Although the Health Security Act contains a provision for aiding providers of essential services, like doctors in rural areas, it does not offer sufficient funds to increase the number of delivery sites or to expand the public health infrastructure. The $2.5 billion per year it earmarks for building new clinics and community-based facilities is half of what the Association of Community Health Centers says is needed for America's 2,147 medically underserved counties. That may seem like a good start, but it has to be viewed against a backdrop of the complete dismantling of Medicaid funding for safety-net hospitals. Hence, it is unclear how the 43 million people in these communities can be adequately served.

Treating the uninsured will change medicine, but no one seems to foresee the implications of this. Without the facilities and providers to deliver the services that the new insurance will cover, there can be no health security. If coverage of the uninsured is really to happen, practitioners, medical schools and insurers will be dealing with disease and people they have heretofore mapped entire institutional strategies to avoid. It is unlikely that this will change, since there is nothing coming out of Washington that will compel providers to do otherwise. The competitive value of cost reduction—the heart of the Clinton plan —is certainly not going to encourage it.

A health care system based on a right to health care would be designed to serve the neediest. It would dictate that health care delivery focus on public health first. Health care delivery could then be designed as a unified system of coherent standards, goals and delivery mechanisms—not a universality of financial plans. Such a system would guarantee both access and equity.

* * *

The problem is that there is no rational structure of health care in the United States, just a marketplace for the buying and selling of life and death. Judging from the narrowness of the current debate, most people seem to have accepted a system that is wholly profit based; in which the pieces of health care they receive—or don't receive—are commodities like all others in a highly developed global economy; in which arguments about decency, justice and responsibility are inappropriate. Hence the focus on controlling costs rather than improving lives. Like a phantom limb, discussion of health care as a social good kicks in at moments but, by and large, it has become an amputated discourse.

Today, most middle-income Americans apparently expect a health care system that responds to public needs about as much as we expect a good public transportation system. Yet individuals also know that something larger, more awful is happening to us: "Medicine" or "health care" is becoming a metaphor for neglect, for what might be monstrous about American life devoid of a belief in the common good. Our caretakers have receded behind institutions with darker, more meanspirited goals. Commodification is one thing; the commodification of medicine is quite another.

Everyone feels the continental shift when the doctor becomes the purveyor, when medicine becomes the corporation and M.B.A.s the moral arbiters. And this does not happen overnight, or directly, though the Clintonian embrace of managed care has accelerated and will complete that process. The American health care system is made up of institutions and entire agencies that function as business managers, executing the financial directives of those providers or regulators. If the institutions in America had a strong health agenda, individual practitioners would not be entrepreneurs. Opportunism and the exploitation of individuals originate within institutions and are hidden by the technical jargon of advanced education. When this happens, as it has in the management mentality that has infected all areas of American life, it is a loss. In health care it is a mortal danger.

The HIV epidemic has taught Americans that getting a catastrophic disease can change one's class status. Poverty begets disease, and disease begets poverty. Both serve as sources of stigmatization within and exclusion from a national health system wholly tuned to profit. The dominant rhetoric of cost containment in health care has so perverted discourse, it is almost impossible to articulate the loss in reasonableness, humaneness, decency.

There are signs of resistance. The very breakdown of social obligation in our institutions has fostered a new set of "informal" relations of obligation. Whether it is between ACT UP [AIDS Coalition to Unleash Power] and the Food and Drug Administration, among providers of health care in shelters or in migrant worker camps, among citizens in cities working on the front line against the invisibility of whole communities, a new health activism across race and class lines is calling for a new shape to the health and social policies of the United States. As the system approaches chaos, individuals—many of them with nothing left to lose—gain sight of their own power to help and be helped. If this new activism among the coalitions representing those at multiple jeopardy becomes a true political movement, it could well gain momentum as the civil rights struggle of the next century.

By invoking universality, the Clinton initiative may yet do something paradoxical. It may raise expectations that its own reform measures cannot but fail to meet. If so, the Beltway may one day be forced to join millions of patients, health care providers, policy-makers, and citizens who sill believe in common human decency. The question is how to forge that belief into a movement for the years ahead.

NO

Irwin M. Stelzer

WHAT HEALTH-CARE CRISIS?

The devil, we are often told, is in the details. When appraising public-policy proposals, look not at the broad caption—"gun control," "reinventing government," "deficit reduction"—but at the minutiae of the legislation aimed at achieving the unexceptionable goal. Therein will the true strengths, or weaknesses, of the proposed policy be revealed.

In accordance with this injunction, the debate over President Clinton's proposals for reforming our health-care system has been dominated by "experts" and policy wonks who, like the President himself, are never so happy as when they are poring over statistics and the details of this or that new arrangement. The net effect has been to confine discussion to the comparative merits of the Clinton plan as against the single-payer option espoused by certain Democrats, or the four or five other rival reforms espoused by other Democrats or Republicans.

Lost in all this has been the large question of whether a massive transformation of our health-care system is in truth either necessary or desirable. And discussion of *that* question has been inhibited, and even for all practical purposes silenced, by the fact that the main participants in the debate—the politicians—have, for fear of seeming callous, accepted the unexamined assumptions that there is a great "crisis" in health care, and that our system is radically flawed and desperately needs to be overhauled.

Therefore I do not propose to analyze the details of Clinton's plan. They will in any event be altered, perhaps beyond recognition, as the bill wends its way through a skeptical Congress. Instead, I wish to ask whether there is something that can legitimately be called a crisis in the provision of health care in America, a crisis so severe as to dictate a thoroughgoing transformation of our system and one which will inevitably involve, at the very least, a huge expansion of government control over a significant sector of our lives and of the American economy.

The idea that there is such a crisis stems, it would appear, from four sources. The first is the insecurity generated by the most recent recession. Most Americans' health insurance is linked to their jobs, with employers paying about 86 percent of the total cost: lose your job, lose your coverage; get a new job and you might not get coverage if you have a health problem. During a period of rising unemployment, enough Americans found this prospect sufficiently unsettling to create a constituency for changes in the way health-insurance coverage is maintained.

Then there is the concern over costs. Already claiming 14 percent of our gross national product—a figure high by international standards—health-care costs have also been rising. Many people have convinced themselves that unless something is done, health care will consume an ever-larger share of GNP [gross national product], leading in the end to the impoverishment of America.

Additional pressure for reform comes from the notion that *everyone*—no exceptions—should have health insurance as a matter of right. Since somewhere between 37 and 39 million Americans are now widely said to be without coverage, the system must be failing and it must be revamped to provide insurance for all.

A fourth contributor to the sense of crisis is the well-documented liberal bias of the major media. This factor helps to explain one of the great anomalies in the health-care debate: although 75 percent of Americans have been persuaded that there is a crisis (32 percent say the system "needs fundamental changes," and 47 percent that it "needs to be completely rebuilt"), 80 percent simultaneously report *themselves* as "very" or "somewhat" satisfied with the quality and cost of their own health care. "This contradiction," writes Fred Barnes in the premiere issue of *Forbes MediaCritic*, "can be attributed to the media-generated myths that have shaped America's view of its health-care system."

All this has added up to a great political opportunity for the Democrats. The President's advisers have long been telling him that the Democrats have no future as the party of the poor because the middle-class majority has had its fill of income transfers to what it sees as excessively prolific welfare mothers and ghetto youngsters who prefer looting to learning. To wed the middle class to the Democrats, to prevent the reemergence of the blue-collar Reagan Democrat, the party needs a modern version of Franklin D. Roosevelt's Social Security system. Enter health-care reform.

Unfortunately for the President's political strategists, however, the crisis on which the case for this reform rests—unlike the Depression of the 30's which made Social Security possible—can be shown to be a synthetic one, and the intended beneficiaries (i.e., middle-class Americans) its biggest losers.

* * *

Take the much-heralded 14-percent figure. The approximately $940 billion Americans spent on health care in 1993 did indeed represent a bit more than 14 percent of the nation's total output of goods and services. By what standard is that too much? Three are generally offered: other nations spend less; in the past we ourselves spent less; and the results we get do not justify the amount of money we put in.

But international comparisons—to begin with them—are notoriously flawed. First of all, we are the richest nation in the world, with more houses, cars, telephones, toilets, parks, and other amenities than most other nations can even imagine. As such, we cannot be expected to deploy increments of our rising incomes in the same way as do, say, the

Japanese, 54 percent of whom in the average-income bracket still lack indoor toilet facilities (whereas only 1.8 percent of America's *poor* are without such facilities). If we prefer to devote a larger portion of our incomes to top-quality health care, what is wrong with that?

After all, we do not settle for the housing standards that prevail in poorer countries: we insist on central heating and air-conditioning, the latter now installed in nearly half of the homes of even those we classify as poor. Nor are tiny cars with mechanical clutches, common elsewhere, the stuff of which the American dream is made. Neither is spartan health care. Hence we afford ourselves the luxury of making much greater use than other countries do of expensive diagnostic techniques like CAT scans and ultrasound tests.

Another reason why international comparisons mean little is that they give no weight to differences in the quality of service. The *Congressional Quarterly* cites the fact that "Japan's government plays a much greater role in private health-care delivery than does the U.S. government" to explain how "Japan keeps its costs considerably lower than those of the United States." No mention of what Fred Barnes calls "Japanese . . . assembly-line treatment from doctors who see an average of 49 patients a day," and who perform gynecological examinations on scores of women assembled in a single nonprivate room, as physicians scramble to maintain incomes in the face of too-low per-capita reimbursements.

Such stringent government controls on physicians' fees do succeed in lowering the recorded cost of Japanese medical care. But because payment is based on patient visits, the doctor keeps the average length of each visit to five minutes, and the Japanese on average make twelve visits per year, or about three times as many as Americans, whose average visit length is fifteen to twenty minutes. These decreases in convenience for patients, and increases in patient time and travel costs, points out Patricia Danzon of the Wharton school, "are excluded from the national health accounts and from public visibility."

International cost comparisons also ignore queuing and other forms of rationing that reduce recorded costs by forcibly limiting the availability of the service. Like consumer goods in the old Soviet Union, medical services in many of the countries with which America's reformers invidiously compare the U.S. are cheap but hard to get.

Joseph White, a Brookings Institution researcher whose comparison of America's system with those of six other nations leads him to conclude that "America's health-care system must be reformed," nevertheless concedes that "Britain has restricted capacity severely and makes people wait much longer for services that Americans would consider necessary, than we would accept." Certainly, the British rule that patients over fifty-five are not eligible for kidney dialysis would not be acceptable here.

We further discover from White that Australia faces both availability restrictions and "spiraling costs," and that there are "stirrings of dissatisfaction" in France. On the other hand, he dismisses Canada's waiting lists as the result of "unexpected increases in demand . . . [rather] than . . . intentional constraints on capacity."

Here White shows no recognition that the shortages caused by government planning and operation are *often* "unintentional"—planners, immunized from the consequences of the shortages they create by preferential access to goods and services (did a Kremlin bureaucrat ever queue for anything?), rarely match demand and supply with any precision. And Canada's recent response to unbearable cost increases—a reduction in the services covered—passes without mention in White's analysis. Nor does he tell us what we learn from Patricia Danzon, who notes that Canadian physicians "work fewer hours as [government-mandated] expenditure ceilings are approached," thereby shifting the risks and costs of waiting for care to patients—and lowering the recorded cost of health care in Canada. This is not a trivial matter in a country in which 1.4 million people are waiting for medical service, and 45 percent of those queuing up for surgery say they are "in pain."

Japan, writes White, "has not yet experienced significant complaints about waiting lists." But that silence may well be due more to stoic acceptance of shortages than to their absence. As for Germany, it achieves its low costs by limiting malpractice suits; by eschewing extraordinary life-prolonging measures for those judged to be terminally ill; by buying fewer pieces of high-technology equipment than Americans typically use; and by price controls. Even so, costs are soaring and the German insurance funds are broke, despite premiums that come to 13 percent of payrolls.

* * *

Yet another reason why international comparisons are misleading is that they omit societal attitudes. A prominent British physician described to me how decisions are reached in that country about whether to expend resources in an effort to save a seriously damaged newborn, or to let nature take its course. A hospital staff conference, a quiet meeting with the parents, a decision. In America, in similar circumstances, draconian efforts would be made to prolong the child's life. So, too, at other stages of life, including extreme old age.

Indeed, it is the very success of these efforts that contributes to the high cost of health care: the dead are no burden to the system; survivors are. The high expenditures incurred thereby do not result from the greed of doctors (real earnings of American doctors have remained constant for the past fifteen years), or the inefficiency of hospitals, or the swollen profits of insurers, or the price-gouging of drug companies. Rather, they reflect a basic American value—mistaken in the view of certain health-policy experts but deeply held: damn the costs, save lives, and use expensive technologies whenever necessary.

Thus, in an interview with the *New York Times*, Dr. William Castelli, the director of the Framingham Heart Study (which has been tracking cardiovascular disease in that Massachusetts town since 1949) observes:

> Since the early 1970's,... there has been nearly a 40-percent drop in the death rate from heart attacks and a 58-percent decline in the death rate from strokes in the United States. But the rate at which people suffer heart attacks and strokes has not fallen to a comparable degree.... Most people who get heart attacks and strokes don't die. They live. This is how our country is going broke, paying for the bypass operations, angioplasties, and truckloads of medicines needed to keep people with cardiovascular diseases alive.

His colleague, Dr. William B. Kannell, adds: "Right now, we're salvaging more and more people with coronary disease who, instead of dying, are living to develop heart failure..., leading to numerous costly hospitalizations and nursing-home care."

These ultimately expensive life-extending techniques are not forced on patients by doctors in love with their high-tech toys and insensitive to the fact that an estimated 30 percent of our health-care costs are incurred in the last six months of patients' lives. Ezekiel Emanuel, an oncologist and medical ethicist at the Harvard Medical School, points out that fewer than one out of ten physicians surveyed would put "Grandma" on a respirator if she had a stroke, whereas 40 percent of family members would.

High health-care costs in America also reflect another distinctive feature of our society—the social pathology of our underclass. None other than President Clinton pointed this out to an assembly of doctors at Johns Hopkins: "We'll never get the cost of health care down to where it is in other countries as long as we have higher rates of teen pregnancies and higher rates of low-birth-weight births and higher rates of AIDS, and, most important of all, higher rates of violence." And, he might have added, nothing in his own health-care plan addresses any of those problems.

Because other nations do not have as many crack babies, or bullet-riddled drug pushers, or members of urban gangs as we do, they spend less on health care. America's relatively high level of medical expenditures on these problems is no more due to faults in our health-care system than Alaska's relatively high expenditure on heating oil is due to inefficient furnaces. Nor would changing our health-care system help, as

the following report in the pro-Clinton *New York Times* vividly suggests:

> In Washington, a sullen young woman named Margaret Williams was dragging her toddler into a medical van. He was more than a year behind on his vaccination shots.
>
> She had no job. She had no husband. She explained in disgust that she had no time to hassle with the social workers and the Medicaid forms that would have given her son free care.
>
> "They want you to run around, and do this or that for nothing," she said. In the meantime, her son had got rickets.

The costs Williams and her offspring will eventually impose on the health-care system will most likely prove significant. And no reform of the system itself will avoid that cost. Which means that the staggering health problems of the urban underclass provide no justification for a radical change in how we deliver health services. If anything, the opposite is true. Since it is a government-administered system—welfare—that is a major contributor to these problems, the case of Margaret Williams would seem to provide a compelling argument against turning the private health-care industry over to the kinds of bureaucracies that have established their incompetence in related fields.

Yet even if international comparisons were corrected to account for these factors, what would they tell us? America spends more per student on higher education than any other country in the world—$13,000 per year as against $6,000–$7,000 for 24 advanced-industrial nations. Do the academics who feel our per-capita health-care costs should be brought into line with those of other countries feel the same way about our outlays for higher education? If so, perhaps they would like to begin by capping academic salaries.

*   *   *

The second basis of comparison offered to support the contention that we are spending too much on health care is our own past. In 1960 we devoted 5 percent of GNP to health care; by 1993 we were up to the famous 14 percent. Yet we do not compare the price of a modern automobile—with automatic transmission, heating, air-conditioning, and stereo tape and CD decks, plus safety features including seat belts, air bags, ABS brakes, and crash-resistant design— with the price of a model-T Ford, and then complain about how much more the new car sells for. So why ignore quality changes in medical care? Indeed, ignoring such quality changes leads to a particularly serious misrepresentation of true costs where medical treatment is concerned.

Most people beyond the age of Washington's current crop of experts can remember when an operation to remove cataracts resulted in a hospital stay of two to four days and an even longer recuperative period at home. That surgery is now typically done on an outpatient basis. Again, as Dr. Ira Cohen, formerly chief of the Division of General Medicine at New York City's Beth Israel hospital, tells us, in the days when the electrocardiogram was the sole diagnostic tool, the victim of a heart attack could count on a four- to six-week hospital stay; now, improved diagnostic techniques and equipment replace guesswork with information about the extent of muscle damage and other problems, permitting the doctor to discharge the typical heart patient in a week or ten days. Or again, a gall-bladder laparoscopy costs roughly 20 percent more than surgical removal, but a hospital stay of perhaps a week is replaced by an outpatient procedure or an overnight stay, and three weeks off the job by about three to five days. Similarly with kidney-stone operations, where the widespread use of extracorporeal shock-wave lithotripsy has also been making surgery unnecessary, cutting the time in lost work to one-tenth of what it used to be.

Yet, astonishingly, the savings in lost wages nowhere appear in our accounting of trends in health-care costs. Nor do we have any way of measuring the savings in suffering and lost output that result from the higher medical outlays these new techniques often entail. If we did, we might find that health-care costs, properly measured, have not risen as much or as rapidly as the unadjusted data suggest.

Nor, so far as the future is concerned, can we credit the projections that bring us from 14 to 26 percent of GNP by 2030. Such projections all assume that recent trends in health-care prices and in the volume of services consumed will continue indefinitely. But this is unlikely. First, the health-care industry, circa 1994, is offering an unprecedented range of new products, from diagnostic tools to treatments. Like most new products, they will go through a cycle of rapid growth, followed by falling prices and costs as competition among suppliers emerges, consumers become more discriminating, and cost-saving production and application techniques are developed.

In addition, if faced with the costs of their decisions, consumers might adjust. Failure to acknowledge such elasticity of demand is what produced the forecasts that led President Carter to proclaim an "energy crisis." But instead of trebling to

$100 per barrel, real oil prices have fallen by more than half, as consumers have learned to conserve and to use other, less expensive fuels.

* * *

So much, then, for the contentions that international comparisons and cost trends demonstrate that we spend too much on health care. What of the argument that our expenditures seem excessive when stacked up against results?

It is, of course, difficult to gauge just what "bang" we get for our health-care "buck." But the most commonly used standards are infant mortality and life expectancy, and by those America does badly: we seem to buy less life with more money than do other countries. For example, both Canada (10 percent) and Britain (6 percent) spend far less on health care than we do, but life expectancy at birth is higher, and infant mortality lower, in those countries.

Leave aside important questions about the comparability of these figures, and concentrate instead on the implicit assumption that these differences are attributable solely to differences in the efficiencies of the various health-care systems. To accept that hypothesis is to ignore all other influences—in the case of life expectancy, the fact that motor-vehicle deaths per 1,000 population are 28 percent higher in the United States than in Canada, and the fact that Americans consume 20 percent more cholesterol-laden beef and veal than do our neighbors to the north. Not to mention the effect on our longevity figures of the frighteningly high rate of homicide among young blacks.

As for infant mortality, Nicholas Eberstadt of the American Enterprise Institute shows conclusively that the low ranking of the U.S. is attributable to our higher illegitimacy rates (since unwed mothers of all races and in all income groups are more likely to give birth to low-weight babies). Add the disinclination of black women to avail themselves of prenatal care even when it is easily available and free, and the result is an infant-mortality rate that cannot be blamed on the structure of the health-care system.

In short, against the risks inherent in a radical transformation of that system, we cannot expect as probable benefits longer lives and increased infant-survival rates. Those goals *are* achievable, but only by major changes in the way Americans live—i.e., by driving, smoking, eating, and shooting less, and marrying more—and in a welfare system that, unlike our health-care system, has a proven record of failure.

Before leaving this discussion of costs, we should keep in mind an important admonition, offered by Robert Reischauer, director of the Congressional Budget Office:

> The conviction that health-care costs are too high, are rising too rapidly, and are creating undesirable repercussions is a major impetus driving health-care reform. But we also care about access and the continuity of insurance coverage; about the quality and quantity of care we receive; about consumer choice; about our ready access to state-of-the-art treatments, and the pace at which medical technology advances; even about the amenities that have little or no impact on health outcomes.

Which is to say that "costs are not everything." A society as affluent as ours properly insists that noneconomic considerations, including steady progress in the use of expensive technologies that reduce suffering, be given weight.

* * *

If there is no crisis in health-care costs, is there one in insurance coverage? Here we come to the second major statistic driving the health-care debate: at some point in 1991, the last year for which comprehensive data are available, 37 million people were without medical insurance. (This figure rose to 38.9 million in 1992, a year of relatively high unemployment, and one for which detailed data of the sort used below are not yet available.)

Note: these citizens are *not* denied health care, nor do they expire on the steps of hospitals because they cannot produce proof of insurance coverage. For hospital emergency rooms provide care to all comers. In fact, nonprofit hospitals, which constitute 88 percent of those in the U.S., cannot legally turn away any patient needing medical care, or unreasonably deny access to all the modern technology hospitals have available. And not just for the duration of the emergency: the hospital that sets a broken arm for an uninsured patient is obliged to see the treatment through. The care may not be luxurious, but neither is it casual. Per-capita health-care spending on the uninsured, pre-Medicare population is about 60 percent of per-capita expenditures on the insured population—a level sumptuous by the standards of other industrial countries.

Nonetheless, if the 37-million figure did mean what it is often taken to mean —that 15 percent (some estimates are as high as 17.4 percent) of our population lives with the unnerving and continual threat of being unable to pay for medical care—there would certainly be grounds for revising the way we provide medical services.

Fortunately, there is less of a problem here than meets the eye. Some of the uninsured are between jobs; some are students entering the labor market. Katherine Swartz, a specialist in health-care statistics at the Harvard University School of Public Health, points out that most of the uninsured are uninsured for only a short period of time. "Almost half of all uninsured spells end within six months and only about 15 percent of all uninsured spells last more than two years," she told *Congressional Quarterly*. The chronically-uninsured group in our society, then, numbers closer to 5.5 million than 37 million people.

And probably fewer than 5.5 million. For not all Americans without insurance find that condition imposed upon them. Only 1 percent of those under the age of sixty-five are uninsurable, according to the Employee Benefit Research Institute. More than half of the uninsured are members of families headed by full-time workers; 40 percent of the uninsured have incomes in excess of $20,000, and 10 percent have incomes in excess of $50,000; only 29 percent are below the poverty level. And those with incomes below $20,000 spend several times as much on entertainment, alcohol, and tobacco as they do on health care, which, says Nicholas Eberstadt, they seem "to treat... as an optional but dispensable luxury good." Furthermore, 37 percent of the uninsured are under the age of twenty-five, a generally healthy group—the University of Michigan's Catherine McLaughlin calls them "the young invincibles"—for whom health insurance is often not a cost-effective buy.

If we put all this together—the 15 percent of the uninsured without coverage for two years, plus some who are uninsured for a shorter time, minus those who choose to be uninsured—we come up with a figure of perhaps 3 percent of the population who—although able to obtain health care—cannot obtain affordable health insurance. The policy question thus becomes: should we perform radical surgery on our health-care system for the sake of that 3 percent?

Before answering with a resounding No, we have to consider the possibility that when the uninsured are treated in a hospital, and cannot pay, the cost of that treatment is loaded onto the rest of us. Hence, says the President, we should get behind a scheme that provides universal coverage, and then hospital charges to the now-insured will decline.

This view may well be wrong. It assumes that hospitals subsidize nonpayers by charging paying customers more than they otherwise would—an assumption that is questioned by, among others, Michael Morrisey of the Department of Health Care Organization and Policy at the University of Alabama. But even if cross-subsidization from the insured to the uninsured does occur—even if, in other words, the uninsured do put a burden on the insured—the cure is simple: subsidize insurance for the truly poor, and compel payment by the voluntarily uninsured. This would be far less risky than an overhaul of the entire system.

* * *

We are left, finally, with a relatively simple set of choices. Everyone agrees that any scheme that would turn 14 percent of the economy over to what the *Economist* calls "a rickety apparatus of new bureaucracies" should be instituted only in response to a major breakdown in the private sector. The proponents of a radical overhaul claim that such a breakdown has occurred. But they are mistaken.

As we have seen, costs are tolerable, all things considered, and results are not unsatisfactory: as Senator Christopher Bond of Missouri observes, kings and sheikhs come here for treatment. And if we compare our private system with the Veterans Health Administration, which is already run by the government, the case against a lurch toward greater state control becomes even stronger. VA patients in need of such care as cardiac or orthopedic diagnosis often wait 60 to 90 days to see a specialist, and months more for surgery. And 55 percent of patients with routine problems wait three hours or longer to be examined for a few minutes by what former Congressman and VA attorney Robert Bauman describes as "an overworked doctor struggling with increasing numbers of patients and piles of government forms, regulations, controls, and policy directives." Is this the direction in which we want to go?

There are, to be sure, reforms that could and should be made within the context of our present system. In addition to subsidizing those who are involuntarily uninsured, the most important is to make coverage "portable," so that the temporary loss of a job does not deprive a worker of his insurance. Such tweaks to the system would certainly help. But even more certainly, they would avoid the disastrous consequences in store for us if we follow the Clintons down the path to a health-care system presided over by a series of government boards inevitably staffed by the same people who are already doing such a wonderful job delivering our mail.

POSTSCRIPT

Is There a Health Care Crisis in the United States?

"An aura of inevitability is upon us," writes George Lundberg, M.D., in *The Journal of the American Medical Association* (May 15, 1991). "It is no longer acceptable morally, ethically, or economically for so many of our people to be medically uninsured or seriously underinsured." Not everyone, however, believes that there is a true health care crisis, despite the large numbers of uninsured Americans.

Even the numbers of uninsured Americans is a point of controversy. The figure of 35–40 million uninsured Americans is the often-cited figure that has convinced many that something must be done to enable these people to have access to health care. But the population of uninsured is not static. According to a 1990 Urban Institute study, more than half of those uninsured millions will be insured in less than four months, and nearly three-fourths will be insured in less than a year. Other estimates have put the number of the "chronically and involuntarily" uninsured at closer to 10–15 million, or about 6 percent of the population. In "The Welfarization of Health Care," *National Review* (February 7, 1994), Dick Armey and Newt Gingrich claim that while this 6 percent should concern us, it does not represent a crisis. A similar viewpoint is expressed in "Washington Perspective: What Health Care Crisis?" *Lancet* (February 5, 1994).

Costs, too, seem to be stabilizing. In "Do We Really Have a Health Care Crisis?" *Kiplinger's Personal Finance* (June 1994), Jane Clark and Joan Goldwasser claim that the health care crisis has lessened due to the sharply lowered inflation rates for health care. Senator Bob Dole agrees in "Dole: No Health-Care Crisis, Clinton on the Wrong Road," *Congressional Quarterly Weekly Report* (January 29, 1994). This viewpoint is further echoed in "Crisis? What Crisis?" *Time* (January 24, 1994), in which Adam Zagorin contends that as medical inflation eases, so does the sense of urgency that President Bill Clinton needs to push his health care reforms through Congress.

The article "Accounting for Health Care," *National Review* (October 4, 1993) claims that President Clinton's health plan and the assumptions underlying it rest upon false beliefs about America's health care and that there has been an exaggeration that the present system is riddled with vast gaps. The author claims, for example, that many parents fail to immunize their children despite the availability of free vaccinations and that life expectancy in the United States is high. In a report in *Health Affairs* (October 1994), the United States was identified as having one of the highest life expectancies in the world.

Other writers disagree, claiming that America does have a genuine health care crisis. For this view, see "Why There Is a Health Care Crisis," *Consumers Research Magazine* (June 1994); "Is There a Crisis? Absolutely!" *Business and Health* (March 1994); "The Horse's Mouth," *New Republic* (October 11, 1993); "Why We Need Health Reform," *U.S. News & World Report* (October 4, 1993); "The Health Care Crisis Hits Home," *Newsweek* (August 2, 1993); "A National Health Program Is Necessary," *Challenge* (May/June 1989); and "The Crisis in Health Care: Sick to Death," *Maclean's* (February 13, 1989).

The issue of medicine being treated as a business rather than as a social service is addressed in the following: "Dangerous to Your Health: The Madness of the Market," *The Nation* (January 9/16, 1995); "Insurers Versus Doctors: Who Knows Best?" *Business Week* (February 18, 1991); "When Healers Are Entrepreneurs: A Debate Over Costs and Ethics," *New York Times* (June 2, 1991); and "Caught in a Trap of Technology," *San Francisco Examiner* (October 9, 1990).

ISSUE 2

Should the Government Require U.S. Medical Schools to Produce More Primary Care Doctors?

YES: **James Nolan,** from "Why We Need Government Regulation: A Conversation With James Nolan, MD," *The Internist: Health Policy in Practice* (March 1994)

NO: **Richard A. Cooper,** from "Regulation Won't Solve Our Workforce Problems," *The Internist: Health Policy in Practice* (March 1994)

ISSUE SUMMARY

YES: James Nolan, physician and chair of the Department of Medicine at the State University of New York at Buffalo, argues that voluntary efforts have been unsuccessful in meeting the need for primary care physicians and that the government should step in to raise their numbers.

NO: Richard A. Cooper, dean of the Medical College of Wisconsin and director of its Health Policy Institute, supports an increased emphasis on primary care medicine but strongly objects to government regulation of the educational process.

Currently, only about one-third of all physicians in America practice primary care medicine. This includes family doctors, pediatricians (baby and children's care), and general internists. The remaining providers practice specialty medicine such as cardiology (heart specialist) and ophthalmology (eye specialist). These doctors provide care pertaining to specific body organs or limit their practices to specific medical skills such as surgery or radiology. Many experts believe that the nations' health care needs would be better met with a 50-50 ratio of general practitioners to specialists.

Study after study has indicated that there is a shortage of primary care physicians in America, or at least a surplus of specialists. Currently, there are 82 recognized medical specialities, half of which have been created since 1980! A surplus of specialty care doctors has been linked to higher medical costs and has been identified as a contributor to the situation of the millions of Americans who do not have access to primary medical care. Although many have concerns over the disproportionate numbers of specialists, some see them as being on the forefront of medicine with their utilization of high-tech research and equipment. And people with chronic and serious diseases such as cancer, kidney failure, and heart disease depend on specialists for their specific needs.

Although specialists provide valuable services, there is a high demand for general practitioners. They are especially needed for those Americans living in medically underserved inner-city and rural communities. Primary care doctors are more likely than specialists to locate in underserved areas; approximately 40 percent of recent graduates of family medicine programs practice in rural communities. Primary care physicians are also needed in managed care programs such as Health Maintenance Organizations (HMOs) and to provide care to the uninsured.

The demand for more doctors practicing primary care is clear. However, it is uncertain that medical costs would decrease or the quality of health care would improve if this demand were met. It is true that specialists are more expensive than primary care physicians: the tests they order cost more, the fees for their services are higher, and they admit patients to hospitals more often than do primary care providers. However, studies comparing costs and quality of care between specialists and primary care providers are contradictory. Primary care providers claim that they can treat almost everything a specialist can for less money. Specialists reply there is no comparison; treating a brain tumor is nothing like treating runny noses.

Why do so many doctors become specialists? In a 1992 American Medical Association study, general practitioners earned the least of any physician—about $100,000 annually. In contrast, radiologists earned the most, or nearly $2^1/2$ times as much as a general practitioner. Specialists also tend to practice in more desirable and affluent areas of the country, where they have access to high-tech equipment. In addition, there is more prestige in being a specialist.

There are obvious advantages to becoming a specialist; however, should the government do more to encourage greater numbers of doctors to forgo specialty medicine to meet the growing demand for primary care physicians? Proponents of government involvement in medical education believe that the free market alone will not lead more doctors to practice primary care medicine. They feel that the government needs to step in and cap the number of specialty practice residencies at medical schools. Furthermore, the government could legislate a fixed number of specialty care doctors and provide financial incentives to medical schools who train primary care physicians.

Echoing this view, physician James Nolan argues that the federal government has to play a lead role in regulating graduate medical education because voluntary efforts have not been successful to date in meeting the primary care workforce needs of the United States. Richard A. Cooper argues that the government has no way of determining the nation's primary care needs in the future, so capping graduate medical education could actually create a shortage of specialists in the twenty-first century.

YES

James Nolan

WHY WE NEED GOVERNMENT REGULATION

The current president of the Association of Professors of Medicine, James Nolan, MD, is one of a number of medical educators who support a role for the federal government in regulating the physician workforce supply. Dr. Nolan chairs the Department of Medicine in the State University of New York at Buffalo. In a recent conversation with [*The Internist's*] Managing Editor Diana Madden, he explained the reasons supporting his view.

INTERNIST: Many critics of a government role in regulating the physician workforce contend that the U.S. can meet its needs through natural shifts in the marketplace, voluntary efforts on the part of medical schools and teaching hospitals, and incentives to individuals (such as improved reimbursement for primary care and loan forgiveness programs). How would you respond to that?

NOLAN: Voluntary efforts on the federal, state and medical-school levels have been unsuccessful to date in meeting the workforce needs of the nation. The number of senior students entering the three primary care specialties in 1992 was 14 percent; only 3.5 percent expressed an interest in general internal medicine. Although the percentage interested in primary care increased slightly in 1993, it is still unacceptably low, and this is after a decade of so-called voluntary efforts through foundations as well as federal and state governments—particularly New York state—to shift this balance.

Certainly, voluntary efforts should be continued. We need to change the culture of medical schools and shift the emphasis toward generalism. But we don't have the time to wait for market forces to take hold. That strategy hasn't worked so far, and we are seeing a decline—or, at best, a stabilization—in the number of students going into general internal medicine. Any legislation aimed at regulating the workforce should have a sunset provision so that if marketplace forces and incentives do have an impact in the future, we can reassess the need for government allocations.

We are not doing our medical students a favor by training them and letting them go into specialties in such great numbers, when we don't believe there's going to be a place for them in the practice community of the future.

From James Nolan, "Why We Need Government Regulation: A Conversation With James Nolan, MD," *The Internist: Health Policy in Practice* (March 1994). Copyright © 1994 by The American Society of Internal Medicine. Reprinted by permission.

INTERNIST: What is your best argument in support of giving the federal government the responsibility to establish national goals for the appropriate supply, specialty mix and distribution of physicians?

NOLAN: The federal government has to play the lead role because it provides the funding for graduate medical education (GME) and probably is the only group that can support GME to the extent that is necessary. But the federal government has to work closely with the states and voluntary organizations such as the Accreditation Council for Graduate Medical Education (ACGME), the specialty societies, and—in internal medicine—the Residency Review Committee (RRC) and the American Board of Internal Medicine (ABIM). The federal government is the only body that can provide the resources and the leadership to bring these groups together.

INTERNIST: You noted that we simply don't have time to let the market forces work. However, some people would contend that even if the federal government were heavily involved in influencing the supply of physicians, those changes wouldn't be seen for 20 or 30 years.

NOLAN: I think that is correct. If, starting tomorrow, our medical schools could turn out a 50:50 ratio in terms of specialists to generalists it would take until the year 2040 to equalize the workforce. But that doesn't seem to be an argument against regulation. We need to reach the 50:50 goal as rapidly as possible. If we stay at the present 20:80 ratio, it will be much longer before we reach any kind of equilibrium.

We need to do other things, too. In the future, as the need for specialists gets smaller and medical schools continue to turn out more specialists into the practicing community, we will need to retrain some of these specialists so they can find a job. Retraining is a short-term answer to our lack of primary care physicians. But retraining is not an argument against starting now to balance the workforce with people who desire to be generalists in the first place.

INTERNIST: We haven't been successful in predicting workforce needs. How can we be sure what the needs will be tomorrow? How sound is the 50:50 estimate?

NOLAN: You've hit on a major problem. The prediction of the future physician supply is an inexact art, and it takes a considerable amount of guesswork. On the other hand, other Western nations that have medical outcomes similar to our own have more primary care physicians than specialists. The 50:50 ratio is a compromise. It is felt to be a reasonable number, but it is certainly not exact. It won't be exact until we can do some well-controlled studies—specialty-by-specialty studies as well as geographical studies—to see the needs of the future.

We have to take into consideration two factors: First, we all seem to agree that managed care is going to be increasingly important in the health care system. We know that managed care companies use fewer specialists than does the fee-for-service sector. If that's the case, then there is going to be less demand for specialists and more demand for primary care physicians. The second factor to be considered is the use of nurse practitioners and physician assistants, which might further reduce the need for primary care physicians. If state health departments, medical schools and specialty societies carefully examine these current trends, we ought to be able to make a rational approximation.

INTERNIST: What type of strategy should the federal government use in terms of setting up goals, achieving those goals and enforcing them?

NOLAN: We will need some sort of a national commission that should report to either the executive or congressional branch. The commission will need to determine workforce needs on the basis of regional input from states and specialty societies. Although quality should be a determining factor whenever possible, the federal government cannot make the decision to keep training programs open or closed strictly on the basis of quality. There has to be a rational geographic distribution of programs. Nevertheless, the commission should work with the ACGME to rate programs in all specialties on quality.

Also, political factors undoubtedly will play a role when programs are recommended for closure. The commission must be insulated from political pressure —perhaps like the present base-closing operation. Enforcement of this allocation could be tied to accreditation programs by the ACGME and certification by the boards. That is the lever that the federal government, or any kind of national commission, would have.

INTERNIST: How flexible should the government's strategy be?

NOLAN: It should be very flexible. In order for it all to work, all interested parties must be at the table. Physicians in practice, educators and the public would have to be represented on this national commission in a meaningful way. Much like Medicare now relies on the Joint Commission on the Accreditation of Healthcare Organizations (JCAHO) to inspect and certify hospitals, this national commission will need to rely heavily on the present voluntary accreditation and certification bodies, such as the RRC in internal medicine and the ABIM. The strategy needs to be flexible so it can be a true partnership between the government and these voluntary bodies.

INTERNIST: What about other strategies that have been discussed—for example, capping the number of residency positions or changing the funding policy for graduate medical education? Are there other steps that ought to be taken?

NOLAN: Well, I think there is some sense in the recommendation by the Council on Graduate Medical Education (COGME) to cap the number of residency positions at the number of U.S. medical graduates plus 10 percent. If we are going to reduce the overall workforce—which we probably will need to do—it doesn't make much sense to allow the number of available residency positions to exceed the number of U.S. medical graduates by 30 percent to 40 percent. International medical graduates who come to the U.S. to fill these positions and remain here after training have been valuable additions. But in the future, they could add to the workforce imbalance. This would make it even more difficult for individuals who are already out there to be able to practice what they have been trained to do. COGME's recommendation is a reasonable figure. It's not a magical figure—maybe it should be 20 percent, maybe it should be 5 percent. But I think that it is a reasonable approximation.

In terms of the funding of graduate medical education, I would favor an all-payer system. Right now, the federal government through Medicare funds most of these positions. The federal government, by its very size, will continue to be the major contributor. But health maintenance organizations and other private insurers benefit from the training of house officers; they should contribute to this training. That would help balance the burden so the federal government won't have to provide all the funding by itself.

If we want to get more people into primary care, then it is critical that—while this allocation process goes on—we take other significant steps to promote careers in generalism and general internal medicine. We need to increase the compensation for generalists. We need to narrow the broad income gap between procedural and cognitive specialties. We need to work on decreasing the hassle, both from the government and private insurers. The burden of this intrusion is placed unfairly on the generalist rather than the specialist. In both the undergraduate and graduate medical education system, we should make primary care a more attractive experience for our medical students and graduate residents. They need to see more of the "real life" of what an internist does, working in ambulatory sites much more than they are now.

INTERNIST: If health system reform does create a larger role for the government in terms of managing graduate medical education, what controls would be needed to protect the legitimate interests of the medical schools, academic medical centers and members of the medical profession?

NOLAN: Clearly, if we create any national commission, we need input from practicing physicians, schools and academic medical centers. They must be at the table in a meaningful role. Indeed, I don't think that the federal government could make these allocation decisions without significant input from these groups because they are the ones who will actually have to carry out the training. I have no doubt that they will be major participants in deciding the future of graduate medical education. As I said before, the government also will need help from the voluntary accrediting and certifying bodies. These organizations can help balance any unfair dominance by the federal government.

INTERNIST: Is there anything you want to add?

NOLAN: The government has to play a role in regulating the physician workforce starting now. We don't have the time to wait any longer. I also believe that the government's role may be temporary. If we make generalism more attractive in the educational and practice settings, then the government may not need to play as much of a role five or 10 years down the line.

When you look at what is happening in the country today—when you look at places where managed care is penetrating—you see that the cardiologists, for example, cannot get into the system. They are looking for patients and for ways to build up their general internal medicine practice. We are doing our medical students a great disservice if we continue to let large numbers of them go into specialties that will not have practice opportunities.

NO
Richard A. Cooper

REGULATION WON'T SOLVE OUR WORKFORCE PROBLEMS

Government regulation of the physician workforce—that's the question. But could the government really do it? Would it have any idea of what the workforce should be? What sort of regulation would make the physician workforce into something it isn't now? Would the government also regulate all of the other workforces that contribute to patient care? And how soon could regulation achieve any real difference?

No subject has engaged medical school deans as much as the physician workforce and the perceived need to expand primary care capacity. Conventional wisdom is that such an expansion is necessary to cure many of the ills of our health care system, including problems of cost, access and geographic distribution. This view has lead to the widely accepted conclusion that half of all medical students must become primary care physicians, twice the current number now entering primary care—the "50 percent solution."

THE '50 PERCENT' SOLUTION

Many organizations... have endorsed the 50 percent solution. Laws now existing or proposed in a number of states either mandate such an outcome or demand that medical schools explain how and when they can achieve it. The president's Health Security Act has called for changes in graduate medical education (GME) financing that would require half of all residents to train in one of the traditional primary care disciplines.

We are caught in a rush to regulate the process of medical education in order to achieve the 50 percent solution. That may be unwise. Although I strongly support an increased emphasis on primary care and, as a dean, have fostered major institutional changes favoring primary care, I do not endorse a primary care target of 50 percent, and I strongly object to government regulation of the educational process. It would be wise to reexamine the premise underlying the 50 percent solution, and reassess whether regulating the physician workforce could help solve our health care problems.

What are the problems of our health care system? A major one is access. This includes access for the uninsured and underinsured; access for the poor, particularly those in America's inner cities; and access for patients in remote towns and rural areas. Many of those people lacking access live within designated health professional shortage areas (HPSAs). The social and political imperative to remedy these shortages is vast, yet the number of physicians needed is proportionately small. It is estimated that 5,000 additional physicians would bring the current HPSAs to minimum standards. Similar needs are now being met by the network of federally designated community health centers that collectively utilize only 2,700 physicians. A doubling or tripling of that number could make a profound difference.

COST, ACCESS AND EQUITY

But these numbers are almost insignificant in comparison with a physician workforce of more than 600,000 and a primary care workforce of more than 200,000. If these comparatively small needs cannot be satisfied by our current abundant supply of physicians, then satisfying them by regulating the size and composition of the physician workforce seems unlikely. Yet the desire to meet the needs of rural America and our inner cities is a major force fueling the legislative drive to increase the total number of primary care physicians. Clearly, other strategies are necessary, such as mandatory service by all medical graduates, greater use of non-physician providers and structural changes in the systems of providing care. Moreover, it is likely that

different strategies will be necessary for different geographic sites.

A second problem is cost. Issues of cost have focused on physicians because physicians have determined the volume of services, and conventional wisdom holds that clinical services have been overused—particularly by specialists. However, the manner in which physicians influence costs is changing, as new, more collaborative organizational models of medical practice develop, and as capitated or contractual models of reimbursement replace fee-for-service medicine. These new models are beginning to contain costs already. They also are demanding more primary care services, and the market is beginning to respond, as both physicians and non-physician providers adapt to fill the void. The rate at which market forces are driving this evolutionary process is astounding.

Finally, there is the problem of equity. We must correct unfair insurance practices and find an equitable way to finance basic health care for all. This is the greatest problem of our health care system, and the one most in need of reform, but it has no relationship to the size or composition of the physician workforce.

Why, then, is there such an intense focus on creating regulations to achieve a workforce in which half of all physicians are primary care physicians?

An important reason is the observation that, in other Western democracies that manage their health care spending better than we do, 50–75 percent of all physicians are primary care physicians, whereas in the U.S. this number is only 37 percent. However, a recent review of the health care systems in a number of European countries has revealed percentages of primary care physicians that are actually much lower and more similar to those in the U.S.[1] The old 50 percent benchmark is simply inaccurate, yet it is an important premise underlying the logic of workforce regulation.

PREDICTABLE NEEDS?

Another premise underlying the regulatory approach is the prediction that shortages in the number of primary care physicians will continue. Unfortunately, the experience with physician workforce predictions has not been good, in either the U.S. or other democracies.[2,3] The study by the Graduate Medical Education National Advisory Committee (GMENAC) is such an example. Conducted almost 15 years ago, it failed to predict the needs for the 1990s, concluding instead that there would be adequate numbers of primary care physicians, general surgeons and specialists in obstetrics/gynecology.

Why is it so difficult to predict a nation's needs for physicians? One reason is the unpredictable but inexorable growth of medical capacity as new drugs, devices and procedures are invented. Medicine today is what Lewis Thomas, MD, called "half-way technology." We can do so much, yet there is so much more we cannot do. Of course, more will become possible in the future, but the process of discovery is nonlinear and unpredictable, and workforce needs are hard to anticipate over several decades.

Another reason that projections are so difficult is that the demographics of our country are hard to predict, as are the needs for physician services within various demographic groups. For example, estimates of the needs of the elderly in the next century vary by as much as 50 percent.[4]

Workforce predictions also are difficult because the work habits of physicians are unpredictable. We are now experiencing a rapid increase in the number of female physicians, as well as an increase in the average age of all physicians. In addition, the age at which physicians are retiring seems to be declining. How all this will affect the physician workforce is unclear. Physicians also are becoming more mobile as fewer physicians engage in solo practice and more become employees of health care organizations. Finally, physicians are free to change what they do —whether by simply shifting emphasis within a specialty or by changing specialties entirely—and they are expressing that freedom more than ever as the dynamics of health system reform impinge upon them. The physician workforce is, in the aggregate, resilient, elastic and unpredictable.

WHO ARE THE PROVIDERS?

An added requirement for workforce predictions is clarity in the definition of terms. There is enormous diversity among specialists, and there is diversity among primary care physicians as well. Some primary care practitioners emphasize well-patient care; others, the care of patients with chronic disease. Some practice obstetrics, and some serve the gatekeeper role. Family practitioners care for patients across the age spectrum and readily serve the needs of patients in rural towns. General internists and pediatricians necessarily serve a more narrow age spectrum, and they tend to practice in metropolitan areas. Some elements of primary care are provided by specialists. Which do we want, and how many of each?

Moreover, physicians are not the only providers of primary care. These services also are provided by advanced-practice nurses and physician assistants, as well as by chiropractors, purveyors of unorthodox remedies, practitioners of Oriental and other ethnic forms of healing, and a range of other helpers and healers who do provide care when the need exists. They also must be factored into the equation.

And there are other important variables affecting physician workforce projections. Together, these variables define a system that is not simple, deterministic and amenable to regulation but—like some other sectors of our economy[5]—is complex, dynamic and evolutionary.

Despite these complexities, many have predicted that it will be necessary for half of all medical graduates to become primary care physicians. Unfortunately, the graduates in question are not yet in medical school. For example, the goals established by the president are for graduating classes beginning in the year 2003, and these graduates would not begin to practice until the year 2006. Incremental changes in workforce composition would occur over the ensuing five to 10 years, but we would not achieve the 50 percent solution until the year 2040.[6]

THE REGULATORY TIME LAG

If a 50–50 mix is as important as those who advocate it claim that it is, then certainly we cannot wait several decades to achieve that goal. Yet, because of the inherent delay in modifying the physician workforce through the professional choices of new graduates, the regulatory approach will take several decades.

The market, on the other hand, will not wait. It will find other ways. Indeed, it is

already. Compensation for primary care providers is increasing, and many physicians are changing their practices to include more primary care. The market also is stimulating the formation of more collaborative practice arrangements, as well as the training of additional advanced-practice nurses and physician assistants. All of these strategies will add to our capacity to provide primary care services. Moreover, all will temper the demand for primary care physicians in the next century.

But is the 50 percent solution even an appropriate target? Should regulatory energy be deployed to achieve a workforce in which half of all physicians practice primary care? Indeed, is it even appropriate to express the size of the primary care workforce as a percentage of the total workforce? Primary care needs are based on demographic considerations, and it seems more appropriate to express them in per capita terms—for example, the number of physicians per 100,000 of the population. Expressed in those terms, a primary care workforce of 80 per 100,000 to 85 per 100,000 should be adequate to meet the primary care needs as currently defined. Within the limits that workforce predictions have, it appears that this number could be assured if approximately 35 percent of medical graduates entered the primary care disciplines.[6] In view of the growing enthusiasm for primary care among current medical students, it does not appear that regulatory action will be required to achieve this goal.

AN APPROPRIATE WORKFORCE

What impact would the 50 percent solution have on specialty medicine? While there may be a surplus of specialists today—particularly in some of the subspecialties of internal medicine—regulations that forced a 50–50 mix would create a specialty physician workforce during the next century that, on a per capita basis, would be smaller than the specialty workforce in the 1980s. Unfortunately, this smaller pool of specialists would come at a time when the technologic demands on specialty medicine are likely to increase substantially. The wisdom of regulations that lead to such an outcome should be reconsidered.

There is an even more pervasive and overriding reason to question the wisdom of regulation. It has to do with the nature of the system being regulated. Regulation demands certainty, whereas health care is characterized by uncertainty. Regulation requires bureaucratization, whereas physicians thrive on professionalism. Regulation demands scrutiny, whereas trust dominates the relationship between physicians and patients. Trust, professionalism and dealing with uncertainty are major themes in medical education.

While physicians are not perfect, they cannot be regulated to become more perfect. The rapid adaptation that physicians are now undergoing in response to the almost cataclysmic changes in the structure and financing of health care is a tribute to their professionalism, their ability to deal with uncertainty and their respect for the public trust that they hold.

Neither have medical schools been perfect in anticipating the needs in primary care that are so well appreciated today, but these needs were not fully appreciated by the GMENAC study in the late 1970s either. Nevertheless, medical schools are responding to anticipated needs by increasing ambulatory care education (particularly within primary care community sites), by emphasizing generalist skills and generalist role models, and by promoting research in areas such as health services and ethics. It is the strength of our medical education system that has produced the finest physician workforce in the world, while also fueling the biotechnology revolution that has become both a major economic engine and a major factor in clinical medicine. Moreover, medical school faculties are playing an ever-increasing role in providing care to the underserved.

IMPACT ON THE PROFESSION

There are few entities in our society that achieve the high degree of social responsibility exercised by medical schools. Do we want to see their energy and creativity usurped by regulation?

The U.S. does not need to regulate physician training in order to meet the future needs for primary care. Moreover, regulation could not be expected to meet those needs effectively. Those, I suppose, are reasons enough to reject the regulatory approach. However, there are intangibles at stake as well. Even if, on theoretical grounds, regulation could achieve the intended goals, the adverse consequence of regulation for the profession of medicine and for medical education is a price that is simply too high to pay.

REFERENCES

1. Whitcomb M. "Medical Education/Physician Workforce Issues: England, France and Germany." *Health Professions Analysis and Research Report*, Bureau of Health Professions, November 1993.
2. Martini CJM. "Medical Workforce Planning and Medical Education. Attaining Consensus." *Journal of the American Medical Association (JAMA)*. 270:1101–1104, 1993.

3. Feil EC, Welch HG and Fisher ES. "Why Estimates of Physician Supply and Requirements Disagree." *JAMA*. 269:2659–2553. 1993.

4. Reuben DB, Zwanziger J, Bradley TB, Fink A, Hirsch SH, Williams AP, Solomon OH and Beck JC. "How Many Physicians Will Be Needed To Provide Medical Care For Older Persons? Physician Manpower Needs for the Twenty-first Century." *Journal of the American Geriatric Society*. 41:444–453. 1993.

5. Arthur WB. "Positive Feedbacks in the Economy." *Scientific American*, (February 1990):92–99.

6. Kindig DA, Cultice JM and Mullan F. "The Elusive Generalist Physician. Can We Reach the 50 Percent Goal?" *JAMA*. 270:1069–1073, 1993.

POSTSCRIPT

Should the Government Require U.S. Medical Schools to Produce More Primary Care Doctors?

There is a consensus that there are too many medical specialists and not enough general practitioners in the United States. However, no one is certain exactly how many generalists would be enough. As Nolan and Cooper note, a 50-50 ratio of generalists to specialists is a commonly desired goal. But even if half of all graduating medical students choose to practice general medicine, it would take at least 40 years to achieve this goal. Although there has been an increased interest in primary care medicine, only approximately 22 percent of the 1994 medical graduating class expressed an interest in general medicine, far below the 50-50 goal.

Even though more doctors have been expressing an interest in general medicine, the serious shortage of doctors practicing in inner-city and rural areas will probably continue to grow as more and more physicians opt for more lucrative practices in the suburbs. One interesting question that has arisen is, Can other health providers such as nurse practitioners and physician assistants offer high-quality general medical care to people in underserved areas? A 1986 report by the Congressional Office of Technology Assessment analyzed several earlier studies and found that nurse practitioners, physician assistants, and certified nurse midwives can provide care equal to that of physicians. These providers also seem to do an even better job of preventive care. A 1992 study completed for the American Nurses Association found similar results.

Not only can nurse practitioners and physician assistants provide high-quality basic medical care, but they can also treat patients for less money. Because of their lesser training, their salaries and fees tend to be lower than the average physician. Many experts believe that physician salaries are an important factor in ever-rising health care costs. The following articles debate physician salaries: "Income Survey Spotlights Image Problem: Survey Shows That Americans Think That Physicians Should Earn Less," *American Medical News* (April 1993); "An Emerging Health Care Crisis: Doctors Aren't Paid Enough!" *American Journal of Medicine* (November 1994); "Its Time to Douse Fire on Physician Pay," *American Medical News* (April 26, 1993); and "Why Do Auto Mechanics Make More Than Doctors?" *Medical World News* (January 1992).

While nurse practitioners and physician assistants may help ease both health care costs and the shortage of general practitioners in the United

States, other market forces may actually decrease the supply of generalists. More and more people are taking advantage of primary care services due to the growth of Health Maintenance Organizations (HMOs), or managed health care plans. Ironically, the growth of HMOs may increase the shortage of generalists, especially in inner cities and rural locations. Although they encourage the utilization of general practitioners, large HMOs in the suburbs are attracting many of the limited number of providers. See "Health Care Seems Alive and Well Under HMO Plans," *Time-Picayune* (November 27, 1994).

For an overview of the issue of medical specialists versus primary care providers, see "Primary Care: Will More Family Doctors Improve Health Care?" *CQ Researcher* (March 17, 1995); "Medical Students' Opinions of Health System Reform," *Journal of the American Medical Association* (January 4, 1995); "Encourage Med Students to Be GPs, Not Specialists," *USA Today* (August 9, 1994); "Time to Redirect the Specialist Subsidy for Doctors," *The Boston Globe* (August 28, 1994); "We Shouldn't Phase Out Medical Specialists," *The New York Times* (August 28, 1994);"Shortage of Doctors in Poor Areas Is Seen as Barrier to Health Plans," *The New York Times* (October 18, 1993); and "More Primary Care Doctors Means Healthier Lives—Study," *American Medical News* (January 18, 1993).

The topic of government intervention versus market forces in health care workforce needs is discussed in "Medical Student Career Choice: Will the Market Provide the Solution to Our Health Care Workforce Needs?" *The American Journal of Medicine* (November 1994); "Seeking a Balanced Physician Workforce for the Twenty-first Century," *Journal of the American Medical Association* (September 7, 1994); and "Give Family Docs Free Education," *USA Today* (June 8, 1993).

ISSUE 3

Should Doctors Ever Help Terminally Ill Patients Commit Suicide?

YES: Timothy E. Quill, from "Death and Dignity: A Case of Individualized Decision Making," *The New England Journal of Medicine* (March 7, 1991)

NO: Herbert Hendin and Gerald Klerman, from "Physician-Assisted Suicide: The Dangers of Legalization," *American Journal of Psychiatry* (January 1993)

ISSUE SUMMARY

YES: Timothy E. Quill, M.D., who describes a physician-assisted suicide, believes that doctors have roles other than healing and fighting against death.

NO: Physicians Herbert Hendin and Gerald Klerman argue that there is a great potential for abuse and exploitation if physician-assisted suicide is legalized.

Should doctors ever help their patients die? While doctors should provide every support possible to their dying patients, do they have the right or obligation to actually hasten the process even if a patient requests it? Should hopelessly ill patients be kept alive indefinitely? This topic has been the subject of numerous debates over the past few years.

Some of the practices that were controversial a short time ago in the care of hopelessly ill patients have become accepted and routine. Many doctors now believe that it is ethical to use "do-not-resuscitate" orders on dying patients, while others feel that it is also acceptable to withhold food and water from patients who are hopelessly ill and dying. The word *euthanasia*, which comes from two Greek roots—the prefix *eu*, meaning good, fortunate, or easy, and the word *thanatos*, meaning death—describes a good or easy death. While withdrawing care or treatment (referred to as *passive euthanasia*) may be acceptable to many doctors, *active euthanasia*, or playing an active role in a patient's death, may not. One form of active euthanasia, physician-assisted suicide, has been a subject of controversy in recent years.

In early 1988 the *Journal of the American Medical Association* published a short article entitled "It's Over, Debbie" (January 8, 1988), which was written by an anonymous physician who described administering a lethal dose of morphine to a young woman with end-stage cancer. The doctor claimed her suffering was extreme and that there was absolutely no hope of recovery. The morphine was requested by the patient, who said, "Let's get this over with." The patient died minutes after receiving the drug, while the doctor looked on. This article generated a great deal of criticism because the doctor had only met the patient for the first time that evening and had not consulted with colleagues or family members before making his decision. The doctor did, however, believe he was correctly responding to the patient's request.

Soon after this incident, Dr. Jack Kevorkian assisted in the suicide of an Oregon woman who suffered from Alzheimer's disease. Dr. Kevorkian supplied the woman with a device that he developed—a "suicide machine"—which allowed her to give herself a lethal dose of drugs. Intense criticism followed regarding the ability of Dr. Kevorkian to diagnose the patient's illness (which was not immediately terminal) and whether or not the patient was able to make an informed decision to end her life.

In March 1991 Timothy E. Quill published an editorial in the *New England Journal of Medicine* that described an assisted suicide. A woman, Quill's patient for eight years, was dying of leukemia. She had decided not to undergo chemotherapy, which would have offered her only a 25 percent chance of long-term survival with considerable side effects. In addition to refusing treatment, the patient requested that Quill help her commit suicide.

In the following selection, which is from that editorial, Quill discusses why he believes that an informed patient should have the right to choose or refuse treatment and to die with as much control and dignity as possible. Herbert Hendin and Gerald Klerman, in opposition, argue against physician-assisted suicide and assert that there is potential for abuse if physician-assisted suicide becomes legal. They believe that the elderly, people frightened by illness, and depressed people of all ages would be possible victims of this abuse.

YES

Timothy E. Quill

DEATH AND DIGNITY: A CASE OF INDIVIDUALIZED DECISION MAKING

Diane was feeling tired and had a rash. Her hematocrit was 22, and her white-cell count was 4.3 with some metamyelocytes and unusual white cells. I called Diane and told her it might be serious. When she pressed for the possibilities, I reluctantly opened the door to leukemia. Hearing the word seemed to make it exist. "Oh, shit!" she said. "Don't tell me that." I thought, I wish I didn't have to.

Diane was raised in an alcoholic family and had felt alone for much of her life. She had vaginal cancer as a young woman, and had struggled with depression and her own alcoholism for most of her adult life. I had come to know, respect, and admire her over the previous eight years as she confronted and gradually overcame these problems. During the previous three and a half years, she had abstained from alcohol and had established much deeper connections with her husband, her college-age son, and several friends. Her business and artistic work was blossoming. She felt she was living fully for the first time.

Unfortunately, a bone-marrow biopsy confirmed the worst: acute myelo-monocytic leukemia. In the face of this tragedy, I looked for signs of hope. This is an area of medicine in which technological intervention has been successful, with long-term cures occurring 25 percent of the time. As I probed the costs of these cures, I learned about induction chemotherapy (three weeks in the hospital, probable infections, and hair loss; 75 percent of patients respond, 25 percent do not). Those who respond are then given consolidation chemotherapy (with similar side effects; another 25 percent die, thus a net of 50 percent survive). For those still alive to have a reasonable chance of long-term survival, they must undergo bone-marrow transplants (hospitalization for two months, a whole-body irradiation—with complete killing of the bone marrow—infectious complications; 50 percent of this group survive, or 25 percent of the original group). Though hematologists may argue over the exact percentage of people who will benefit from therapy, they don't argue about the outcome of not having any treatment—certain death in days, weeks, or months.

From Timothy E. Quill, "Death and Dignity: A Case of Individualized Decision Making," *The New England Journal of Medicine*, vol. 324, no. 10 (March 7, 1991), pp. 691–694. Copyright © 1991 by The Massachusetts Medical Society. Reprinted by permission.

Believing that delay was dangerous, the hospital's oncologist broke the news to Diane and made plans to begin induction chemotherapy that afternoon. When I saw her soon after, she was enraged at his presumption that she would want treatment and devastated by the finality of the diagnosis. All she wanted to do was go home and be with her family. She had no further questions about treatment and, in fact, had decided that she wanted none. Together we lamented her tragedy. I felt the need to make sure that she and her husband understood that there was some risk in delaying, that the problem would not go away, and that we needed to keep considering the options over the next several days.

Two days later Diane, her husband, and her son came to see me. They had talked at length about the problem and the options. She remained very clear about her wish not to undergo chemotherapy and to live whatever time she had left outside of the hospital. Her family wished she would choose treatment but accepted her decision. She articulated very clearly that it was she who would be experiencing all the side effects of treatment and that one-in-four odds were not good enough for her to undergo so toxic a course of therapy. I had her repeat her understanding of the treatment, the odds, and the consequences of forgoing treatment. I clarified a few misunderstandings, but she had a remarkable grasp of the options and implications.

* * *

I have long been an advocate of the idea that an informed patient should have the right to choose or refuse treatment, and to die with as much control and dignity as possible. Yet there was something that disturbed me about Diane's decision to give up a 25 percent chance of long-term survival in favor of almost certain death. Diane and I met several times that week to discuss her situation, and I gradually came to understand the decision from her perspective. We arranged for home hospice care, and left the door open for her to change her mind.

Just as I was adjusting to her decision, she opened up another area that further complicated my feelings. It was extraordinarily important to Diane to maintain her dignity during the time remaining to her. When this was no longer possible, she clearly wanted to die. She had known of people lingering in what was called "relative comfort," and she wanted no part of it. We spoke at length about her wish. Though I felt it was perfectly legitimate, I also knew that it was outside of the realm of currently accepted medical practice and that it was more than I could offer or promise. I told Diane that information that might be helpful was available from the Hemlock Society.

A week later she phoned me with a request for barbiturates for sleep. Since I knew that this was an essential ingredient in a Hemlock Society suicide, I asked her to come to the office to talk things over. She was more than willing to protect me by participating in a superficial conversation about her insomnia, but it was important to me to know how she planned to use the drugs and to be sure that she was not in despair or overwhelmed in a way that might color her judgment. In our discussion, it was apparent that she was having trouble sleeping, but it was also evident that the security of having enough barbiturates available to commit suicide, if and when the time came, would give her the peace of mind she needed to live fully in the present. She was not despondent and, in fact, was making deep, personal connections with her family and close friends. I made sure that she knew how to use the barbiturates for sleep, and how to use them to commit suicide. We agreed to meet regularly, and she promised to meet with me before taking her life. I wrote the prescriptions with an uneasy feeling about the boundaries I was exploring—spiritual, legal, professional, and personal. Yet I also felt strongly that I was making it possible for her to get the most out of the time she had left.

The next several months were very intense and important for Diane. Her son did not return to college, and the two were able to say much that had not been said earlier. Her husband worked at home so that he and Diane could spend more time together. Unfortunately, bone weakness, fatigue, and fevers began to dominate Diane's life. Although the hospice workers, family members, and I tried our best to minimize her suffering and promote comfort, it was clear that the end was approaching. Diane's immediate future held what she feared the most: increasing discomfort, dependence, and hard choices between pain and sedation. She called her closest friends and asked them to visit her to say good-bye, telling them that she was leaving soon. As we had agreed, she let me know as well. When we met, it was clear that she knew what she was doing, that she was sad and frightened to be leaving but that she would be even more terrified to stay and suffer.

Two days later her husband called to say that Diane had died. She had said her final good-byes to her husband and son that morning, and had asked them to leave her alone for an hour. After an hour, which must have seemed like an eternity, they found her on the couch, very still and covered by her favorite shawl. They called me for advice about how to proceed. When I arrived at their house we talked about what a remarkable person she had been. They seemed to have no doubts about the course she had chosen, or about their cooperation, although the unfairness of her illness and the finality of her death were overwhelming to us all.

I called the medical examiner to inform him that a hospice patient had died. When asked about the cause of death, I said acute leukemia. He said that was fine and that we should call a funeral director. Although acute leukemia was the truth, it was not the whole story. But any mention of suicide would probably have brought an ambulance, efforts at resuscitation, and a police investigation. Diane would have become a "coroner's case," and the decision to perform an autopsy would have been made at the discretion of the medical examiner. The family or I could have been subjected to criminal prosecution; I could have been subjected to a professional review. Although I truly believe that the family and I gave her the best care possible, allowing her to define her limits and directions, I am not sure the law, society, or the medical profession would agree.

Diane taught me about the range of help I can provide people if I know them well and if I allow them to express what they really want. She taught me about taking charge and facing tragedy squarely when it strikes. She taught me about life, death, and honesty, and that I can take small risks for people I really know and care about.

NO

**Herbert Hendin and
Gerald Klerman**

PHYSICIAN-ASSISTED SUICIDE: THE DANGERS OF LEGALIZATION

There are situations when helping a terminally ill patient end his or her life seems appropriate. For centuries physicians have helped such patients die. Why should we not protect them and at the same time make it easier for the terminally ill to end their lives by legalizing physician-assisted suicide? The movement to do so represents such a drastic departure from established social policy and medical tradition that it needs to be evaluated in the light of what we now know about suicide and terminal illness.

We know that 95% of those who kill themselves have been shown to have diagnosable psychiatric illness in the months preceding suicide (1–4). The majority suffer from depression, which can be treated. This is particularly true of the elderly, who are more prone than younger victims to take their lives during the type of acute depressive episode that responds most effectively to modern available treatments (3). Other diagnoses among the suicides include alcoholism, substance abuse, schizophrenia, and panic disorder; treatments are available for all of these illnesses.

Advocates of physician-assisted suicide try to convey the impression that in terminally ill patients the wish to die is totally different from suicidal intent in those without terminal illness. However, like other suicidal individuals, patients who desire an early death during a terminal illness are usually suffering from a treatable mental illness, most commonly a depressive condition (5). Strikingly, the overwhelming majority of the terminally ill fight for life to the end. Some may voice suicidal thoughts in response to transient depression or severe pain, but these patients usually respond well to treatment for depressive illness and pain medication and are grateful to be alive.

Studies of those who have died by suicide have pointed out the nonrational elements of the wish to die in reaction to serious illness. More individuals, particularly elderly individuals, killed themselves because they feared or *mistakenly* believed they had cancer than killed themselves and actually had cancer (6, 7). In the same vein, preoccupation with suicide is greater in those

From Herbert Hendin and Gerald Klerman, "Physician-Assisted Suicide: The Dangers of Legalization," *American Journal of Psychiatry,* vol. 150, no. 1 (January 1993), pp. 143–145. Copyright © 1993 by The American Psychiatric Association. Reprinted by permission.

awaiting the results of tests for HIV [human immunodeficiency virus] antibodies than in those who know that they are HIV positive (8).

Given the advances in our medical knowledge and treatment ability, a thorough psychiatric evaluation for the presence of a treatable disorder may literally make the difference between choosing life or choosing death for patients who express the wish to die or to have assisted suicide. This is not an evaluation that can be made by the average physician unless he or she has had extensive experience with depression and suicide (9).

Even the highly publicized cases that have been put forward by the advocates of legalizing assisted suicide dramatize the dangers and abuses we would face when those who are not qualified to do so evaluate such patients or when we accept at face value a patient's assertion that he or she prefers death. Perhaps the first such case was featured in a front-page story more than a decade ago (10). It concerned a woman who, after being diagnosed as having breast cancer, brought together her friends and her husband (who was a psychologist), filmed her farewells, and took a lethal overdose. For years the woman had been an advocate of the "right to suicide." Her film became a television documentary, and media stories portrayed her as something of a pioneer. A pioneer for what? Does her story contain a message we wish to send to the thousands of women facing possible breast surgery? The woman was not terminally ill; her cancer was operable. Although her psychologist husband supported her decision and felt it was appropriate, surely he was not the person to evaluate her. Was her choice as rational as everyone claimed?

Suicidal individuals are prone, just as this woman was, to make conditions on life: "I won't live if I lose my breast," "if this person doesn't care for me," "if I don't get this job" or "if I lose my looks, power, prestige, or health." Depression, often precipitated by discovering a cancer, exaggerates the tendency toward rigid thinking, toward seeing problems in black-and-white terms (11).

More recent cases are equally troubling. In the *New England Journal of Medicine,* a physician published the case of a woman whom he helped to commit suicide (12). The woman had a past history of both alcoholism and depression and had recently been diagnosed as having acute leukemia. Her chances of surviving painful chemotherapy and radiation were assessed as one in four. She told her doctor that "she talked to a psychologist she had seen in the past" and implied that the psychologist supported her decision to commit suicide. The physician helped her to implement her decision to end her life. He then published an account of what transpired in an attempt to persuade the medical community of the need for legal sanction for his actions.

The fact that this or any patient may find relief in the prospect of death is not necessarily a sign that the decision is appropriate. Many who are depressed and suicidal appear less depressed after deciding to end their lives. It is coping with the uncertainties of life and death that agitate and depress them. One would need a far more extended examination by someone knowledgeable about suicide to evaluate this woman.

Depression, which is often covert and can coexist with physical illness, is, together with anxiety and the wish to die, often the first reaction to the knowledge of serious illness and possible death.

This demoralizing triad can usually be treated by a combination of empathy, psychotherapy, and medication. The decision whether or not to live with illness is likely to be different with such treatment.

The publications of groups like the Hemlock Society, who advocate a more general "right to suicide," make clear that physician-assisted suicide for patients who have less than 6 months to live (as in the recently defeated California and State of Washington proposals) is but a first step in their campaign. Only a small percentage of the people they are trying to reach are terminally ill. The terminally ill, in fact, constitute only a small portion (less than 3%) of the total number of suicides (1, 3, 9). Right-to-suicide groups have been joined in their efforts by well-meaning physicians concerned with the plight of the terminally ill.

Discussions of the right to suicide or the rationality of suicide in particular cases have tended to ignore the potential for abuse were physician-assisted suicide to be legalized. Particularly vulnerable potential victims would be the elderly, those frightened by illness, and the depressed of all ages.

The elderly are often made to feel that their families would prefer that they were gone. Societal sanction for physician-assisted suicide for the terminally ill is likely to encourage family members so inclined to pressure the infirm and the elderly and to collude with uninformed and unscrupulous physicians to provide such deaths. Some advocates of changing social and medical policy toward suicide concede that such abuses are likely to occur but feel that this is a price we should be willing to pay (13).

Those whose terror of illness persuades them that quick death is the best solution may be willing victims of physicians who advocate assisted suicide. A woman in the early stages of Alzheimer's who was fearful of the progress of the disease was seen briefly by Dr. Jack Kevorkian, a retired pathologist in Michigan with a passionate commitment to promoting assisted suicide and the use of his "suicide machine." After a brief contact he decided she was a suitable candidate. He used the machine to help her kill herself. Is he the person who should be making such a determination? No Michigan law prohibits assisted suicide (19 states do not have such laws), but Dr. Kevorkian was admonished by the court not to engage in the practice again. Disregarding the admonition, he subsequently provided machines to two more women who were seriously but not terminally ill (14). They used the machines to kill themselves. Dr. Kevorkian's license to practice medicine has since been "summarily suspended," but a Michigan judge ruled that he could not be prosecuted for murder in the absence of a state law prohibiting assisting a suicide.

Societal sanction for physician-assisted suicide is likely to encourage assisted suicide by nonphysicians, rendering those who are depressed, with or without physical illness, vulnerable to exploitation. Such abuse already exists. For example, a young man gave a depressed young woman he knew a lethal quantity of sleeping pills. He sat with her and fed them to her as she ate ice cream. While she was doing so, he persuaded her that, since she was going to die, she should write out a will leaving him her possessions. He went home and told his roommate what he had done; the roommate called the police and the young woman was saved. The young man went unpunished because he did what he did in a state with no law prohibiting assisted suicide (11).

So-called suicide pacts, often romanticized by the press, provide another example of such abuse. Published case reports confirm our own clinical experience, which indicates that such pacts are usually instances where a man who wishes to end his life coerces a woman into joining him as proof of her love (11, 15, 16). In her book, her taped suicide note, her letters, and conversations with friends, the former wife of Derek Humphry, the founder of the Hemlock Society, made clear that she was tormented by having actively participated with Humphry in the suicide pact of her parents. Although her 92-year-old father may have been ready to die, she was aware that her 78-year-old mother was not (17–19).

Surely there is a price to be paid for current policy where physicians, patients, and family members must act secretly or may be unwilling to act even in situations where it seems appropriate. The protection of the honorable physician does not now warrant legalizing physician-assisted suicide in a society where the public is relatively uninformed of present abuses involving assisted suicide and the potential for much greater abuses if legalization occurs. It took us several decades to become knowledgeable about when it may be appropriate to withdraw life support systems. We are not close to that point with physician-assisted suicide.

Nor by itself can evaluation of the patient by psychiatrists knowledgeable about suicide, depression, and terminal illness provide us with a simple solution to a complex social problem. Certainly, the individual physician confronted with someone requesting assisted suicide should seek such consultation.

There is still too much we do not know about such patients, too much study yet to be done before we could mandate psychiatric evaluation for such patients and define conditions under which assisted suicide would be legal. We are likely to find that those who seek to die in the last days of terminal illness are a quite different population from those whose first response to the knowledge of serious illness is to turn to suicide.

Not all problems are best resolved by a statute. We do not convict or prosecute every case in which someone assists in a suicide, even in states where it is illegal. Given the potential for abuse, however, to give assisted suicide legal sanction is to give a dangerous license.

In some cultures (the Alorese are perhaps the most famous example), when people became seriously ill, they took to their beds, stopped eating, and waited to die. How we deal with illness, age, and decline says a great deal about who and what we are, both as individuals and as a society. The growing number of people living to old age and the increasing incidence of depression in people of all ages present us with a medical challenge. Our efforts should concentrate on providing treatment, relieving pain for the intractably ill, and, in the case of terminal illness, helping the individual come to terms with death.

If those advocating legalization of assisted suicide prevail, it will be a reflection that as a culture we are turning away from efforts to improve our care of the mentally ill, the infirm, and the elderly. Instead, we would be licensing the right to abuse and exploit the fears of the ill and depressed. We would be accepting the view of those who are depressed and suicidal that death is the preferred solution to the problems of illness, age, and depression.

REFERENCES

1. Robins E, Murphy G, Wilkenson RH Jr, Gassner S, Kayes J: Some clinical considerations in the prevention of suicide based on a study of 134 successful suicides. Am J Public Health 1959; 49:888–899

2. Dorpat TL, Ripley HS: A study of suicide in the Seattle area. Compr Psychiatry 1960; 1:349–359

3. Barraclough B, Bunch J, Nelson B, Sainsbury P: A hundred cases of suicide: clinical aspects. Br J Psychiatry 1974; 125:355–373

4. Rich DC, Young D, Fowler RC: San Diego Suicide Study, I: young vs old subjects. Arch Gen. Psychiatry 1986; 43:577–582

5. Brown JH, Henteleff P, Barakat S, Rowe CJ: Is it normal for terminally ill patients to desire death? Am J Psychiatry 1986; 143:208–211

6. Conwell Y, Caine ED, Olsen K: Suicide and cancer in later life. Hosp Community Psychiatry 1990; 41:1334–1339

7. Dorpat TL, Anderson WF, Ripley HS: The relationship of physical illness to suicide, in Suicidal Behaviors: Diagnosis and Management. Edited by Resnick HLP. Boston, Little, Brown, 1968

8. Perry S: Suicidal ideation and HIV testing. JAMA 1990; 263:679–682

9. Conwell Y, Caine ED: Rational suicide and the right to die: reality and myth. N Engl J Med 1991; 15:1100–1103

10. Johnston L: Artist ends her life after ritual citing "self-termination" right. New York Times, June 17, 1979, P A1

11. Hendin H: Suicide in America. New York, WW Norton, 1982

12. Quill TE: Death and dignity—a case of individualized decision making. N Engl J Med 1991; 324:691–694

13. Batten MP: Manipulated suicide, in Suicide: The Philosophical Issues. Edited by Batten M, May D. New York, St Martins Press, 1980

14. Doctor in suicides assails US ethics. New York Times, Nov 3, 1991, p A1

15. Noyes R, Frye S, Hartford C: Single case study: conjugal suicide pact. J Nerv Ment Dis 1977; 165:72–75

16. Mehta D, Mathew P, Mehta S: Suicide pact in a depressed elderly couple: case report. J Am Geriatr Soc 1978; 26:136–158

17. Wickett A: Double Exit. Eugene, Ore, Hemlock Society, 1989

18. Gabriel T: A fight to the death. New York Times Magazine, Dec 8, 1991, p 46

19. Abrams G: A bitter legacy—angry accusations abound after the suicide of Hemlock Society co-founder Ann Humphry. Los Angeles Times, View section, p 1

POSTSCRIPT

Should Doctors Ever Help Terminally Ill Patients Commit Suicide?

As our population ages and the incidence of certain diseases, such as cancer and AIDS, continues to increase, it appears that the ranks of the dying and suffering will grow. In the past, there were limited means of prolonging life; however, due to advances in modern medicine and technology, the dying can sometimes be kept alive for lengthy time periods. As a result, some doctors are beginning to speak more often of euthanasia. Euthanasia is already being practiced in the Netherlands, but in the United States the American Medical Association has unequivocally reaffirmed its opposition to the practice. It refers to euthanasia as a euphemism for intentional killing and claims that "this is not part of the practice of medicine, with or without the consent of the patient."

The Dutch have taken a different viewpoint: In the past several years, thousands of Dutch have died by their own choice with the help of their doctors. While Dutch law still refers to euthanasia as a crime, the highest courts there have determined that doctors may practice it if they follow specific guidelines set up by the Royal Dutch Medical Association. Currently, it is estimated that 11 percent of Dutch AIDS patients die in this manner. An article in *Hippocrates*, "The Gentle Death" (September/October 1989), discusses this ability of the Dutch to have their wish to die granted by their physicians. "Is It Time for Mercy Killing?" *The Washington Post* (August 15, 1989) debates the euthanasia issue. Susan Wolf, an associate for law at the Hastings Center, argues that the consequences of easing the restrictions against euthanasia are unacceptable in "Holding the Line on Euthanasia," *Hastings Center Report* (January/February 1989).

Many doctors seem to be uncertain as to whether or not they should have a role in a patient's death. Articles that support euthanasia include "The Physician's Responsibility Toward Hopelessly Ill Patients," *The New England Journal of Medicine* (March 30, 1989); "Suicide: Should the Doctor Ever Help?" *Harvard Health Letter* (August 1991); "The Physician Can Play a Positive Role in Euthanasia," *Journal of the American Medical Association* (December 1, 1989); "Mercy Mission," *U.S. News & World Report* (March 18, 1991); "Physicians' Aid in Dying," *The New England Journal of Medicine* (October 31, 1991); "Intentional 'Death with Dignity' Raises Moral, Ethical, Legal Issues," *Des Moines Register* (March 5, 1989); and "Assisted Suicide—Is It Acceptable?" *The Washington Post* (April 4, 1989).

Opponents of euthanasia and physician-assisted suicide argue that all life has value and that doctors do not have the right to end it. Leon R. Kass, in "Neither for Love nor Money: Why Doctors Must Not Kill," *The Public Interest* (December 1989), maintains that under no circumstances should doctors take a life. Philosophy professor Richard Momeyer of Miami University asserts that not only are the arguments against physician-assisted suicide paternalistic but they rely on inappropriate notions of what ideal medicine is in "Does Physician Assisted Suicide Violate the Integrity of Medicine?" *Journal of Medicine and Philosophy* (vol. 20, 1995).

Other articles that discuss the issue of physician-assisted suicide include "Holding the Line on Euthanasia," *Hastings Center Report* (January/February 1989); "Coming Soon: Your Neighborhood T.S.C.," *America* (April 30, 1994); and "They Shoot Horses, Don't They?" *New Scientist* (September 14, 1991). Additional readings on the topic include "Should Physicians Aid Their Patients in Dying?" *Journal of the American Medical Association* (May 20, 1992); "Assisted Suicide: Should Doctors Help Hopelessly Ill Patients Take Their Lives?" *CQ Researcher* (February 21, 1992); "Are Laws Against Assisted Suicide Unconstitutional?" *Hastings Center Report* (May/June 1993); "The Euthanasia Follies," *Commonweal* (June 3, 1994); "Attitudes Toward Assisted Suicide; Euthanasia Among Physicians in Washington State," *The New England Journal of Medicine* (July 14, 1994); and "Assisted Suicide Controversy: Should Physicians Help the Dying to End Their Lives?" *CQ Researcher* (May 5, 1995).

ISSUE 4

Should Health Care for the Elderly Be Limited?

YES: Daniel Callahan, from "Setting Limits: A Response," *The Gerontologist* (June 1994)

NO: Ezekiel J. Emanuel and Linda L. Emanuel, from "The Economics of Dying: The Illusion of Cost Savings at the End of Life," *The New England Journal of Medicine* (February 24, 1994)

ISSUE SUMMARY

YES: Hastings Center director Daniel Callahan believes that medical care for elderly people who have lived their natural life expectancy should consist only of pain relief rather than expensive health care services that serve only to forestall death.

NO: Physicians Ezekiel J. Emanuel and Linda L. Emanuel argue that cost savings due to limitations in medical care at the end of life are not likely to be substantial and that health care costs would be reduced if changes were made in the overall delivery of health care.

In 1980, 11 percent of the U.S. population was over age 65, but they utilized about 29 percent ($219 billion) of the total American health care expenditures. By the end of the decade, the percentage of the population over 65 had risen to 12 percent, which consumed 31 percent of total health care expenditures, or $450 billion. The costs of Medicare, the government insurance for the elderly, is expected to increase to $114 billion by the year 2000. It has been projected that by the year 2040, people over 65 will represent 21 percent of the population and consume 45 percent of all health care expenditures.

Medical expenses at the end of life appear to be extremely high in relation to other health care costs. Studies have shown that nearly one-third of annual Medicare costs are for the 5–6 percent of beneficiaries who die that year. Expenses for dying patients increase significantly as death nears, and payments for health care during the last weeks of life make up 40 percent of the medical costs for the entire last year of life. Some studies have shown that up to 50 percent of the medical costs incurred during a person's entire life are spent during their last year!

Many surveys have indicated that most Americans do not want to be kept alive if their illness is incurable and irreversible, for both economic and humanitarian reasons. Many experts believe that if physicians stopped using high technology at the end of life to prevent death, then we would save billions of dollars, which could be used to insure the uninsured and provide basic health care to millions.

In England, the emphasis of health care is on improving the quality of life through primary care medicine and well-subsidized home care and institutional programs for the elderly and those with incurable illnesses, rather than through life-extending acute care medicine. The British seem to value basic medical care for all rather than expensive technology for the few who might benefit from it. As a result, the British spend a much smaller proportion of their gross national product (6.2 percent) on health services than do Americans (10.8 percent) for a nearly identical health status and life expectancy.

In the following selection, Daniel Callahan argues that using medical technologies to extend the lives of the hopelessly ill and/or individuals who have lived out their natural life spans is an expensive and inappropriate use of modern medicine. Technology, he feels, should be used to avoid premature death and to relieve suffering, not to prolong full and complete lives. He believes that most elderly and hopelessly ill people agree with these principles: they indicate a wish that their lives not be aggressively extended beyond a point at which they still possess a good level of physical and mental functioning and a certain degree of value and meaning. Callahan also states that the attempt to indefinitely extend life can be an economic disaster. This goal also fails to put health in its proper place as only one among many human values, and it discourages the acceptance of aging and death as part of life.

Ezekiel J. Emanuel and Linda L. Emanuel counter that the actual savings from withholding treatment at the end of life would be minimal. They claim that high-quality care, such as providing pain medications and helping in the activities of daily living, requires skilled and expensive personnel. Even low-technology medical care is costly. They also argue that since death is often unpredictable, it is not always possible to say accurately which patients will benefit from high-technology treatment and which will not.

YES

Daniel Callahan

SETTING LIMITS: A RESPONSE

Some six years ago, in the fall of 1987, I published *Setting Limits: Medical Goals in an Aging Society* (Callahan, 1987). I argued that we would have to rethink once again the place of aging in the life cycle and that, in the future, scarcity of resources could force an age limit on medical entitlements for the elderly. That was not a popular thesis. I expected controversy and I got it, ranging from scholarly debates conducted with academic decorum to nasty public and media exchanges. Some six books of commentary and criticism, and an issue of a law review, were directly or indirectly inspired by *Setting Limits* (St. Louis University Law Journal, 1989; Homer & Holstein, 1990; Binstock & Post, 1991; Jecker, 1991; Barry & Bradley, 1991; Winslow & Walters, 1993; Hackler, in press).

The birth of *Setting Limits* came about because, beginning in the mid-1980s, I became aware of the striking demographic trends being reported, often accompanied by worries about their economic and social impact in the decades ahead (Preston, 1984). I saw us moving—through no one's fault, and surely not the elderly—toward a potential tragic dilemma of the first order. Something would have to give somewhere. We could not possibly guarantee indefinitely to the growing number and proportion of the elderly all of the potentially limitless fruits of medical progress at public expense without seriously distorting sensible social priorities. Where and how could we set some sensible and fair limits?

WHAT I TRIED TO SAY

Setting Limits was the result of my effort to think through that problem. I argued that we should begin now, *before* the crisis is fully upon us, to change our expectations about elderly care in the future. I stressed in the book the *trend* in the development of expensive technologies, not their present costs, and the likely need for *future* change in entitlement policies, not at present. As a way into these likely changes, I said that we need to rethink two deeply imbedded ideas, widely if not universally held. The first is the cherished notion that we should try endlessly through medical progress to modernize

From Daniel Callahan, "Setting Limits: A Response," *The Gerontologist*, vol. 34, no. 3 (June 1994), pp. 373–398. Copyright © 1994 by The Gerontological Society of America. Reprinted by permission.

old age, to turn it into a more or less permanent middle age. We should instead accept aging as a part of life, not just another medical obstacle to be overcome. The valuable and necessary campaign against ageism, highly individualistic in its premises, runs the risk of emptying age as a stage in life of meaningful content and, with the help of science, trying to turn it into a kind of repairable biological accident. The second idea I criticized was the view that there should be no limits to the claims of the elderly as a group to expensive life-extending medicine under *public* entitlement programs, that only their individual needs should count, and count in an age-blind way.

After criticizing those two ideas, I offered a different picture of what a future health care policy for the elderly might look like, one designed to balance the new limits with some enriched entitlements. I was seeking a public policy that: (1) would guarantee the elderly, along with everyone else, access to universal health care; (2) would help everyone to avoid an early, premature death; (3) would achieve a better balance of caring and curing to overcome the powerful bias toward the latter (whose effect is to undermine the former), and in particular to greatly strengthen long-term and home care support; and (4) would use age as a categorical standard to cut off life-extending technologies under the Medicare entitlement program—but using it as a standard *if and only if the* other reforms were put in place first.

I proposed the idea of a "natural life span" as a rough way of determining such a cut-off point. I would have been wise to have chosen a different word than "natural," since I meant by that concept a biographical not a biological standard,

that is, a notion of when it might be said that most people will have lived an adequately full, if not necessarily totally full, life. I drew that notion from my own experience, and the traditions of most cultures, which perceives an important moral and social distinction between the sadness but fittingness of death in old age and the tragedy or outrage of an avoidable early, particularly, childhood death. I did not specify an exact age but suggested that the "late 70s or early 80s" would be an appropriate age range in which to look for it.

The great need is to find a type of limit that would dampen the potent trend to apply ever more expensive technologies to saving and extending the life of the elderly. That trend has seen a steady rise in the age of various surgical and other medical procedures, and in particular a rise often marked by successful results (Hosking, Warner, Lobdell, Offord, & Melton, 1989; Latta & Keene, 1989; Breidenbaugh, Sarsitis, & Milam, 1990). But it is the success, I argued, that was creating the problem for us, not the failures, and I did not foresee us going backwards in care for the elderly, but radically slowing up and eventually plateauing the forward march of expensive medical progress.

I held, finally, that the needed changes should be effected, not by compulsion —the young imposing it by force on the unwilling old—but democratically, preceded by a decades-long period of changing our thinking, attitudes, and expectations about elderly health care. Those of us still reasonably young should be prepared in the future to impose an age limit on ourselves. As I noted in the Preface to my book, in a passage often overlooked, "what I am looking for is not any quick change but the beginning of a long-term discussion, one that will lead people to change their thinking and, most important, their expectations, about old age and death" (Callahan, 1987, p. 10).

RESPONSES TO CRITICS

Let me take up, in turn, the major objections leveled at my argument. Since there were well over 100 papers written about the book, and I was given the back of someone's hand in at least that many more, I will consolidate here the criticisms.

The Use of Age as a Standard for Limiting Health Care Would Be Ageist and Unjust.   There are two discordant ways of thinking about the place and relevance of age from an individual and from a policy perspective. From an individual perspective, it is said, age as such should have no place in resource allocation. It is not a good predictor of health, mental or physical. True. Yet the difficulty here is obvious from a policy perspective: Age *is* a relevant and conspicuous variable in health care costs, and the elderly are more costly as a group than people of younger ages. The fact that many elderly people remain healthy most of their final years—and that there is a heterogeneous pattern of health care usage—does not change the fact that the average per capita costs of the elderly are significantly higher than for younger people. Public policy must take account of, and work with, those averages. They are what count in devising programs, in projecting future costs, and in estimating different health care needs. Age matters.

If age matters, how does it matter? It matters when, as we can now see, meeting the health care costs of the elderly as a group begins to threaten the possibility of meeting the needs of other age groups. In the nature of the case, moreover, there are no fixed boundaries to the amount of money that can be spent combating the effects of biological aging and attempting to forestall death in old age. It is an unlimited frontier. One could say exactly the same thing about trying to save the life of low birthweight infants. We can go from the present 450–500 grams and 24–25 weeks gestation to 400 to 300 grams, and 20–21 weeks gestation, and so on. There are no end of possibilities there as well, and thus some very good reasons to set limits to those efforts, using either weight or gestational age as a categorical standard (Callahan, 1990). It is no more an anti-aging act than it is an anti-baby act to set limits (for instance, on neonatal care) in order to avoid pursuing unlimited, potentially ruinous possibilities.

Aging and death in old age are inevitable, and there should be no unlimited claim on public resources to combat them. But premature death, and bad schools, and blighted urban areas of great poverty, are not inevitable. The first health task of a society is that the young should have the chance to become old. That should always take priority over helping, at great cost, those who are already old from becoming still older. That is exactly what we can look forward to, as we throw more and more money into the fight to cure the chronic and degenerative diseases of aging, but not to care well for those who cannot be saved.

But if we set a limit on public entitlement for the elderly would this not be unfair and ageist? I believe we cannot achieve perfect equality in this world, much less in a health care system, without some harmful consequences. No country in the world, save the communist countries, has achieved any such goal, and the price they paid was rampant corruption and bribery; the wealthy and powerful still got better care. An age limit on entitlement benefits would of course perpetuate a two-tier system, with the rich able to buy health benefits not available to the poor, but that need not be the disaster many fear. The test should not be whether everyone receives exactly the same level of care. It should instead be whether the poorest and worst off receive decent health care. I believe the system I propose, guaranteeing universal care, a powerful effort to beat back premature death, a full range of health services through the late 70s or early 80s, a good range of social and caring services thereafter for one's entire life, and then (and only then) an age limit on expensive life-extending therapies, would be decent. If combined, moreover, with other kinds of limits in the health care systems for all groups, it would not be ageist even if it used age as a standard. It would use age as a standard simply because, as argued above, age does matter from a policy perspective.

It Is Unduly Pessimistic to Take Seriously the Projections That Show a Steadily Increasing Burden of Elderly Health Care Costs. "Callahan," one commentator said, "is overly alarmist about the relative burden of older persons..." (Lawlor, 1992, p. 132). I have never known quite what to make of that charge. I have used the standard research available on demographic trends and projected health care costs. I have never been able to find *any* optimistic projections based on historical and current demographic and economic projections. Even the critic who said I was "alarmist" concluded that paragraph by criticizing the optimists for failing to note that "the arithmetic of compound growth is at work in the increase of health expenditures (prices, demographic change, and increasing intensity of care)" (Lawlor, 1992, p. 132). Since I wrote *Setting Limits*, moreover, the "pessimistic" data have continued to pour forth, even from those who are my critics on other grounds (Schneider & Guralnik, 1990).

Since I have been unable to locate *any* optimistic data and reassuring projections, nor have any been cited in rebuttal, I can only observe that those who find me pessimistic rely on hopeful, but essentially still imaginary, scenarios about the future. One scenario is that in the future there will be a "compression of morbidity" and thus a decrease in the costs of elderly morbidity. That is a most invigorating hope, but the present evidence has moved in exactly the opposite direction, to greater not lesser morbidity, even if there is at least one recent report suggesting a slight amelioration of that trend (Manton, Corder, & Stallard, 1993). The second scenario is that advances in medical research will find cures or inexpensive treatments for the degenerative diseases of aging (Schneider & Guralnik, 1990). I hope that is true, but there is no evidence so far to support that hope as a likely outcome. The third scenario is that the elderly in the future will retire later and work longer, thus contributing more and much later to their health care costs. That could surely happen, and may by force happen, but it will as such not do a great deal about the disproportion of resources that could go to the elderly, although it surely might help. It is not likely to be helpful with the large number of people who live beyond 85, a rapidly growing group.

It Is Only Because Our Health Care System Is Wasteful, Capitalistic, and Paternalistic That We Are Even Thinking of Rationing and Limits on Care for the Elderly. There is no doubt that ours is a wasteful, fragmented, and excessively costly system, and that we could spend more on the elderly if we reduced waste elsewhere (Estes, 1988). The amount of money we spend in comparison with other developed countries, which get as good and often better outcomes for considerably less money, establishes that point well enough (though it does not establish that the money saved should go to the elderly as distinguished, say, from improving the schools). There are two points to consider here. The first is that, after more than 20 years of trying, we have not discovered in this country how, short of the universal health care and global budgeting we have been slow to embrace, to significantly control our costs; they just keep rising.

The second point is that, even if we can achieve those needed reforms, the problem will still not go away. The experience of other developed countries is already showing how an aging population can continue to push costs and demand up even in efficient, cost-effective, non-market health care systems (Hollander & Becker, 1987; Loriaux, 1990; Jouvenel, 1989). Those countries, controlling the fees of health care workers, rationing technology, keeping a lid on drug and equipment costs, still have a growing age-related problem even so. Better health care systems can delay the problem, or ameliorate it; but they are not going to be a solution to it.

A popular proposal to reduce elderly costs is the promotion of "advance directives" to allow the elderly to voluntarily forgo expensive, useless, and undesired care at the end of life. Could that make a difference? The evidence is mixed on that point and still scanty. One study found that advance directives made no difference in the medical treatment or in the medical costs (Schneiderman, Kronick, Kaplan, Anderson, & Langer, 1992), while another found evidence of dramatic savings (Chambers, Diamond, Perkel, & Lasch, 1994). My own guess is that advance directives will in the long run make some economic difference in relatively clear-cut cases of terminal illness for some classes of patients. There are two problems, however, which will make the greatest difference over time. One of them is the number of people who will execute advance directives, now still a significant minority. The other is the extent of expensive medical treatments that successfully avert the need to invoke advance directives, putting them off to another day; that's where the real bill is likely to add up, even if money can be saved in the last illness. To save money in the last days of life is not identical with saving money in the last years of life.

Even If It Becomes Necessary to Set Limits on Public Expenditures for Elderly Health Care, That Should Be Done on a Case-by-Case Basis Rather Than Categorically by Age. Should rationing or limits be necessary, almost everyone's ideal would be a system that was simultaneously individualized, fair, and effective. Each patient would be considered on his or her medical merits, not on the basis of some categorical standard. Rejecting categorical standards, "the impersonal application of a rule to a faceless group," Dr. Norman G. Levinsky has written that "society must not insulate itself from the agony of each decision to forgo beneficial treatment as it is experienced by patients, families, and care givers" (Levinsky, 1990, p. 1815).

I can well understand the sentiment behind Dr. Levinsky's thinking, but I have simply never been able to understand how it would be possible to limit health care in general while individualizing it in particular. If the assumption is that people should receive care on the basis of its individual efficacy for them, then we will run afoul of what I would call the "efficacy fallacy," that is, the notion that those treatments that are individually efficacious are therefore socially affordable. But precisely the problem we are likely to face is this: It will be the efficacious, not wasteful, treatments that will cause us the most financial grief, simply because it will be all the harder to deny people such treatment. There is a related fallacy, what I will dub the "hidden hand fallacy," that is, the view that the aggregate impact of meeting individual needs will turn out to be identical with the available common resources. Why should that be the case?

My assumption, by contrast—using the available projections—is that we will be forced to limit some proven, efficacious treatments, of a kind that people will want and that would extend their lives. The choices we will have to make will then be genuinely tragic choices. The pain of such choices is that they allow us no happy way out. It is an easy exercise to measure age-limit proposals against the standard of unlimited resources and no hard choices; and, naturally, an age limit looks terrible by that standard. But if we understand that we may one day be faced only with nasty options, then our task will be to compare those options with each other, not compare them against a world where no unpleasant choices are needed.

The Idea of Using a "Natural Life Span" as a Basis for Setting an Age Limit is Too Vague, and Too Controverted, to Be Useful. With great frequency I felt my proposal ran up against the individualism of our culture, not only in the repeated assertion about the heterogeneity of the elderly, but also in the rejection of a use of the life cycle as a place to look for an age limit. Yet I find it hard to know where else we might fruitfully look. If our standard is simply individual benefit, regardless of age, then there is no possible way we could effectively limit elderly health care costs; they will inexorably rise as technology improves. My alternative approach is to ask: How can we design a health care and entitlement system that would allow each of us to live a long and full life, but would not entail unlimited public support for whatever technology turned up at whatever cost?

I turned to the idea of a "natural life span" in order to capitalize on a common culture sentiment, still alive in the United States. It is that, while all death is a cause for sadness, a death in old age after a long and full life is, given the inevitability of death, the most acceptable kind of death. Unlike the death of a child, or a young adult, death in old age is part of our biology and part of the life cycle. It is no accident, think, that there is less weeping at the death of a very old person than at the death of a child. Although the idea of a "natural life span" as a biographical notion was thoroughly assaulted by many of my critics, a recent survey indicates that the idea is still strong in our society, even if most people would at present probably resist using it for rationing purposes (Zweibel, Cassel, & Karvison, 1993). Increased financial pressure, certain in the years ahead, may perhaps change the public bias against an age-based rationing standard.

I come back to a fundamental question. Do the elderly have an unlimited medical claim on public resources? No, they have only a reasonable and thus limited claim. What is a "reasonable" claim? I take it to be a claim to live a long life with public support, but not indefinitely long, and not at the price of potential harm to others. If we can agree with that proposition, then a "natural life span" is one that is highly useful—though admittedly not precise —allowing us a way of talking about what should count as a premature death, and as the basis for a claim on the public purse. It will surely work better than, say, "individual need," which is subject to technological escalation and intractable subjective desires. If we agree, for instance, that the preservation of life is a basic medical need, then in the nature of the case with the aging person there are no necessary limits at all, scientific or economic, to what can be done to achieve that goal. To be sure, any specific age to invoke as a limit will be arbitrary, but not necessarily capricious. That was true of age 65 when Medicare was established. It could have been 66 or 64. The point is that it was within a generally acceptable range of choices, and that is sufficient for fair public policy.

SOME TELLING POINTS

My response so far might indicate that I have been unwilling to give way to my critics or to admit any validity to what they say. Up to a point that is true. Nonetheless, on the old principle that much of life and policy lies in the details, some telling points have been made against me. They are worth further thought.

The most powerful criticism is political: Whatever the rational arguments in its favor, neither the public nor legislators would ever accept an open, explicit use of age as a criterion for cutting off life-extending medical care. One critic called this assumption on my part a "blunder," and (in some sympathy with my general argument about the need for limits) said that we might be forced to covertly have an age standard (Moody, 1991). I have no doubt that an age limit would, politically, be obnoxious to politicians, at least at present. Even those countries known for using age as a norm (such as England and Switzerland) have done so tacitly and quietly, out of the public eye. Yet, if it is true that an explicit age standard is now and will remain for some time politically unacceptable as public policy, then we will be left with another dilemma. We will either have to come up with some other standard, bound to be unwanted also if it has any bite, or resign ourselves to euphemism and evasion, using age privately but never admitting it publicly.

There is a telling scientific criticism also. One of my goals with an age limit is to discourage the kind of scientific "progress" that endlessly generates new, almost always expensive, ways of extending the lives of elderly people. If those modalities were not going to be reimbursed, that would be a powerful disincentive to developing them in the first place. The problem here, as many noted, is that most of the technologies now used with the elderly were first developed with younger people in mind; few life-extending technologies are created for the elderly as such.

I cannot deny the force of those contentions. But that leaves us with another dilemma: If scientific progress moves along in an unchecked fashion, generating still more expensive ways of saving life, our tragic dilemma will become all the more painful. The gap between what we know we can or could do to save life will all the more harshly and conspicuously clash with our economic limitations. My own preference would be for a sharp increase in research designed to decrease morbidity and disability, discouraging when possible explicit efforts to develop more life-extending technologies.

Still another criticism might, for lack of a better name, be called the repugnance argument. It takes a number of forms. One of them is that we would find it repugnant to deny reimbursement to someone for a form of care that would clearly save that person's life; we could not just stand by and let the person die for lack of money. Another form is that, however nice my theory of justice between age groups, it would *look* like we were devaluing the worth of the elderly if we used age as an exclusive standard for denying care; we would find that hard to stand.

I agree that most people would find these consequences of an age limit repugnant. But again we are left with a dilemma, indeed more than one. What will we do about the repugnance that could well result from seeing a larger and larger, and even more disproportionate, share of resources going to the elderly while the needs of younger groups are going unmet? Or placing heavier and heavier economic burdens on the young to sustain the old? If we leave all choices about resource allocation to doctors and families at the bedside, what will we do about the repugnance regarding the variations in treatment that method will bring, with some getting too much treatment and others getting too little? If we find the open use of an age limit repugnant, will we feel any better about a covert use, one that could be forced by a shortage of money?

Another telling point, in some ways the most fundamental, leaves me with a deep and unresolved problem. In an unpublished paper Per Anderson suggests that the "high quality aging that Callahan wants medicine and society to support will serve to make the idea of the life cycle increasingly implausible ... one can wonder whether Callahan would have us adopt an ethic of limits because it is the human good or because it is the grim necessity to which we must be resigned" (Anderson, 1991, p. 3). On this point, a profound one for medicine in general and not just for care of the aged, I am deeply ambivalent.

My own reading of history is that those people and cultures who live with some sense of intrinsic limits, whether natural or culturally inspired, better adapt to the human situation, and to aging and mortality, than do those who want to carry out endless warfare against human finitude. Yet I cannot ignore the other side of that coin, which is that we have enormously benefited from many efforts to transcend what earlier generations took to be fixed limits. I might not now be alive but for those efforts. How do we find the right balance here, between acceptance and acquiescence and the desire to struggle against our human condition? It is open to my critics to make a good case for fighting the ravages of age and to seek to further postpone death. I will respond by asking: Why should we believe that will necessarily increase our human satisfaction and sense of well-being? We will, I am sure, go back and forth on that point—and no doubt so will future generations.

WHAT ABOUT THE FUTURE?

There were three reasons why I was drawn to the use of an age limit as a likely way to eventually control health care allocation to the elderly. One reason was that it seems to me better in general for human beings to live with a strong sense of their mortality and to be willing to understand that their lives must come to an end. A second reason is that it seems to me merely the prejudice of an affluent, hyper-individualistic, technologically driven society to think that a denial of reimbursement for life-extending care beyond a certain point is tantamount to a denial of value and dignity to the elderly. The third reason for being drawn to age was that I simply could not imagine—and still cannot imagine—any other way of decisively and effectively and uniformly drawing a clear policy line than the use of age. It is precisely because it cuts through, and transcends, our individual differences that it is attractive for policy purposes.

That of course is precisely its greatest liability in the eyes of my critics, and I am more persuaded than I was initially that, for both symbolic and practical reasons, an age-based policy will appear, and well could be, obnoxious. Yet, having conceded that, I must then add: Show me an equally decisive alternative, one that will work to hold down costs, that does not depend upon variable bedside judgments, and that takes with full seriousness the need to find a solution —and a solution that does not depend on evading the problem altogether by invoking some yet-to-be-seen hopeful scientific or economic miracle.

If we agree on the eventual need for limits, does it follow that only an age limit would work? Not at all, and it may well be that the various repugnances I noted above will stand forever in the way of using an age limit. But in that case it will be necessary to come up with some plausible alternatives. Robert Veatch and Norman Daniels have suggested some interesting and alternative ways of using age, less stark than mine. They can be debated. Nancy S. Jecker and Robert A. Pearlman, after criticizing Harry R. Moody, Norman Daniels, and myself for our willingness to consider an age limit, conclude their article with a brief review of some possible alternatives—and find them full of problems as well! (See Jecker & Pearlman, 1989). No doubt anyway, as they say, we will have to explore those alternatives. I offer a simple test as we try to think about one alternative or another: If it seems to avoid the need for nasty choices altogether, or seems painless and congenial (like just cutting out unwanted treatment), we should have a hard time taking it seriously. In the best of all possible worlds, what the elderly want and need would fit perfectly with the available resources. Ours is not, nor is likely to be, such a world. Any solution that seems to imply such a world merits the same suspicion as offers of free trips to Europe or Florida just by placing a phone call.

Time and again I was accused of "blaming the elderly" for our present allocation problems. How nice it would be to find identifiable villains here, but I see no fault here *at all* with the elderly. Instead, we are only now beginning to see some of the costs and pitfalls of the great medical advances that have been made in recent decades, and some of the unforeseen and probably unforeseeable hazards of pursuing medical progress. It is the success of medicine, not its failures, that has created the problem of sustaining and paying for decent health care for the elderly. It is the success of the campaign against ageism, increasing the expectations of everyone for a medically and socially transformed old age, that have added to that problem. If there is any blame to be apportioned it should be directed at our dreams, some of which have come true. It is just that we did not know what that would mean. Now we are finding out.

REFERENCES

Anderson, P. (1991). On the "ragged edge" of medical progress: Daniel Callahan and problems of limits. Unpublished paper.

Barry, R. L., & Bradley, G. V. (Eds.). (1991). *Set no limits: A rebuttal to Daniel Callahan's proposal to limit health care for the elderly.* Urbana: University of Illinois Press.

Binstock, R. H., & Post, S. G. (Eds.). (1991). *Too old for health care: Controversies in medicine, law, economics, and ethics.* Baltimore: The Johns Hopkins University Press.

Breidenbaugh, M. Z., Sarsitis, I. M., & Milam, R. A. (1990). Medicare end stage renal disease population, *Health Care Financing Review, 12,* 101–104.

Callahan, D. (1987). *Setting limits: Medical goals in an aging society.* New York: Simon and Schuster.

Callahan, D. (1990). *What kind of life: The limits of medical progress.* New York: Simon and Schuster.

Callahan, D. (1993). *The troubled dream of life: Living with mortality.* New York: Simon and Schuster.

Chambers, C. V., Diamond, J. J., Perkel, R. L., & Lasch, L. A. (1994). Relationship of advance directives to hospital charges in a Medicare population. *Archives of Internal Medicine, 154,* 541–547.

Estes, C. L. (1988). Cost containment and the elderly: Conflict or challenge? *Journal of the American Medical Association, 36,* 68–72.

Hackler, C. (Ed.). (In press). *Health care for an aging population: Planning for the twenty-first century.* Albany: State University of New York Press.

Holahan, J., & Palmer, J. L. (1988). Medicare's fiscal problems: An imperative for reform. *Journal of Health, Politics, Policy and Law, 13,* 53–81.

Hollander, C. F., & Becker, H. A., (Eds.). (1987). *Growing old in the future.* Dordrecht: Martinius Nijhoff Publishers.

Homer, P., & Holstein, M., (Eds.). (1990). *A good old age: The paradox of setting limits.* New York: Simon and Schuster.

Hosking, M. P., Warner, M. A., Lobdell, C. M., Offord, K. P., & Melton, J. L. (1989). Outcome of surgery in patients 90 years of age and older. *Journal of the American Medical Association, 261,* 1909–1915.

Jecker, N. S., (Ed.). (1991). *Ethics and aging.* Clifton, NJ: Humana Press.

Jecker, N. S. (1991). Age-based rationing and women. *Journal of the American Medical Association, 266,* 3012–3015.

Jecker, N. S., & Pearlman, R. A. (1989). Ethical constraints on rationing medical care by age. *Journal of the American Geriatrics Society, 37,* 1067–1075.

Jouvenel, H. de. (1989). *Europe's ageing population: Trends and challenges to 2025.* Special co-publication of *Futures and Futuribles.* Guildford, UK: Butterworth.

Latta, V. B., & Keene, R. E. (1989). Leading surgical procedures for aged Medicare beneficiaries. *Health Care Financing Review, 11,* 99–100.

Lawlor, E. F. (1992). What kind of medicine? *The Gerontologist, 32,* 131–133.

Levinsky, N. G. (1990). Age as a criterion for rationing health care. *New England Journal of Medicine, 322,* 1813–1815.

Loriaux, (1990). Il Sera une fois... la revolution gruse jeux at enjeux autour d'une profunde mutation societale (Someday it will happen... the revolution of aging and the profound social change at stake). Université Catholique de Louvain. Louvain-la-Neuve, Claco: Institut de Démographie.

Manton, K. G., Corder, L., & Stallard, S. (1993). Changes in the use of personal assistance and special equipment from 1982 to 1989: Results from the 1982 and 1989 NLTCS. *The Gerontologist, 33,* 168–176.

Moody, H. R. (1991). Allocation, yes; Age-based rationing, no. In R. H. Binstock & S. G. Post, (Eds.), *Too Old for Health Care.* Baltimore: The Johns Hopkins University Press, pp. 180–203.

Preston, S. (1984). Children and the elderly: Divergent paths for America's dependents. *Demography, 21,* 455–491.

St. Louis University. (1989). Health care for the elderly. Symposium in the *St. Louis University Law Journal, 33,* 557–710.

Schneider, E. L., Guralnik, J. M. (1990). The aging of America: Impact on health care costs. *Journal of the American Medical Association, 263,* 2335–2340.

Schneiderman, L., Kronick, R., Kaplan, R. M., Anderson, J. P., & Langer, R. D. (1992). Effects of offering advance directives on medical treatment and costs. *Annals of Internal Medicine, 117,* 599–606.

Winslow, G. R., & Walters, J. W. (Eds.). (1993). *Facing limits: Ethics and health care for the elderly.* Boulder, CO: Westview Press.

Zweibel, N. R., Cassel, C. K., & Karvison, T. (1993). Public attitudes about the use of chronological age as a criterion for allocating health care resources. *The Gerontologist, 36,* 74–80.

NO

**Ezekiel J. Emanuel and
Linda L. Emanuel**

THE ECONOMICS OF DYING:
THE ILLUSION OF COST SAVINGS
AT THE END OF LIFE

For more than a decade, health policy analysts have noted—and some have decried—the high cost of dying.[1-7] With the acceleration of pressures on health care costs and calls for reform, considerably more attention has been focused on proposals to control costs at the end of life.[8] One proposal would require persons enrolling in a health care plan to complete an advance directive.[9,10] Others would require hospitals to establish guidelines to identify and reduce futile care.[11-13] Similar ideas have been expressed by members of President Bill Clinton's Health Care Task Force and by Joycelyn Elders, the surgeon general.[14]

Advance directives and hospice care were developed to ensure patients' autonomy and to provide high-quality care at the end of life. Compassion and dignity are sufficient justification for their use. Nevertheless, the persistent interest in saving money at the end of life through the use of advance directives and hospice care makes it imperative to assess how much money might realistically be saved.

COST AT THE END OF LIFE AND REASONS FOR COST CONTROL

Expenditures at the end of life seem disproportionately large. Although the precise numbers vary, studies consistently demonstrate that 27 to 30 percent of Medicare payments each year are for the 5 to 6 percent of Medicare beneficiaries who die in that year.[15-17] The latest available figures indicate that in 1988, the mean Medicare payment for the last year of life of a beneficiary who died was $13,316, as compared with $1,924 for all Medicare beneficiaries (a ratio of 6.9:1).[15] Payments for dying patients increase exponentially as death approaches, and payments during the last month of life constitute 40 percent of payments during the last year of life.[15] Identical trends and ratios have been found since the early 1960s.[6,15-17]

From Ezekiel J. Emanuel and Linda L. Emanuel, "The Economics of Dying: The Illusion of Cost Savings at the End of Life," *The New England Journal of Medicine*, vol. 330, no. 8 (February 24, 1994), pp. 540–544. Copyright © 1994 by The Massachusetts Medical Society. Reprinted by permission. All rights reserved.

Many people believe that these expenditures are for the care of patients known in advance to be dying. The time of death is usually unpredictable, however, except perhaps when the patient has advanced cancer. There is no method to predict months or weeks in advance who will live and who will die. Consequently, it is difficult to know in advance what costs are for care at the end of life and what costs are for saving a life.[6,7] Only in retrospect, after a patient's death, can we identify the last year or month of life. Nevertheless, to many people, reducing expenditures at the end of life seems an easy and readily justifiable way of cutting wasteful spending and freeing resources to ensure universal access to health care.[9–11,18] General rules intended to curtail the use of unnecessary medical services have been shown to reduce both effective and wasteful services.[19] Consequently, there is some reluctance to limit interventions for relatively healthy people. Many believe, however, that interventions for patients whose death is imminent are inherently wasteful, since they neither cure nor ameliorate disease or disability.

Advance directives and hospice care have been proposed as methods of reducing medical costs at the end of life; both can transform "good ethics [into] good health economics."[9] In survey after survey, Americans indicate that they do not want to be kept alive if their disease is irreversible. If doctors would stop using high-technology interventions at the end of life, the argument goes, then we could simultaneously respect patients' autonomy and save tens of billions of dollars.[8–11,14] When we link ethics and economics to prevent futile care, it is claimed, "everyone wins—the patient, the family, and society as a whole."[11]

Despite the allure of these arguments, we are skeptical. Before making major changes in policy regarding the care of dying patients and formulating budget projections on the basis of cost savings of billions of dollars, we should review the economics of care at the end of life. The cost savings that could be achieved through the wider use of advance directives, hospice care, and curtailment of futile care have not been well studied. The available data suggest, however, that such savings would be less than many have imagined.

ADVANCE DIRECTIVES FOR HEALTH CARE AND COST SAVINGS

One study evaluating the effect of advance directives on costs randomly assigned outpatients to either a physician-initiated discussion of advance directives and encouragement to use them or no intervention.[20] There was no difference in medical costs or other variables between the groups: as the authors stated, "executing the California Durable Power of Attorney for Health Care and having a summary copy placed in the patient's medical record had no significant positive or negative effect on a patient's well-being, health status, medical treatments, or medical treatment charges."[20] Although this study involved small numbers of patients at only two hospitals and measured hospital charges rather than actual costs, similar preliminary results were reported in another study involving 854 patients who died at five medical centers.[21] Executing an advance directive did not significantly affect the cost of patients' terminal hospitalizations. The average hospital bill for those without an advance directive was $56,300, as compared with $61,589 for those with a living will and $58,346 for those with a durable power of attorney.[21] Additional studies are certainly needed, but these reports suggest that the wider use of advance directives is unlikely to produce dramatic cost savings.

HOSPICE CARE AND COST SAVINGS

Hospice patients refuse life-sustaining interventions, favor palliative care, and are often treated at home; they serve as another source of information on the magnitude of the potential savings from the reduced use of high-technology interventions at the end of life. A series of studies comparing hospice care and traditional care of terminally ill patients estimated that in the last month of life, home hospice care saves between 31 and 64 percent of medical care costs.[22–27] The difference is accounted for mostly by the reduced use of hospital services. Consequently, the savings for hospital-based hospice care are lower. However, the longer patients receive hospice care, the smaller the savings. As the National Hospice Study reported, for hospice patients "the longer the stay in hospice, the more likely [it was that] costs incurred exceeded those of conventional care patients in the last year of life; the economies associated with hospice occur primarily in the last weeks of life."[28] During the last six months of life, the mean medical costs for patients receiving hospice care at home are 27 percent less than for conventional care, and the savings with hospital-based hospice care are less than 15 percent.[22,24,26]

These studies may systematically overstate the savings associated with hospice care. Most have not been randomized and may have incorporated a selection bias, since hospice patients by definition want less aggressive care. The one randomized study of hospice care found no cost savings for long-term hospice patients.[23] Patients receiving care in a hospice also tend to be from higher socioeconomic groups and to have informal support structures that enable them to obtain additional services, such as personal attendants not covered by Medicare, that are invisible in most cost estimates.[29] As rates of hospitalization decline, so, too, may the savings from hospice care.[22] Finally, an overwhelming majority of hospice patients have cancer, a fact that limits the generalizability of these data.[28]

FUTILE CARE AND COST SAVINGS

A related proposal to save money at the end of life is to reduce "futile care."[10,11] What constitutes futile care is controversial,[30–33] but the paradigmatic case is cardiopulmonary resuscitation for patients dying of cancer.[30–34] Unfortunately, there have been no studies of the financial consequences of eliminating resuscitation for patients with cancer. In a study of the cost of care for all patients with do-not-resuscitate (DNR) orders at a tertiary care hospital, almost 25 percent of whom had cancer, it was found that among patients who died, medical care for those with DNR orders cost about the same as for those without DNR orders: a mean of $62,594 for 616 patients with DNR orders as compared with $57,334 for 219 patients without DNR orders.[35]

Advocates of cost cutting have suggested extending the concept of futility to curtail marginally beneficial care.[10,11] Chemotherapy for unresectable [not removable] non-small-cell lung cancer is an example of marginal if not entirely futile therapy; it does not systematically enhance longevity, improve the quality of life, or palliate pain.[36,37] A randomized trial in Canada, comparing chemotherapy with high-quality supportive care for patients with non-small-cell lung cancer, found that the average cost of the supportive care was $8,595 (in 1984 Canadian dollars), whereas one chemotherapy regimen cost less ($7,645) and another regimen cost more ($12,232).[38] Some aspects of this study are controversial, and some costs were approximated because they were "not routinely identified in the Canadian health care system."[38,39] Nevertheless, the authors concluded that even if chemotherapy is expensive, "a policy of supportive care for patients with advanced non-small-cell lung cancer was associated with substantial costs."[38]

CAN WE SAVE ANY MONEY ON CARE AT THE END OF LIFE?

Can we realize any savings by the more frequent use of advance directives, hospice care, and less aggressive care at the end of life? We can estimate the proportion of health costs that might be saved in a best-case scenario—that is, if every American who died had executed an advance directive, refused aggressive care at the end of life, and elected to receive hospice care at home. The only reliable cost data for the last year of life are Medicare costs for patients 65 years of age or older; there are no reliable data on the total costs of health care for patients either over or under 65 who die. Consequently, many approximations are necessary in calculating the savings that can be realized.

In 1988, the mean annual cost per Medicare beneficiary who died during that year was $13,316.[15] Medicare primarily pays for acute care, however, and ac-

counts for only 45 percent of total health care costs for those 65 years old or older; the bulk of the excluded costs are for nursing home care.[49] The simplest way to estimate the additional health care costs for Medicare beneficiaries who die is to assume they use the same fraction of these other services that they do of services covered by Medicare. This means that patients 65 or older who die in a given year account for 27 percent of total health care expenditures—Medicare costs, nursing home costs, and the costs of other services for all patients 65 or older. Thus, we estimate that patients 65 years old or older who died in 1988 spent $29,295 for all their health care services, of which $13,316 was covered by Medicare.

How should we estimate costs during the last year of life for patients less than 65 years of age? Although costs for younger patients who die of cancer and the acquired immunodeficiency syndrome (AIDS) are probably substantially higher than costs for dying Medicare patients,[41] the costs for those who die of accidents, suicide, and homicide are probably less. Scitovsky showed that among a group of California patients who died, the mean total medical costs for the last year of life were about the same for those under 65 years of age as for those 65 to 79 years of age.[42] In 1988, the mean Medicare cost for 65-to-79-year-old patients who died was $15,346 (Lubitz J: personal communication). Assuming that this is 45 percent of total health care expenditures, we can estimate that the mean annual medical cost for patients under 65 who died in 1988 was $34,102.

We know that 2.17 million Americans died in 1988, of whom 1.49 million were Medicare beneficiaries. Using the hospice data, and assuming that the maximum we might save in health care costs during the last year of life by reducing interventions is 27 percent,[22,24,26] we can calculate how much could be saved if each of the 2.17 million Americans who died executed an advance directive, chose hospice care, and refused aggressive, in-hospital interventions at the end of life. As Table 1 shows, the total savings in health care expenditures would have been $18.1 billion in 1988, or 3.3 percent of all health care spending. In 1988, the savings in Medicare costs would have been $5.4 billion, or 6.1 percent of expenditures.[43] Since the percentage of health dollars spent on patients who died has been constant over 30 years, the savings as a percentage of total national health care costs and Medicare spending is unlikely to change over time.[6,15,44]

This calculation relies on best-case assumptions that err on the side of overestimating savings. We have extrapolated the savings for patients who receive hospice care to the use of advance directives and to the reduced use of futile interventions. Yet not everyone would refuse life-sustaining interventions in their advance directives, and futile interventions are hard to define, let alone stop. Moreover, achieving savings of any considerable magnitude depends on decreasing the numbers of days spent in the hospital, yet over the past decade there has already been a significant decline in both the number of hospital days for all patients and the proportion of costs for patients who die that are allocated to hospital care.[15] Furthermore, curtailing care at the end of life is likely to affect acute care and thus Medicare costs, but unlikely to decrease nursing home and other outpatient costs; indeed, it may even increase such costs. (Excluding nursing home costs would reduce the total savings from $18.1 billion to $15.9 billion, or 2.9 percent of total health care spending.)

Reducing health care expenditures by 3.3 percent cannot be dismissed lightly. Yet even with the most generous assumptions possible, the savings will be less than the scores of billions of dollars predicted by many commentators and the savings estimated from cutting administrative waste.[8-11,14,45]

WHY IS THERE NOT MUCH MONEY TO BE SAVED AT THE END OF LIFE?

Why, despite the high cost of dying documented for Medicare beneficiaries, is there not likely to be much in the way of cost savings from the use of advance directives, hospice care, and fewer high-technology interventions? One explanation is that the Medicare data produce a distorted image of the cost of dying. Commentators extrapolate the data for Medicare patients who die to the entire population.[8,10,11,14] Using 1990 expenditures, for example, Singer and Lowy calculate that "the care of patients who died" cost $184 billion (27 percent of the $661 billion spent on health care in 1990).[8] They suggest that $55 billion to $109 billion might be saved "from a policy of asking all patients about their wishes regarding life-sustaining treatment and incorporating those wishes into advance directives."

Although Medicare data on mortality and expenditures may be the only reliable figures available, they cannot be extrapolated without adjustment to the whole health care system. Less than 1 percent of the total American population dies each year, yet 5 to 6 percent of Medicare beneficiaries die. Five percent of Medicare patients may account for 27 percent of Medicare payments, but it is improbable that the less than 1 percent of the American population who die account for 27 percent of the total national spending on health care. We estimate that the 2.17 million Americans who die annually account for about 10 to 12 percent of health care expenditures.

It may be difficult to reduce substantially the percentage of health care expenditures spent on patients who die because humane care at the end of life is labor-intensive and therefore expensive. Even when patients refuse life-sustaining interventions, they do not necessarily require less medical care, just a different kind of care. High-quality palliative care —providing pain medications, helping in the activities of daily living, using radiation therapy for pain relief, and so on —requires skilled, and costly, personnel. Thus, even low-technology health care that is administered outside hospitals to terminally ill patients is not cheap.

Another explanation is related to the unpredictability of death. Since there are no reliable ways to identify the patients who will die,[6,44,46] it is not possible to say accurately months, weeks, or even days before death which patients will benefit from intensive interventions and which ones will receive "wasted" care. Retrospective cost studies will inflate costs at the end of life as compared with costs for patients known in advance to be dying because they include many patients receiving expensive care who are not expected to die yet do die. This clinical uncertainty also means that resources are initially expended until a patient's prognosis becomes clearer and physicians, patients, and the family are sure about either forging ahead with aggressive treatment or withdrawing it. This process is both ethically correct and what most Americans seem to desire.[47] Advance direc-

tives are unlikely to reduce this type of care, since physicians, patients, and family members are hesitant to discontinue therapy when there is a real chance of survival.

In addition, medical practice has changed over the past decade. For the vast majority of patients who die, DNR orders are already in place and other interventions are terminated. For instance, at Memorial Sloan-Kettering Cancer Center, 85 percent of patients with cancer who have cardiac arrest have DNR orders[48]; other institutions have reported rates of DNR orders among patients with cancer that are as high as 97 percent.[35] Currently, in tertiary care hospitals, between 60 and 80 percent of dying patients have DNR orders.[49-51] Admittedly, the decision to give a DNR order or withdraw life-sustaining treatment is usually made late in the course of a patient's illness. Nevertheless, given the steep rise in costs as death approaches, reducing care in these final days of life should yield the most savings.[15,35] As the data on hospice care demonstrate, there may be additional— but smaller—cost savings if the decision to stop treatment is pushed back several weeks.[22,24,26,28]

Finally, the increased use of living wills and health care proxy forms may not necessarily curtail the use of life-sustaining treatment. We have no empirical evidence that patients are getting substantially more treatment than they or their families want. Although there have been a few well-publicized cases in which physicians have treated patients against their wishes, these are probably unrepresentative.[52] Studies consistently show that physicians are more willing than patients and family members to withhold or withdraw life-sustaining treatments.[53,54] A large minority of people consistently want treatment even after they become incompetent or have a low chance of survival. For instance, about 20 percent of patients want life-sustaining therapy even if they are in a persistent vegetative state.[47] Similarly, about half of patients with AIDS want aggressive life-sustaining treatment, including admission to an intensive care unit and cardiopulmonary resuscitation, in circumstances in which they have a relatively poor chance of survival.[55,56] Thus, patients who complete advance directives may request more life-sustaining treatment than they currently receive, precluding any cost savings. In addition, studies demonstrate that family members are consistently more hesitant to withhold or withdraw life-sustaining treatment than the patients themselves.[53,54,57,58] Thus, if patients are encouraged to select proxy decision makers by executing durable powers of attorney, the cost savings may be minimal.

CONCLUSIONS

None of the individual studies of cost savings at the end of life associated with advance directives, hospice care, or the elimination of futile care are definitive. Yet they all point in the same direction: cost savings due to changes in practice at the end of life are not likely to be substantial. The amount that might be saved by reducing the use of aggressive life-sustaining interventions for dying patients is at most 3.3 percent of total national health care expenditures. In 1993, with $900 billion going to health care, this savings would amount to $29.7 billion. It is important to note that achieving such savings would not restrain the rate of growth in health

care spending over time.[59] Instead, this amount represents a fraction of the increase due to inflation in health care costs and less than the $50 billion to $90 billion needed to cover the uninsured population.

The unlikeliness of substantial savings in health care costs does not mean, however, that there are no good reasons to use advance directives, fund hospice care, and employ less aggressive life-sustaining treatments for dying patients. Respecting patients' wishes, reducing pain and suffering, and providing compassionate and dignified care at the end of life have overwhelming merit. But the hope of cutting the amount of money spent on life-sustaining interventions for the dying in order to reduce overall health care costs is probably vain. Our alternatives for achieving substantial savings seem limited to major changes in the financing and delivery of health care, difficult choices in the allocation of services, or both. Whatever we choose, we must stop deluding ourselves that advance directives and less aggressive care at the end of life will solve the financial problems of our health care system.

We are indebted to James Lubitz, M.P.H., Dan Brock, Ph.D., Joseph P. Newhouse, Ph.D., Rashi Fein, Ph.D., David Kidder, Ph.D., and Jane Weeks, M.D., for their comments on earlier drafts of the manuscript, and to the members of President Clinton's Health Care Task Force who discussed these issues with us.

REFERENCES

1. Leaf A. Medicine and the aged. N Engl J Med 1977;297:887–90.

2. Turnbull AD, Carlon G, Baron R, Sichel W, Young C, Howland W. The inverse relationship

between cost and survival in the critically ill cancer patient. Crit Care Med 1979;7:20–3.

3. Ginzberg E. The high costs of dying. Inquiry 1980;17:293–5.

4. Shroeder SA, Showstack JA, Schwartz J. Survival of adult high-cost patients: report of a follow-up study from nine acute-care hospitals. JAMA 1981;245:1446–9.

5. Bayer R, Callahan D, Fletcher J, et al. The care of the terminally ill: mortality and economics. N Engl J Med 1983;309:1490–4.

6. Scitovsky AA. "The high cost of dying": what do the data show? Milbank Mem Fund Q Health Soc 1984;62:591–608.

7. Scitovsky AA, Capron AM. Medical care at the end of life: the interaction of economics and ethics. Annu Rev Public Health 1986;7:59–75.

8. Singer PA, Lowy FH. Rationing, patient preferences and cost of care at the end of life. Arch Intern Med 1992;152:478–80.

9. d'Oronzio JC. Good ethics, good health economics. New York Times. June 8, 1993:A25.

10. Fries JF, Koop CE, Beadle CE, et al. Reducing health care costs by reducing the need and demand for medical services. N Engl J Med 1993;329:321–5.

11. Lundberg GD. American health care system management objectives: the aura of inevitability becomes incarnate. JAMA 1993;269:2354–5.

12. Schneiderman LJ, Jecker N. Futility in practice. Arch intern Med 1993;153:437–41.

13. Murphy DJ, Finucane TE. New do-not-resuscitate policies: a first step in cost control. Arch Intern Med 1993;153:1641–8.

14. Godec MS. Your final 30 days—free. Washington Post. May 2, 1993:C3.

15. Lubitz JD, Riley GF. Trends in Medicare payments in the last year of life. N Engl J Med 1993;328:1092–6.

16. Lubitz J, Prihoda R. The use and costs of Medicare services in the last 2 years of life. Health Care Financ Rev 1984;5(3):117–31.

17. McCall N. Utilization and costs of Medicare services by beneficiaries in their last year of life. Med Care 1984;22:329–42.

18. Siu AL, Brook RH. Allocating health care resources: how can we ensure access to essential care? In: Ginzberg E, ed. Medicine and society: clinical decisions and societal values. Boulder, Colo.: Westview Press, 1987;20–33.

19. Siu AL, Sonnenberg FA, Manning WG, et al. Inappropriate use of hospitals in a randomized trial of health insurance plans. N Engl J Med 1986;315:1259–66.

20. Schneiderman LJ, Kronick R, Kaplan RM, Anderson JP, Langer RD. Effects of offering advance directives on medical treatments and costs. Ann Intern Med 1992;117:599–606.

21. Teno J, Lynn J, Phillips R, et al. Do advance directives save resources? Clin Res 1993;41:551A. abstract.

22. Kidder D. The effects of hospice coverage on Medicare expenditures. Health Serv Res 1992;27:195–217.

23. Kane RL, Wales J. Bernstein L, Leibowitz A, Kaplan S. A randomised controlled trial of hospice care. Lancet 1984;1:890–4.

24. Spector WD, Mor V. Utilization and charges for terminal cancer patients in Rhode Island. Inquiry 1984;21:328–37.

25. Hannan EL, O'Donnell JF. An evaluation of hospices in the New York State Hospice Demonstration Program. Inquiry 1984;21: 338–48.

26. Mor V, Kidder D. Cost savings in hospice: final results of the National Hospice Study. Health Serv Res 1985;20:407–22.

27. Brooks CH, Smyth-Staruch K. Hospice home care cost savings to third-party insurers. Med Care 1984;22:691–703.

28. Greer DS, Mor V. An overview of National Hospice Study findings. J Chronic Dis 1986;39: 5–7.

29. Moinpour CM, Polissar L. Factors affecting place of death of hospice and non-hospice cancer patients. Am J Public Health 1989;79:1549–51.

30. Schneiderman LJ, Jecker NS, Jonsen AR. Medical futility: its meaning and ethical implications. Ann Intern Med 1990;112:949–54.

31. Tomlinson T, Brody H. Futility and the ethics of resuscitation. JAMA 1990;264:1276–80.

32. Lantos JD, Singer PA, Walker RM, et al. The illusion of futility in clinical practice. Am J Med 1989;87:81–4.

33. Loewy EH, Carlson RA. Futility and its wider implications: a concept in need of further examination. Arch Intern Med 1993;153:429–31.

34. Blackhall LJ. Must we always use CPR? N Engl J Med 1987;317:1281–5.

35. Maksoud A, Jahnigen DW, Skibinski CI. Do not resuscitate orders and the cost of death. Arch Intern Med 1993;153:1249–53.

36. Ihde DC. Chemotherapy of lung cancer. N Engl J Med 1992;327:1434–41.

37. Ruckdeschel JC. Is chemotherapy for metastatic non-small cell lung cancer "worth it"? J Clin Oncol 1990;8:1293–6.

38. Jaakkimainen L, Goodwin PJ, Pater J, Warde P, Murray N, Rapp E. Counting the costs of chemotherapy in a National Cancer Institute of Canada randomized trial in nonsmall-cell lung cancer. J Clin Oncol 1990;8:1301–9.

39. Rapp E, Pater JL, Willan A, et al. chemotherapy can prolong survival in patients with advanced non-small-cell lung cancer—report of a Canadian multicenter randomized trial. J Clin Oncol 1988;6:633–41.

40. Waldo DR, Sonnefeld ST, McKusick DR, Arnett RH III. Health expenditures by age group, 1977 and 1987. Health Care Financ Rev 1989;10(4):111–20.

41. Riley G, Lubitz J, Prihoda R, Rabey E. The use and costs of Medicare services by cause of death. Inquiry 1987;24:233–44.

42. Scitovsky AA. Medical care in the last twelve months of life: the relation between age, functional status, and medical care expenditures. Milbank Q 1988;66:640–60.

43. Levit KR, Lazenby HC, Cowan CA, Letsch SW. National health expenditures, 1990. Health Care Financ Rev 1991;13(1):29–54.

44. Newhouse JP. An iconoclastic view of health cost containment. Health Aff (Millwood) 1993;12: Suppl:152–71.

45. Woolhandler S, Himmelstein DU. The deteriorating administrative efficiency of the U.S. health care system. N Engl J Med 1991;324:1253–8.

46. Schapira DV, Studnicki J, Bradham DD, Wolff P, Jarrett A. Intensive care, survival, and expense of treating critically ill cancer patients. JAMA, 1993;269:783–6.

47. Emanuel LL, Barry MJ, Stoeckle JD, Ettelson LM, Emanuel EJ. Advance directives for medical care—a case for greater use. N Engl J Med 1991;324:889–95.

48. Vitelli CE, Cooper K, Rogatko A, Brennan MF. Cardiopulmonary resuscitation and the patient with cancer. J Clin Oncol 1991;9:111–5.

49. Gleeson K, Wise S. The do-not-resuscitate order: still too little too late. Arch Intern Med 1990;150:1057–60.

50. Smedira NG, Evans BH, Grais LS, et al. Withholding and withdrawal of life support from the critically ill. N Engl J Med 1990;322: 309–15.

51. Bedell SE, Pelle D, Maher PL, Cleary PD. Do-not-resuscitate orders for critically ill patients in the hospital: how are they used and what is their impact? JAMA 1986;256:233–7.

52. Emanuel EI. Who won't pull the plug? Washington Post. January 2, 1994:C3.

53. Seckler AB, Meier DE, Mulvihill M, Cammer Paris BE. Substituted judgment: how accurate are proxy predictions? Ann Intern Med 1991;115: 92–8.

54. Uhlmann RF, Pearlman RA, Cain KC. Physicians' and spouses' predictions of elderly patients resuscitation preferences. J Gerontol 1988;43(5):M115–M121.

55. Steinbrook R, Lo B, Moulton J, Saika G, Hollander H, Volberding PA. Preferences of homosexual men with AIDS for life-sustaining treatment. N Engl J Med 1986;314:457–60.

56. Haas JS, Weissman JS, Cleary PD, et al. Discussion of preferences for life-sustaining care by persons with AIDS: predictors of failure in patient-physician communication. Arch Intern Med 1993;153:1241–8.

57. Emanuel EJ, Emanuel LL. Proxy decision making for incompetent patients: an ethical and empirical analysis. JAMA 1992;267:2067–71.

58. Steiber SR. Right to die: public balks at deciding for others. Hospitals 1987;61:72.

59. Schwartz WB. The inevitable failure of current cost-containment strategies: why they can provide only temporary relief. JAMA 1987;257: 220–4.

POSTSCRIPT

Should Health Care for the Elderly Be Limited?

In October 1986 Dr. Thomas Starzl of Pittsburgh, Pennsylvania, transplanted a liver into a 76-year-old woman at a cost of over $200,000. Soon after that, Congress ordered organ transplantation to be covered under Medicare, which ensured that more older persons would receive this benefit. At the same time these events were taking place, a government campaign to contain medical costs was under way, with health care for the elderly targeted.

Not everyone agrees with this means of cost cutting. Sociologist Amitai Etzioni argues that rationing health care for the elderly would encourage conflict between generations and would invite restrictions on health care for other groups in "Spare the Old, Save the Young," *The Nation* (June 11, 1988). In agreement with Etzioni is James F. Childress in "Ensuring Care, Respect, and Fairness for the Elderly," *Hastings Center Report* (October 1984). In "Public Attitudes About the Use of Chronological Age as a Criterion for Allocating Health Care Resources," *The Gerontologist* (February 1993), the authors report that the majority of older people surveyed accept the withholding of life-prolonging medical care from the hopelessly ill but that few would deny treatment on the basis of age alone. Two publications that express opposition to age-based health care rationing are Robert L. Barry and Gerard V. Bradley, eds., *Set No Limits: A Rebuttal to Daniel Callahan's Proposal to Limit Health Care for the Elderly* (University of Illinois Press, 1991) and Gerald R. Winslow and James W. Walters, eds., *Facing Limits: Ethics and Health Care for the Elderly* (Westview Press, 1992).

Currently, about 40 million Americans have no medical insurance and are at risk of being denied basic health care services. About 20 percent of all children have not had proper immunizations, and one-third of all pregnant women do not receive prenatal care during their first trimester. Richard Lamm, writing in the *New York Times* (February 19, 1987), claims that the federal government pays 50 percent of the health care costs of the elderly. While it may not meet the needs of all older people, the amount of medical aid that goes to the elderly is greater than any other demographic group, and the elderly have the highest disposable income. Daniel Callahan, in "Limiting Health Care for the Old?" *The Nation* (August 15/22, 1987), maintains that we must confront the realities of economics and limit health care. Callahan also writes on the allocation of health resources in "Allocating Health Resources," *Hastings Center Report* (April/May 1988) and "Debate: Response to Roger W. Hunt," *Journal of Medical Ethics* (vol. 19, 1993).

Most Americans have access to the best and most expensive medical care in the world. As these costs rise, some difficult decisions may have to be made regarding the allocation of these resources, whether by age, probability of beneficence, income, or other criteria. As the population ages and more health care dollars are spent on care during the last years of life, medical services for the elderly or the dying may become a natural target for reduction in order to balance the health care budget. Additional readings on this subject include "Rationing, Patient Preferences and Cost of Care at the End of Life," *Archives of Internal Medicine* (vol. 152, 1992); "A Critique of Using Age to Ration Health Care," *Journal of Medical Ethics* (vol. 19, 1993); "Trends in Medicare Payments in the Last Year of Life," *The New England Journal of Medicine* (vol. 328, 1993); "Who Won't Pull the Plug," *Washington Post* (January 2, 1994); and "What Do We Owe the Elderly: Allocating Social and Health Care Resources," *Hastings Center Report* (March/April 1994).

ISSUE 5

Is Gun Control a Public Health Issue?

YES: Jerome P. Kassirer, from "Guns in the Household," *The New England Journal of Medicine* (October 7, 1993)

NO: J. Neil Schulman, from *Stopping Power: Why 70 Million Americans Own Guns* (Synapse-Centurion, 1994)

ISSUE SUMMARY

YES: Physician Jerome P. Kassirer argues that guns, particularly guns in the household, are a major public health threat and that meaningful gun control legislation is an important first step in reducing gun-inflicted deaths and injuries.

NO: Journalist and author J. Neil Schulman maintains that guns in the household are used mostly in self-defense and that most gun owners are honest citizens, not criminals. He further argues that the issue of gun control is not an epidemiological concern but a criminological one.

More and more people in the United States are buying guns to protect themselves and their families in response to increasing crime rates. There are currently over 216 million firearms—including close to 900,000 assault weapons —in private hands in the United States, more than double the number in 1970. Also, each year more than 24,000 Americans are killed with handguns in homicides, suicides, and accidents (an average of 65 people each day). Firearms are used in 70 percent of all murders committed in the United States. These statistics raise important questions: Does gun ownership afford protection against crime, or does it increase the risk of gun-related death? And are gun control and gun ownership public health concerns? Gun owners and opponents of gun control claim that weapons kept in the home will prevent crime. Proponents of gun control claim that weapons kept in the home are involved in too many domestic fights resulting in injury or death, accidental shootings, and suicides.

To attempt to resolve some of these issues, Dr. Arthur Kellermann, an emergency room physician at the University of Tennessee, and his associates conducted a study, "Gun Ownership as a Risk Factor for Homicide in the Home," *The New England Journal of Medicine* (October 7, 1993). Dr. Kellermann's study indicated that people who keep guns in their homes are much more likely to kill or injure another family member than to use the gun in self-defense against a criminal. Dr. Kellermann believes that a gun almost automatically makes any fight potentially more dangerous and that the risks of having a gun outweigh the benefits. Many supporters of gun control claim that this study confirms their warnings about the basic dangers of owning guns and keeping them in the home.

The contention that gun ownership is more dangerous than beneficial is not without its critics. Some have pointed out, for instance, that the Kellermann et al. study only measured *risks* associated with gun ownership; they did not study cases in which guns actually deterred crime. Kellermann et al. also did not discuss the possibility that the guns may not have caused the violence; the violence may have caused the use of the guns. For instance, in areas with high crime rates, citizens may be more likely to arm themselves for self-protection.

Although it is unclear whether guns deter crime or cause it, gun control in one form or another has been around since the early part of the twentieth century. The first major gun control act strengthening restrictions on handguns followed the assassinations of President John F. Kennedy, Dr. Martin Luther King, Jr., and Robert Kennedy in the 1960s. Other laws banning the sale of handguns and the manufacture and sale of certain types of assault weapons followed. In 1993 President Bill Clinton signed the Brady Bill, which imposed a five-day waiting period for handgun purchases. (The bill was named for James Brady, a press secretary to President Ronald Reagan. Both Brady and Reagan were shot during an assassination attempt in the early 1980s.)

Gun control is a controversial issue in the United States. Its opponents claim that it infringes on the constitutional rights of Americans to bear arms as granted by the Second Amendment. The gun lobby also pictures America under stricter gun controls as a country where honest citizens would be helpless against well-armed criminals. Many advocates of gun control, however, regard the deaths and injuries related to guns as a public health problem that can be treated only by getting rid of guns themselves.

In the following selections, physician Jerome P. Kassirer asserts that guns are definitely a public health issue and supports stricter gun control. He feels that guns offer no protective benefit, even in homicide cases that follow forced entry. Journalist J. Neil Schulman does not believe that there is merit for stricter gun control. He claims that criminologists are the best people to study homicide and guns, not doctors or public health researchers who he feels support a political agenda that will ultimately increase violence in our society by preventing people from defending themselves against violent offenders. Schulman further contends that violence is not a matter of honest citizens killing simply because a gun is nearby but of "criminals committing violence because violence is their way of life."

YES
Jerome P. Kassirer

GUNS IN THE HOUSEHOLD

[In] October [1992] several bizarre coincidences led to the death of a 16-year-old Japanese exchange student in a suburb of Baton Rouge, Louisiana. The student and his American friend, looking for a Halloween party, missed the correct house by a few doors and rang the wrong doorbell. The exchange student, in the spirit of the holiday, was moving around in mimicry of John Travolta in the movie *Saturday Night Fever,* and the frightened woman who answered the door called to her husband to get his gun. The husband mistook a camera in the student's hand for a weapon, and when the student failed to respond to the command "Freeze!" he shot the boy in the chest with a .44 Magnum.[1-3]

We could be resigned about this unusual sequence of events; perhaps it is inevitable that unlikely coincidences from time to time create just the right circumstances for such a tragedy. But we should not forget that the Japanese student would almost certainly be alive today if not for the presence in that house of a loaded handgun. Given the circumstances and the local penchant for having such guns available for protection, the jury's decision to acquit the husband was not surprising, and perhaps it was even appropriate. In the United States accidental and intentional deaths due to guns in and around the home are commonplace in most major cities, and a substantial proportion of an entire generation of young people are armed and prepared to shoot with little or no provocation.[4] People in Japan, however, lacked a framework for understanding either the shooting or the verdict; with few exceptions, private ownership of guns is not permitted in their country.[3]

The study reported in this issue of the *Journal* by Kellermann and his colleagues[5] is the second of two population-based case–control studies that have focused on the home as a site of gun-related deaths. The current study focuses on homicides; the same authors reported on suicides about a year ago.[6] In the current study, carried out in three counties in Tennessee, Ohio, and Washington, interviews with proxies of homicide victims and matched controls disclosed that homes where homicides occurred were significantly more likely to contain firearms than neighboring homes that were not the scenes of homicides. After matching for four potentially confounding variables (age range, sex, race, and neighborhood) and controlling for five other variables, the investigators found that keeping a firearm in the home was associated with a risk of homicide nearly three times as high. Almost all of this increase was due to a greater risk of homicide by a family member or close acquaintance. Not unexpectedly, illicit drug use and domestic violence were important independent risk factors for homicide. In the earlier study, of suicide, there was nearly fivefold increase in the risk of suicide in homes where guns were kept.[6] These are not the first studies to document the risk associated with having guns in the home, but they are among the most persuasive and, I believe, justify routine warnings about this risk by physicians and other health workers.

If we know that keeping handguns around the house is so dangerous, why do millions of people continue to do so? Paradoxically, the primary reason is for protection. Surveys of gun owners indicate that they believe guns protect them from intruders,[7,8] and the enormous increase in gun sales in the Los Angeles area following the riots in the spring of 1992 is further evidence of that conviction. Yet, we actually know little about the collective efficacy of guns in the home in warding off attacks. Estimates of the number of times per year that guns protect citizens (not necessarily only in the home) vary widely, from 80,000 to a million,[7,9] but neither statistics kept by law-enforcement agencies nor any existing polls of citizens have provided accurate data. And the anecdotal reports of crime rates that fall after part or all of the populace of small towns is armed are badly flawed.[7,10] We do know that when guns are readily available, children accidentally kill their siblings and friends,

depressed people impulsively kill themselves (they are more successful when the weapon is a gun), teenagers settle minor arguments with guns rather than with words or fists, drive-by shootings are reported nearly every week, and psychologically scarred people kill fellow workers and others seemingly at random. The study by Kellermann and his colleagues found no protective benefit of gun ownership in the home even in the homicide cases that followed forced entry.[5]

Meanwhile, Congress is idle on gun control. The Brady bill, which mandates a five-day waiting period and background checks before a gun may be purchased, failed to be enacted last year, but it will be introduced again this fall. I doubt that the Brady bill is strong enough to make a difference in handgun-associated deaths, and I favor more stringent regulations and restrictions on handguns and assault weapons. Although assault rifles account for less than 3 percent of the privately owned firearms in this country, they are used in a proportionately larger fraction of crimes.[11,12] Despite the limitations of the Brady bill, it is a reasonable beginning. Might passage of this bill be the beginning of a series of more restrictive statutes? Yes, it could be and should be.

How can we get meaningful gun-control legislation passed given the putative power of the gun lobby, which uses its funds to support national and local political candidates who oppose gun control, harasses gun-control advocates with thousands of letters and telephone calls, and carries out public relations campaigns to persuade citizens to support its views?[13] There are promising signs. The National Rifle Association (NRA) is not the monolith its popular image projects; instead, it is chronically beset by internal squabbling over power.[13] Even more encouraging, the popular movement to control the availability of guns is gaining acceptance. Many citizens have now concluded that we have exceeded the "killing threshhold,"[14] and a great many have decided that something must be done about private ownership of handguns and assault weapons.[15] Polls for the past 15 years have consistently shown that about two thirds of citizens support stricter gun-control laws,[16] and in a nationwide poll of adults reported only a few months ago, 52 percent favored a federal ban on handgun ownership, 63 percent supported a federal ban on the sale of automatic and semi-automatic weapons, and 82 percent favored handgun registration by federal authorities.[15] Nearly 90 percent of those sampled (and 68 percent of NRA members) declared their support for the Brady bill.[15]

Many parts of society have begun to act. In recent years police departments across the country have led a campaign against possession of certain types of weapons and ammunition, and at least five states (California, Connecticut, Hawaii, New Jersey, and New York) have banned assault rifles.[17,18] In some states (Arkansas, Missouri, and Texas) legislation has been defeated that would have allowed citizens to carry concealed weapons,[19] and other states have defeated attempts to turn back gun-control legislation already on the books. Some cities have mounted gun buy-back programs. In 1993 alone, gun-control advocates have scored victories in 11 states (Arkansas, California, Connecticut, Indiana, Minnesota, Missouri, New Jersey, New York, Ohio, Texas, and Virginia).[19] Even the Federal Bureau of Investigation has broken its tradition of neutrality on gun control and proposed national restrictions, including a five-day waiting period before a gun could be purchased, regulation of gun dealers, and restrictions on the possession of assault rifles and certain kinds of ammunition.[20] And finally, Attorney General Janet Reno recently urged the American people to rise up against the gun lobby's unswerving opposition to gun control.[21]

High-quality epidemiologic research is the latest challenge to the gun lobby. Although a cadre of gun advocates (some of them physicians) try hard to discredit all research of this kind, solid data are accumulating on the populations at risk for injury from firearms, the kinds of weapons involved, and the trade-off between the risks and benefits of private gun ownership.[22-24] Fortunately, the facts speak for themselves, as the two studies of Kellermann and his colleagues[5,6] illustrate. Considerably more federal support for research of this kind is warranted.

Although the gun lobby has deep pockets, its resources are not infinite. Over the past two years the NRA has posted multimillion-dollar losses, and it anticipates a continued large loss this year.[25] In two local political battles alone (New Jersey and Virginia), the NRA spent close to a million dollars[26] (and Katz L: personal communication). Some of its members have expressed serious concern about its deficit spending.[25] As an index of its financial status, the NRA has had to shift funds out of its education and sport-shooting divisions over the past decade into its political arm.[13] Resourceful advocates of gun control might consider enlisting the help of more courageous politicians, such as Governors Florio and Wilder, Congressman Andrews, and Senator DeConcini, and mounting campaigns to introduce gun-control legislation around the country. Countering such efforts could be quite expensive for the NRA.

Gun-control advocates should not be unrealistic, however. Rather than set their sights next on a total ban on gun possession, they might try first to craft proposals that would receive wide public support. They could espouse new design standards for firearms, for example, mandating devices that indicate whether a gun is loaded and requiring locks on guns that can be unlocked only by those knowing the code. They could support the registration of firearms and licensing of all gun owners to make it easier for police to trace stolen weapons. They could introduce federal legislation that would proscribe bringing a gun into a school. And they could support a federal ban on the sale of automatic and semi-automatic weapons. If such laws were implemented we could assess their efficacy; if we still found them wanting we would be justified in supporting even more stringent restrictions.

No matter how reasonable some of these less restrictive proposals seem, the gun lobby in recent years has regularly taken an absolutist position, attempting to thwart all gun-control legislation and trying not only to maintain the status quo but also to roll back existing legislation. The efforts of this lobby should not be underestimated. One of their spokesmen, promising to use funds to unseat legislators in New Jersey who "betrayed" him, declared, "We're in this forever because we're fighting for freedom. You don't quit on freedom."[26] Even more compelling is a letter I received from a surgeon on the West Coast after publication of my 1991 editorial[14] (Hunt TK: personal communication). He said, "Guns are single simple answers for situations they (members of the NRA) fear they will face. If any-

one asks you, send them to me. I once had to go from the operating room to tell a young couple that their little boy was dead—shot while playing with his father's handgun. The mother collapsed into tears. The father, who told me he was an NRA member, did not cry, but became visibly angry, saying, 'I taught the dumb kid how to use it right.' That kind of passion dies hard."

REFERENCES

1. Defense depicts Japanese boy as 'scary.' New York Times. May 21, 1993:A10.
2. Acquittal in doorstep killing of Japanese student. New York Times. May 24, 1993:A1.
3. Reid TR. Japanese media disparage acquittal in 'freeze case': commentators see America as a sick nation. Washington Post. May 25, 1993:A14.
4. A survey of experiences, perceptions, and apprehensions about guns among young people in America. New York: LH Research, July 1993.
5. Kellermann AL, Rivara RP, Rushforth NB, et al. Gun ownership as a risk factor for homicide in the home. N Engl J Med 1993;329:1084–91.
6. Kellermann AL, Rivara FP, Somes G, et al. Suicide in the home in relation to gun ownership. N Engl J. Med 1992;327:467–72.
7. Cook PJ. The technology of personal violence. In: Tonry M, ed. Crime and justice: a review of research. Vol. 14. Chicago: University of Chicago Press, 1991:1–71.
8. Kleck G. Point blank: guns and violence in America. New York: Aldine de Gruyter, 1991.
9. Pratt L. Little guns, big equalizers. Wall Street Journal, April 3, 1992:A11.
10. McDowall D, Lizotte AJ, Wiersema B. General deterrence through civilian gun ownership: an evaluation of the quasi-experimental evidence. Criminology 1991;29:541–59.
11. Edel W. Assault weapons are designed for murder. New York Times. September 23, 1992:A26.
12. O'Harrow R Jr, Miller B. Power, price and availability make assault weapons popular. Washington Post. January 28, 1993:B4.
13. Davidson OG. Under fire: the NRA and the battle for gun control. New York: Henry Holt, 1993.
14. Kassirer JP. Firearms and the killing threshold. N Engl J Med 1991; 325:1647–50
15. A survey of the American people on guns as a children's health issue. New York: LH Research, June 1993.

16. Schneider W. Why such trouble now for gun lobby? Boston Herald. March 13, 1993:17.

17. Sack K. Gun-control battles reveal gradual shifts. New York Times. June 13, 1993:37, 41.

18. Handguns, politics and people. Washington Post. June 16, 1993:A20.

19. Gunfighting: state by state. Newsweek. June 21, 1993:8.

20. Johnston D. F. B. I., in shift, proposes backing gun control. New York Times. July 8, 1993:A13.

21. Engardio JP. Reno calls on NRA lobby to get lost. Boston Globe. August 13, 1993:1, 10.

22. Goldsmith MF. Epidemiologists aim at new target: health risk of handgun proliferation. JAMA 1989;261:675–6.

23. Cotton P. Gun-associated violence increasingly viewed as public health challenge. JAMA 1992;267:1171–4.

24. Taubes G. Violence epidemiologists test the hazards of gun ownership. Science 1992;258:213–5.

25. Stone PH. Is the NRA bleeding internally? National Journal. March 13, 1993:626.

26. Gladwell M. New Jersey gun ban survives repeal vote. Washington Post. March 16, 1993:A3.

NO

J. Neil Schulman

MEDICAL MALPRACTICE

Anybody who has studied the stock market knows that when women's hemlines go up, the prices of stocks go up also, but no one is foolish enough to claim that by shortening skirts we can cause a stock-market boom. That sort of common sense, however, doesn't seem to hold when the subject is the so-called epidemiology of "gun violence."

The point at issue is the contention that medical researchers can study firearms-related violence as a matter of epidemiology apart from the motives of the people who pull the trigger—which is the proper study of that branch of sociology known as criminology. By this premise alone, epidemiologists deny the fundamental difference between microbic cultures and human cultures: microbes don't act on their value-judgments; people do.

The latest outbreak of statisticitis emerges from a study led by Arthur L. Kellermann, MD, published in the October 7, 1993, issue of the *New England Journal of Medicine*, and financed by the Centers for Disease Control [CDC]. A previous Kellermann-led study, published in the June 12, 1986, *NEJM* and also financed by the CDC, gave us the factoid that you are 43 times as likely to die from a handgun kept in the home—through homicide, suicide, or accident —as you are to kill a burglar with it.[1] By the time this factoid turned into mega-soundbite of gun-control advocates in the media and Congress, you were supposedly 43 times as likely to die from a handgun kept in the home as to *protect* yourself from a burglar with it.

Dr. Kellermann himself cautioned against that conclusion, saying, "Morality studies such as ours do not include cases in which burglars or intruders are wounded or frightened away by the use or display of a firearm. Cases in which would-be intruders may have purposely avoided a house known to be armed are also not identified. We did not report the total number of nonlethal firearm injuries involving guns kept in the home. A complete determination of firearm risks versus benefits would require that these figures be known."

ON THIN ICE

Kellermann's latest "population-based case-control study" of homicides throws such caution to the winds. He attempts to quantify "firearms risks versus benefits" by comparing households where a homicide occurred with households were no homicide occurred —in three counties, chosen for the convenience of their location to the researchers. After correcting for several other risk factors such as use of alcohol or illicit drugs, previous domestic violence, and previous criminal records in the 316 matched households ultimately compared, Kellermann determined that households where "homicide at the hands of a family member or intimate acquaintance" occurred were almost three times as likely to have kept a loaded handgun in the home as control households where such a homicide did not occur. From this determination Kellermann concludes, "Although firearms are often kept in the home for personal protection, this study shows that the practice is counterproductive. Our data indicate that keeping a gun in the home is independently associated with an increase in the risk of homicide in the home."

An immediate technical problem with Kellermann's methods was raised by David N. Cowan, PhD, in a letter to the NEJM. Dr. Cowan charged that Kellermann grouped socially dysfunctional people—for example, the chronically unemployable—with normal people, and thus *any* other risk factors would be inseparable.

Another problem is that by performing a case study of households with homicide victims, Kellermann is looking at almost twice as many black households as white, and only a handful of Asian households—far too few to be statistically useful. African-Americans are far more likely to be homicide victims than other racial or ethnic groups. Thus studying homicide within the African-American culture may not produce conclusions that can be generalized to other racial or ethnic groups. According to Don Kates, a criminologist with the Pacific Research Institute, "African-Americans have greater death rates than other population groups for drowning, other accidents, and diseases." Other sociological studies note crude differences between African-Americans and Asian-Americans in divorce rates, school-drop-out rates, proportion of households from which the father is absent, and so forth.

A more basic problem with Kellermann's conclusion is that it attempts to draw a reverse implication from a set of facts. Let me explain the general point: It will be true that people who own parachutes will die more frequently in falls from airplanes than people who don't. But does that mean that parachute-ownership constitutes an increased risk factor for death by falling from an airplane? Wouldn't logic tell us that the risk of dying is greater for people who fall from airplanes but *don't* have a parachute?

Dr. Kellermann tells us, "We found no evidence of a protective benefit from gun ownership in any subgroup, including one restricted to cases of homicide that followed forced entry into the home and another restricted to cases in which resistance was attempted."

This is where Kellermann's study is completely disingenuous, and indicates —as does his financing and publication by gun-control zealots James Mercy at the Centers for Disease Control and Jerome P. Kassirer, editor of *The New England Journal of Medicine*—that the intent of these studies is to produce soundbites for Sarah Brady rather than science.

Dr. Kellermann is studying only cases where a handgun *failed* to save the victim's life. We're being shown only the *murder victims*, not the successful resisters. Kellermann didn't even document whether a firearm used in a homicide was the home-owner's or the intruder's. And he still doesn't raise the points he himself said would be necessary for "a complete determination of firearms risks versus benefits": "cases in which burglars or intruders are wounded or frightened away by the use or display of a firearm.... Cases in which would-be intruders may have purposely avoided a house known to be armed."

Dr. Kellermann can't study such questions because these are the proper focus not of doctors, but of criminologists. And when we shift from the medical paradigm of "gun violence" as a health issue, to the criminological paradigm of "offenders and victims," we get a completely different vision.

Immediately we discover that the cases in which Kellermann perceives an increased risk factor—what he terms "homicide at the hands of a family member or intimate acquaintance"—are only around 10 per cent of the yearly homicides. This is according to both the FBI's *Crime in the United States*, 1992, and *Murder Analysis*, 1992, by the Detective Division of the Chicago Police. Most murders do not take place in the home to begin with. In the Chicago study, only 36.8 per cent of the homicides occurred in or around the home—and that includes public housing, where hallway drug-dealer shootouts are common. Dr. Kellermann himself tells us that in the three counties in which his study was conducted, only 23.9 per cent of homicides took place in the home of the victim. Then, driving home his study's limited scope, he also tells us: "Guns were not significantly linked to an increased risk of homicide by [non-intimate] acquaintances, unindentified intruders, or strangers."

What this adds up to is that you are unlikely to be murdered at home by an intimate; that you are still less likely to be murdered at home by a stranger (not surprising, since homes usually have locks to keep strangers out); but that the great majority of the few murders that *do* take place at home are at the hands of those who have a key. The caution here might well be that if you live with someone who you fear might murder you, you might want to move out if he also keeps a loaded handgun. Or, if the loaded handgun is yours, you might want to keep it somewhere where you can get to it faster than he can. This advice does not become more useful if we call it medical advice.

The answer which Kellerman says we need to discover—the overall usefullness of firearms in self-defense—is to be found in the definitive analysis of a dozen studies in the book *Point Blank: Guns and Violence in America* (Aldine De Gruyter, 1991), by Gary Kleck, professor of criminology at Florida State University. Unlike Dr. Kellermann, Professor Kleck has carefully avoided taking funding from advocates in the gun-control debate, and his impeccable liberal credentials—membership in Common Cause and Amnesty International—preclude a presumption of conservative or pro-NRA bias. Kleck's analysis produced an estimate of around 650,000 handgun defenses per year and over a million gun defenses if one included all firearms.

Kleck's latest research, his Spring 1993 National Self-Defense Survey of 4,978 households, reveals that previous studies underestimated the number of times respondents used their firearms in defense. The new survey suggests 2.4

million gun defenses in 1992, 1.9 million of them with handguns; and about 72 per cent of these gun defenses occurred in or near the home. This indicates a successful gun defense about 1,728,000 times a year with no body for Dr. Kellermann to find.

So who is doing the killing? *Murder Analysis*, 1992, tells us that 72.39 per cent of the murderers the Chicago Police studied in 1992 had a criminal history and, interestingly, 65.53 per cent of the victims did as well. A recent National Institute of Justice analysis finds, "It is clear that only a very small fraction of privately owned firearms are ever involved in crime or [unlawful] violence, the vast bulk of them being owned and used more or less exclusively for sport and recreational purposes, or for self-protection."

Criminologist Don Kates concurs: "It has been estimated that 98.32 per cent of owners do not use a gun in an unlawful homicide (over a 50-year, adult life span)."

Overwhelmingly, violence isn't a matter of ordinary people killing because a firearm is handy, but of criminals committing violence because violence is their way of life. When the Centers for Dis-ease Control starts defining bullets as "pathogens" and declares honest gun owners the Typhoid Marys of a "gun-violence epidemic," the medical profession has lent its scientific credibility to a radical political agenda which threatens to increase the overall violence in our society by shifting the balance of power toward the well-armed psychopath.

Oddly enough, even Dr. Kellermann agrees. In the March/April 1994 issue of *Health*, he is quoted as saying: "If you've got to resist, your chances of being hurt are less the more lethal your weapon. If that were my wife, would I want her to have a .38 special in her hand? Yeah."

In this particular gunfight, the best ammunition is the truth.

NOTES

1. Of those 43 deaths 37 were suicide; eliminating suicide immediately drops the claimed figure to a 6 times as likely. We can eliminate suicide from our analysis of gun-effects immediately. *The American Journal of Psychiatry* (March 1990) reported in a study by Rich, Young, Fowler, Wagner, and Black that gun-suicides, which were statistically reduced in the five years following Canada's imposition of handgun restrictions in 1976, were replaced 100 per cent by suicides using other methods, mostly jumping off bridges.

POSTSCRIPT

Is Gun Control a Public Health Issue?

Between 1960 and 1970, both the murder rate in the United States and the rate of handgun ownership doubled. Was it a coincidence that violence and gun ownership grew at nearly the same pace? Can it be assumed from this fact that more guns cause more violence? The conventional wisdom is that guns and violence are related in the sense that owning a gun increases the risk that the *gun owner* will be hurt rather than the criminal. Dr. Arthur Kellermann, quoted in "Should You Own a Gun?" *U.S. News & World Report* (August 15, 1994), says, "Most gun homicides occur in altercations among family members, friends or acquaintances. In a heated dispute, few carefully weigh the legal consequences of their actions. They are too busy reaching for a weapon. If it's a gun, death is more likely to result." In *Mother Jones* (May/June 1993), Dr. Mark Rosenberg maintains that violence is a public health problem and that violence prevention should be pushed to the top of the public health agenda.

Is violence really a *health* issue? Each year, more than 500,000 Americans, including children, are brought to hospital emergency rooms for treatment of a violent injury. These injuries, which include shootings and assaults, add over $5 billion dollars in direct medical costs to health care expenditures. Lifetime costs of violent injuries, which include medical care and loss of productivity, is over $45 billion dollars. And since many gunshot victims are uninsured, the public at large often pays the bill. Articles on the relationship between guns and public health include "Homicide, Handguns, and the Crime Gun Hypothesis: Firearms Used in Fatal Shootings of Law Enforcement Officers, 1980 to 1989," *American Journal of Public Health* (April 1994); "Firearm Violence and Public Health: Limiting the Availability of Guns," *Journal of the American Medical Association* (April 27, 1994); and "Loaded Guns in the Home," *Journal of the American Medical Association* (June 10, 1992).

A majority of gun owners and the general public favor stricter gun controls, including safety classes for gun owners. Only 39 percent of the American public backs a total ban on handguns, according to an article in *USA Today* (December 17, 1993). And although gun control may save some lives, there is a general consensus that it can never truly stem the availability of guns. Articles that argue against gun control include "Security," *Forbes* (November 25, 1991); "The NRA: It's Not Pro-Gun, It's 'Anti-Crime,'" *Newsweek* (December 6, 1993); and "Gun Owners, YOU Are the Target," *American Hunter* (May 1994).

PART 2

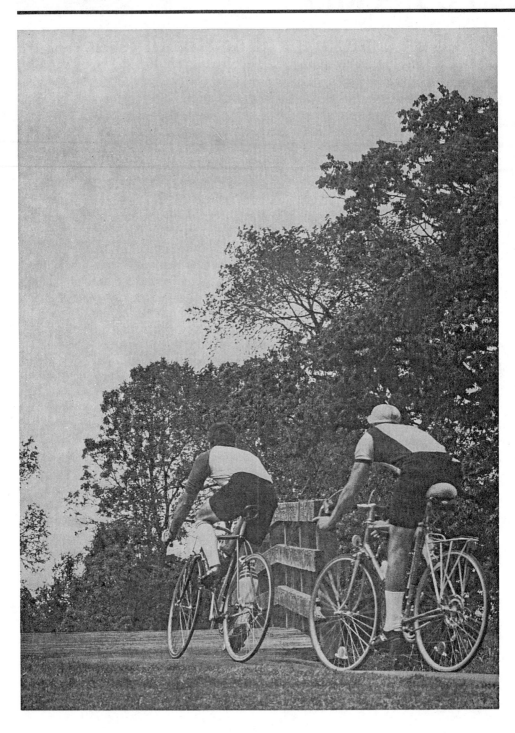

Mind/Body Relationship

Humans have long sought to extend life, eliminate disease, and prevent sickness. In modern times, people depend on technology to develop creative and innovative ways to improve health. However, as cures for diseases such as AIDS, cancer, and heart disease continue to elude scientists and doctors, many people question whether or not modern medicine has reached a plateau in improving health. As a result, over the last decade emphasis has been placed on prevention as a way to improve health. Although millions of people have made changes in their lifestyles in hopes of preventing the onset of disease, some scientists argue that people will always be plagued by illness and that overzealous emphasis on prevention and control is misplaced. The relationship between mind and body is the key to the issues debated in this section.

■ Should Healthy Behavior Be Mandated?

■ Can a Positive Mental Attitude Overcome
    Disease?

ISSUE 6

Should Healthy Behavior Be Mandated?

YES: Michael F. Jacobson, from "Prevention's the Issue: Your Money or Your Life Style," *The Nation* (July 13, 1992)

NO: Faith T. Fitzgerald, from "The Tyranny of Health," *The New England Journal of Medicine* (July 21, 1994)

ISSUE SUMMARY

YES: Michael F. Jacobson, a microbiologist and the director of the Center for Science in the Public Interest, claims that federal policies emphasizing healthy behavior would not only improve public health but reduce health care spending.

NO: Physician Faith T. Fitzgerald argues that there is a "dark side" to the emphasis on healthy lifestyles and a need to reassess the role of preventive medicine, which she feels should not try to control people's behavior for their own good.

During the past decade, there has been a movement toward self-care and prevention as a means to improve health. This movement has been based on several factors: Many diseases, such as cancer or heart disease, have no "magic bullet" cure; health care costs have been spiraling; and it is cheaper, more humane, and more sensible to try and prevent a disease rather than to attempt to cure it. If individuals could be encouraged to quit smoking, exercise, and eat low-fat diets, a significantly lower number of cancers, heart disease, and other illnesses would develop.

While it makes sense to try to prevent a disease rather than to place emphasis on treatment, prevention may not always be possible. To prevent disease, health behavior changes are often necessary, but these changes may be beyond the ability of some individuals, however motivated they may be. Not everyone, for instance, is physically capable of exercising or able to afford healthy food. Other factors can also contribute to disease, many not modifiable. Individuals cannot change their age, gender, or heredity, which are all potential disease risk factors. There is also a limit as to how much an individual can avoid environmental health risks, such as air pollution, pesticides, and toxic waste.

In the following selections, Michael F. Jacobson contends that the United States spends far too little on disease prevention. He states that every year, hundreds of thousands of deaths would be avoided and billions of dollars would be saved if Americans practiced healthier behaviors and if government policies were oriented toward health and disease prevention.

Faith T. Fitzgerald argues that there is a risk that an emphasis on healthy lifestyles will lead to a "tyranny of health" in which individuals who become ill will be accused of having misbehaved. She also maintains that we "must beware of developing a zealotry about health, in which we take ourselves too seriously and believe that we know enough to dictate human behavior, penalize people for disagreeing with us, and even deny people charity, empathy, and understanding because they act in a way of which we disapprove."

YES

Michael F. Jacobson

PREVENTION'S THE ISSUE: YOUR MONEY OR YOUR LIFE STYLE

To listen to the presidential hopefuls, including those who fell by the wayside earlier this year, you'd think that America's health care crisis is solely one of access and payment. Lost in the duels over "play or pay," "single payer" and "small-group-market insurance reform" is the fact that a good chunk of our health costs are preventable. Every year, hundreds of thousands of deaths could be avoided and billions of dollars saved if Americans lived a little differently and if federal tax and other policies were reoriented toward health. But we hear nothing about this from Bush, Clinton or Perot.

Consider booze. Alcoholic beverages cause more devastation in our society than any other product. For starters, booze accounts for 100,000 deaths each year due to cancer, auto crashes, liver cirrhosis, stroke, etc. According to the National Institute on Alcohol Abuse and Alcoholism, drinking is a factor in half of all homicides and in three out of ten suicides. Alcoholism is a major cause of family violence, birth defects, workplace injuries and other tragedies. Cigarettes may kill more people, but alcohol ruins more lives, beginning even in grade-school years, and destroys millions of families. For candidates who claim to be "pro-family," attention to alcoholism is mandatory.

The direct and indirect costs to society of alcohol problems total more than $100 billion each year. By contrast, state and federal excise taxes on alcohol amount to only about $15 billion. Should taxpayers be subsidizing the booze barons?

Former Surgeon General C. Everett Koop's 1988 Workshop on Drunk Driving reported that raising excise taxes "could have the largest long-term effect on alcohol-impaired driving of all policy and program options available." The workshop recommended raising beer and wine taxes to equal the higher liquor rate and to make up for the inflation that since 1970 has severely eroded the value of tax revenues.

The Koop workshop's recommendation would generate more than $16 billion in new revenues annually. Part of that sum could be applied to treating and preventing alcoholism, with the remainder funding critical health and social programs. But even if not one dime were applied to alcohol programs, the higher prices caused by the tax hike would slash alcohol consumption by almost 10 percent—and by even more among grade school and high school students. That's a lot fewer car crashes and teen pregnancies, less mental retardation and lower health care costs.

While tax hikes are generally considered political poison, polls show that the vast majority of Americans support higher alcohol and tobacco taxes. Any regressiveness could be cured by lowering income-tax rates for low-income families.

On another front, a broad coalition, which includes groups ranging from the Christian Life Commission of the Southern Baptist Convention to Public Citizen, from the National P.T.A. to the American Medical Association, is calling for reforms of alcohol advertising. With support from such unlikely bedfellows as Senator Strom Thurmond [R-South Carolina] and Representative Joseph Kennedy [D-Massachusetts], the coalition is seeking legislation that would require health information in all alcohol ads. Currently, TV commercials imply that beer is the elixir of health and key to social and sexual success, while magazine ads and billboards suggest that the road to economic success is paved with empty liquor bottles.

Beyond supporting higher excise taxes and restrictions on advertising, the presidential candidates should be calling for educational programs in schools and the mass media, universally available treatment for alcoholism and other drug addictions, and the prohibition of alcohol purchases and alcohol advertising as tax-deductible business expenses (the last measure alone would raise $2 billion annually).

* * *

As with alcoholic beverages, higher taxes and comprehensive educational campaigns could save billions in medical treatment for victims of tobacco smoke. In a 1988 referendum, Californians voted to boost the state tax on cigarettes from 10 cents per pack to 35 cents. One-fourth of the revenues—$115 million in 1991—was earmarked for tobacco research and aggressive antismoking campaigns. The result: Cigarette smoking declined by 17 percent between 1987 and 1990, a far sharper decline than in any other state. One-third of California's quitters said the state's antismoking ads were the main reason they stopped.

The Canadians, too, have gotten serious about smoking. They raised taxes so that an average pack now costs U.S. $4.72, compared with $1.73 in the United States. As a direct result, 16 percent fewer Canadians smoked in 1991 than in 1990; a decline in lung-cancer, emphysema and heart-disease death rates will surely follow.

Although Congress has voted modest increases in tobacco taxes, they barely keep up with recent inflation. Boosting the tax from the current 20 cents a pack to, say, $1.20 a pack would generate about $21 billion in needed revenues and cut smoking rates by more than 15 percent. Boosting the tax by $2 would still leave the price of a pack less than it is in Canada and bring in more than $30 billion in new revenues.

As for cigarette advertising, Congress has considered tighter restrictions, but without presidential leadership that notion has died a quiet death on Capitol Hill.

* * *

Diet is a third area where federal action could save untold lives and dollars. Fatty, salty diets promote obesity, diabetes, stroke, heart disease and certain cancers. Those diet-related diseases cause hundreds of thousands of premature deaths each year. Surgeons perform about 400,000 coronary bypass operations annually at a cost of more than $13 billion.

If we really wanted to cut health care costs we'd be better off training dietitians than surgeons. If more people followed a diet based on grains, beans and vegetables rather than on meat, eggs and dairy products, we could save thousands of lives and billions of dollars. But the federal government is doing precious little to convey that critical information to Americans. President Bush's only comment on health and nutrition has been to ridicule broccoli and carrots. The Agriculture Department now facilitates programs that enable the meat, dairy and egg industries to spend tens of millions of dollars each year on advertising and public-relations campaigns intended to boost sales. (The department also gave $200 million last year to McDonald's, Gallo, Seagram and dozens of other companies to promote sales abroad of their sometimes less than salubrious products.)

The government could be, but isn't, serving healthy meals to employees and others in government cafeterias, federal prisons, military bases, senior citizen centers and school food programs. While the Food and Drug Administration has sought to implement a law that would require better nutrition labeling on thousands of foods and that would cut down on diet-related illnesses, the food industry, with the help of Vice President Quayle's Competitiveness Council, is seeking a one-year delay.

* * *

The need to prevent serious health problems extends into many spheres of our lives and our economy. Workers need to be far better protected from dangerous machinery and chemicals. Farmers need to be encouraged to reduce their use of dangerous pesticides, veterinary drugs and chemical fertilizers in order to safeguard their health and that of consumers. Manufacturing facilities and hazardous-waste dumps threaten the health of nearby communities. The life-saving Special Supplemental Food Program for Women, Infants and Children must be extended to every needy mother and child. Childhood immunization campaigns, a fundamental aspect of public health, must be fully funded to reverse, for example, the sixfold increase in measles cases that occurred between 1985 and 1989.

Even more broadly, poverty itself correlates with poor health and must be eliminated. A concern for health must be factored into every aspect of a government's policies. All Cabinet secretaries, not just the Secretary of Health and Human Services, must realize that their actions can improve or worsen the public's health.

Yet the presidential candidates are totally neglecting the prevention side of the health issue. It is certainly true that a disease-based economy provides thousands of jobs for physicians, nurses, advertising executives, ranchers, candy manufacturers, tobacco growers, cigarette makers, brewers, vintners, broadcasters, athletes, medical-equipment manufacturers and other potential political supporters.

The long list of industries nourished by, and that nurture, Americans' pathogenic life style makes it difficult for many political candidates to advocate cutting health care costs by improving the public's health. PAC [political action committee] contributions speak louder than words. For instance, in the 1989–90 election cycle, alcoholic-beverage companies, trade associations and executives doled out more than $2.8 million in the form of PAC contributions, honorariums and private donations to members of Congress.

In 1991 Americans spent almost $738 billion on health. Thirty-six million of us lacked health insurance. We certainly do need to obtain universal insurance coverage and control skyrocketing costs of drugs, exorbitant doctors' bills, superfluous operations and unnecessary insurance agents and bill collectors. But disease prevention is even more important, whether you're a cold-blooded economist concerned about the budget or a parent concerned about a child's health. Some individuals, without any encouragement from Uncle Sam, will discard their cigarettes, double cheeseburgers and liquor. But many millions more would do so—leading to a healthier populace and a healthier economy—if our political candidates and elected officials advocated policies that advanced the most sensible way to control the costs of illness: promoting health.

NO

Faith T. Fitzgerald

THE TYRANNY OF HEALTH

There has recently been much in both lay and medical literature on the promotion of healthy lifestyles. Once upon a time people did not have lifestyles; they had lives. Those lives were filled with work and play, battle and respite, excitement and boredom, but principally with the day-to-day struggle for existence, centered largely around the family, birth, death, disease, and health. What is the difference between a lifestyle and a life? Central to it, I believe, is the concept that lifestyle is something one chooses, and life is something that happens to one. This distinction will affect the future of medicine, and certainly health care reform, in this country. The emphasis on healthy lifestyles, although salutary in many ways, has a very dark side to it and has led to the increasing peril of a tyranny of health in the United States. To explain the potential dangers of the emphasis on healthy lifestyles, I here review the concept of health and its role in the fabric of our society.

THE CONCEPT OF WELLNESS

A healthy lifestyle is said to be essential to the promotion of wellness. What is wellness? In 1946, the World Health Organization, largely in revulsion against the activities of Nazi physicians and the creatures who worked with them, redefined health as "a state of complete physical, mental, and social well being, and not merely the absence of disease or infirmity."[1] This has become known as "wellness," a highly desirable state. A well or healthy person is one who is not only physically whole and vigorous, but also happy and socially content. What a good idea! It is generous with implied promise, and many of us in the medical profession eagerly switched from being doctors and nurses (who take care of disease and infirmity) to being health care providers, engaging ourselves in a variety of efforts to make people both physically well and also happy and socially content. We broadened our horizon from physical problems to character flaws, poverty, crime, unhappiness, and even unattractiveness. Internal medicine, surgery, preventive medicine, family practice, pediatrics, neonatology, and especially plastic surgery, genetic engineering, prenatal diagnosis, nutrition, and psychiatry promised potential perfection.

Concurrently, and perhaps naively, both the lay public and the medical profession began to confuse the ideal of health with the norm for health. That is, we went from "Wouldn't it be great to have this be the definition of health" to "This *is* the definition of health." Having accepted the view that health should be a perfect state of wellness, we went on to declare that it was. But if one accepts the idea that physical vigor and emotional and social contentment are not only desirable, but also expected, there is a problem. If health is normal, then sickness and accidents are faults. Who or what is at fault varies: environmental pollution, for example, or government plots, doctors themselves, diet, radon, or political bias. We now act as if we really believe that disease, aging, and death are unnatural acts and all things are remediable. All we have to do, we think, is know enough (or spend enough), and disease and death can be prevented or fixed.

SOCIAL RESPONSIBILITY FOR HEALTH

In the 19th and early 20th centuries, if a person fell ill, had alcoholism or tuberculosis, or abused a spouse or child, it was a pity, but it was a pity for the person and a sadness for his or her family; it was their business. Over the past several decades, however, both the existence of these imperfections and the remedies for them have become society's business, particularly since society began to accept the responsibility to pay for the consequences of the imperfections. Now treatment of drug addiction, prevention of domestic violence, handgun control, and the use of seat belts and helmets are society's responsibility.

Concurrently, however, because the imperfections are unhealthy, they are also the responsibility of doctors and nurses. Both health care providers and the commonweal now have a vested interest in certain forms of behavior, previously considered a person's private business, if the behavior impairs the person's "health." Certain failures of self-care have become, in a sense, crimes against society, because society has to pay for their consequences. And society now looks to health care providers for the education and direction to eliminate behavior that leads to disease.

What harm can all this do? Much harm. If health (physical, mental, and social) is normal and the failure to be healthy is someone's fault, then when a person becomes ill he or she may have done something wrong. If we root out that wrongness, or better yet, prevent it, we can restore that person to normal health and can benefit society. In effect, we have said that people owe it to society to stop misbehaving, and we use illness as evidence of misbehavior. This is clearest in the issues of "self-abuse": obesity, alcoholism, smoking, heart disease, intravenous drug abuse, and human immunodeficiency virus (HIV) infection. Yet our understanding of self-abuse is subject to uncertainty and to arbitrary social fashion. Clearly, our understanding of the scientific basis of health and disease changes over time. Many older people remember when sunshine, milk, bread, butter, and meat were good for you and were recommended by physicians. Shall we recommend antioxidants or proscribe them in patients at risk for lung cancer? Is obesity the consequence of self-indulgent overeating or of genetics?

Why do we make a distinction between socially unacceptable and socially acceptable lifestyles, even though both may lead to disease and dysfunction? We excoriate the smoker but congratulate the skier. Yet both skiing and smoking may lead to injury, may be costly, and are clearly risky. We have created a new medical specialty to take care of sports injuries, an acknowledgment of the hazardous sequelae [secondary results]. And though there are no doubt benefits to exercise and sports, the literature on the complications of some activities is such that were they drugs, they would probably have been banned by the Food and Drug Administration years ago.

So we select certain forms of self-abuse as deserving of opprobrium, and some of us have even seen colleagues refuse to care for certain self-abusers (such as fat people, smokers, drinkers, intravenous drug abusers, or those afflicted with HIV infection), since these victims brought it on themselves by not behaving as we told them to. In this way we can blame patients for their illnesses and deny them both our compassion and our services. The thrust toward the rationing of health care is making the association between vice and disease a public policy.

Is there indeed a risk that we will establish a tyranny of health in which those who are unwell are assumed to have misbehaved (with certain areas of misbehavior forgiven and others condemned)? Will we speak of people as innocent victims only when we can, after thorough exploration, find nothing in their lifestyles to account for their disabilities? And if health involves not only physical disarray but also emotional and social disarray, how far will we go in establishing laws to regulate "healthy behavior," arguing that it is for the individual's own good as well as for the public good? Furthermore, when illness and culpability are so intertwined, it is not surprising that genuinely antisocial behavior is often viewed as an illness, as well as the reverse. Thus, not only is heart disease often seen as the result of a faulty lifestyle, but domestic abuse may also be seen as an illness. The boundaries become hopelessly blurred.

In his paper "Medical Nemesis," Illich[2] wrote in 1974 that classifying all the troubles of humanity as medical problems is actually antithetical to true health, in that it limits the ability of people to learn to cope with pain, sickness, and death as integral parts of life. Health, he maintained, is not freedom from the inevitability of death, disease, unhappiness, and stress, but rather the ability to cope with them in a competent way. If this is true, then the more medicine and society direct individual behavior, the less autonomous, and therefore the less healthy, the individual may become.

We must beware of developing a zealotry about health, in which we take ourselves too seriously and believe that we know enough to dictate human behavior, penalize people for disagreeing with us, and even deny people charity, empathy, and understanding because they act in a way of which we disapprove. Perhaps the health care crisis could be resolved, in part, if we debated more openly the definition of health. We should not abandon modern preventive medicine, but we should undertake a brutally honest assessment of its proper purview. In particular, given our training and expertise, we health care professional are no more competent to treat social distress than other citizens. We cannot fix everything (though we do some things marvelously well), nor can our patients—

no matter how intelligent or attentive—prevent all disease and death. We may be trying to do too much and thus diluting an awareness and application of what we can do well. If we redefine health, I hope we can discover a definition that does not include a medical or social mandate to control people's behavior for the sake of their mortal bodies; this would seem to me particularly compelling in a nation founded on the belief that one should not legislate behavior even for the sake of the immortal soul.

REFERENCES

1. World Health Organization. Constitution of the World Health Organization. In: Beauchamp TL, Childress JF. Principles of biomedical ethics. New York: Oxford University Press, 1979:284–5.
2. Illich I. Medical nemesis. Lancet 1974;1:918–21.

POSTSCRIPT

Should Healthy Behavior Be Mandated?

Fitzgerald does not claim that smoking and high-fat diets are safe and un-related to disease, but she believes that arguments emphasizing disease pre-vention through individual health behaviors are misused and exaggerated. Professors Lenn E. Goodman and Madeleine J. Goodman indicate agree-ment in their article "Prevention—How Misuse of a Concept Undercuts Its Worth," *Hastings Center Report* (April 1986). The Goodmans feel that shift-ing the responsibility of health and well-being onto the individual relieves the government and health care industry of their responsibility to provide education, a clean environment, research into disease causes, and adequate health care for everyone. They also believe that a healthy lifestyle does not guarantee good health and longevity. Paul Marantz makes similar points in "Blaming the Victim: The Negative Consequences of Preventive Medicine," *American Journal of Public Health* (October 1990).

Although a good diet and exercise may help prevent disease, they clearly do not guarantee health. Many other, unmodifiable risk factors can also pro-duce disease. Cardiologist Henry Solomon, in *The Exercise Myth* (Harcourt Brace Jovanovich, 1984), argues that even exercise will not necessarily pre-vent diseases or improve longevity. Solomon believes that heredity is as much responsible for a long life as are healthy behaviors. Thomas Moore makes the same point with regard to cholesterol reduction in *Heart Failure* (Random House, 1989). He claims that diet does not reduce serum cholesterol for many people and that heredity is as important as lifestyle in maintaining and controlling cholesterol. These writers all argue that disease prevention via a healthy lifestyle may not be a valid way to maintain wellness.

Professor Lawrence Green, in "When Health Policy Becomes Victim Blam-ing," *The New England Journal of Medicine* (December 17, 1981), argues against the premise that individuals must always be responsible for their own health. He agrees with the Goodmans that government must not abandon its role in maintaining social conditions that support behavior conducive to health. Green believes that without this social dimension of health promotion, plac-ing responsibility of health solely on the individual has the effect of blaming the victim for his or her poor health. He also claims that a greater emphasis on health promotion and disease prevention often has been limited to budget cuts in old health programs rather than investments or new initiatives. A similar viewpoint can be found in "The Politics of Cancer: Why the Medical Establishment Blames Victims Instead of Carcinogens," *Detroit Weekly Metro Times* (May 19, 1993).

A good example of victim blaming relates to the current increase in breast cancer rates. Since the mid-1930s, the number of diagnosed cases has risen by about 1 percent each year. Currently, one in nine women will develop breast cancer in her lifetime. Researchers hypothesized that controllable health behaviors such as diet and childbearing patterns were responsible for the increased number of cases. As a result, many women felt that their breast cancer was caused by something they did, such as eating too much fat or postponing childbearing.

New evidence suggests that the increasing number of breast cancers might be related more to environmental contaminants and less to health behaviors. A class of fat-soluble chemicals known as organochlorines, which include the substances DDT and PCBs, are especially suspect. Although both have been banned from sale or production in the United States, they remain in the environment. Recent studies have shown that women with the highest traces of these chemicals stored in their bodies have four times the risk of developing breast cancer as women with the lowest levels. Readings on the relationship between breast cancer and environmental contaminants include "One in Nine," *Ms.* (July/August 1994); "Breast Cancer: The Toxin Trail," *Lear's* (April 1994); "Breast Cancer's Deadly Masquerade?" *U.S. News & World Report* (February 7, 1994); and "The Environmental Link to Breast Cancer," *Ms.* (May/June 1993).

While it is clear that we cannot always keep ourselves well via healthy behaviors, many writers claim that individuals, not doctors or government, can maintain health. Donald B. Ardsell, in *High Level Wellness* (Ten Speed Press, 1986), maintains that individuals can join the ranks of those who look to themselves rather than to their physicians for the maintenance of their health. He claims that what an individual can do for his or her own benefit is enormous; what medicine can do is quite limited. Other readings related to individual health behaviors and wellness are "Managing Stress and Living Longer," *USA Today Magazine* (May 1990); "Pressure Treatment: How Exercise Can Help You Control Your Blood Pressure," *Walking* (June 1992); and "Are We Meeting Our Goals for Health?" *New Choice* (March 1994).

ISSUE 7

Can a Positive Mental Attitude Overcome Disease?

YES: Marc Barasch, from "A Psychology of the Miraculous," *Psychology Today* (March/April 1994)

NO: Ellen Switzer, from "Blaming the Victim," *Vogue* (September 1987)

ISSUE SUMMARY

YES: Author Marc Barasch asserts that there is such as thing as a "miracle-prone" personality that enables one to self-heal using the mind.

NO: Freelance writer Ellen Switzer argues that state of mind does not significantly affect the outcome of an illness.

Practitioners of holistic medicine believe that people must take responsibility for their own health by practicing healthy behaviors and maintaining positive attitudes instead of relying on health providers. They also believe that physical disease has both behavioral and psychological components. These psychological components can be explained by the relationship between mental attitude and the immune system.

In 1979 the late journalist Norman Cousins published *Anatomy of an Illness.* In it, Cousins discusses how he cured himself of a serious illness that affected his collagen—*ankylosing spondylitis*—by taking massive doses of vitamin C (which aids in the synthesis of collagen) and keeping a positive mental attitude. He kept his spirits up by watching comedy movies. Since Cousins's book was published, more articles and books have been devoted to the idea that people can control their immune systems, and therefore their health, with their minds. Sufferers of various illnesses have been told to have positive thoughts in order to assist their immune systems. Some studies have found that cancer patients with certain personality traits and those with a sense of helplessness are less likely to survive their disease than patients who maintain a cheerful, positive attitude.

Research over the past 20 years has shown that disease is not only an organic process but also a psychological one and that some personality types are more susceptible to disease than others. Research has also indicated that people are most at risk for disease when exposed to certain types of stress, such as major life changes. It is as if our personalities determine what types of diseases we are most likely to suffer. According to these studies, our health behaviors decide the levels of risk, and stress causes the outcome, which is disease.

In the following selections, Marc Barasch asserts that the mind can have a significant influence over the body. He cites numerous examples of people who have overcome disease through the human psyche, and he contends that an individual's own power of healing can cure. Ellen Switzer argues that people do not become ill because their mental states, psyches, or attitudes negatively affect their biological systems; nor do these qualities affect whether or not an individual is cured. Switzer acknowledges that stress can aggravate illness, but she maintains that there is no conclusive proof that it *causes* disease.

YES

Marc Barasch

A PSYCHOLOGY OF THE MIRACULOUS

A few years ago, something changed my life. It was a violent change —a diagnosis of cancer. Yet when my doctor sat me down on the edge of his padded table, I had felt not fear but a kind of weird exhilaration—like the moment the rollercoaster crests its first hump and you slowly begin the gravity-abducted swoosh to earth.

Something would now require me to draw on every resource I possessed, on whatever I thought I knew about myself and Life in General. As my doctor strove for the right balance between dolor and reassurance, up within me sprang a fugitive hope; a hope familiar to all who find themselves in such circumstances, and which made the drone of his recitative fade momentarily like an FM station in a car leaving town: Who knows? I thought to myself: Maybe there'll be a miracle.

At the time, I was the editor of *New Age Journal*. I had often heard stories around the office of patients who got well after the doctor did everything but pronounce them dead. But such tales have the ring of wistful folklore when your own life seemingly hangs in the balance. I eventually had the doctor's surgery, and was pronounced cured.

Still, I was amazed at how sickness had affected me; how it had seemed to plunge me into a separate reality that, despite years of self-analysis, was as unfamiliar as the dark side of the moon. I had sensed the stirring of great forces I could scarcely begin to fathom. I had felt at once mortality imperiled and embarked on a great adventure; cheated of my life yet restored to some deeper selfhood. My dreams had been infused with a crystalline, terrible immediacy; emotions had swept through me in torrents. The voice of the psyche had never been so stentorian, nor so incomprehensible. I wondered afterward: Had the luminosity I had seen in the throes of illness just been the delirium of the shipwrecked? Or was there some way that disease may summon barely suspected healing powers into existence?

Under a compulsion to sort out my own strange experiences, I spent years interviewing dozens of people who claimed to have had unusual healings. This was no academic pursuit, but a survival exercise; a way to ride out the aftershocks of a catastrophe still rumbling through my life. I was oddly gratified to discover that many of those I spoke to had also undergone inward shiftings of tectonic magnitude. Their crisis of the flesh had become, as had mine, a dilemma of the spirit.

* * *

A few people I met seemed to have had a spontaneous emission of an incurable condition, such a *rara avis* [rarity] of an event that its every sighting is doubted. They ply the circuit, these grateful, sometimes baffled beneficiaries of healing: the man trimmed out in polyester making televised couch-chat out of his vanished polyps; a woman telling Joan Rivers how the tumor-the-size-of-an-orange that once straddled her left ovary just... disappeared. "Incredible," Rivers brays. "You hear these stories, you just go... unbe*liev*able!"

As well you might, if you retain a phosphor of native skepticism. But if you also possess a scintilla of innate curiosity, you cannot help but wonder, *Could it be? Do miracles really happen?* It is only lately that you might hear science reply, with quiet, uncomprehending vehemence, B*eliev*e it.

The evidence, as it turns out, has been there all along, literally hidden between the lines. An eye-opening encyclopedic compilation by California's Institute of Noetic Sciences lists hundreds of case reports unearthed from worldwide medical journals, where they had lain moldering like so many Dead Sea Scrolls.

A typical account, culled from the journal *Cancer*, describes a 51-year-old patient with a "fist-sized" abdominal tumor with metastases to the liver—a fast-progressing, invariably fatal condition. The man's stomach was operated on, but when his surgeons saw the spread of cancer's malign domain, they could only close him up and send him home to die. Inconveniently, 12 years later the left-for-dead man appeared in the emergency room of a Boston-area veterans hospital and presented himself to Dr. Steven Rosenberg.

Rosenberg was a bona fide Doogie Houser: college at 16, an M.D. and Ph.D. by his early twenties. This case, one of his very first as a junior surgical resident, looked routine enough if a little depressing. The man, named Mr. DeAngelo, whose symptoms led Rosenberg to correctly surmise he was now suffering an infected gall bladder, was a grizzled old vet down on his luck.

Yet Mr. DeAngelo, with what Rosenberg would later remember as "an aura of secret triumph," regaled him with an outlandish story the young doctor was sure came from the befuddlements of age and alcohol. Mr. DeAngelo insisted he had had terminal cancer and it had just... gone away. Digging out the man's original pathology report, a skeptical Rosenberg was nonplussed to discover it was true—the man before him with the graying stubble and self-congratulatory mien was a species of medical freak, consigned to the grave and yet risen.

Rosenberg performed the gall-bladder operation, taking time to probe the man's liver for the cancer he was sure was still there, if perhaps inexplicably slowed in its usual growth. There was nothing.

"I rushed out of the operating room," Rosenberg was later to write in his book, *The Transformed Cell*, "still dressed in green, still encrusted in drying blood. This didn't seem possible. There had been only four documented cases—not four a year in the United States, but four ever, in the world—of spontaneous and complete remission of stomach cancer."

Mr. DeAngelo, he immediately realized, "presented a mystery of ultimately enormous dimensions. Something began to burn in me, something that has never gone out."

From that moment on, Rosenberg dedicated himself to a quest to uncover the body's secret cancer-fighting mechanisms. By the relatively tender age of 34, he was made chief of surgery at the National Cancer Institute. Three years ago, he devised a highly experimental cancer treatment for advanced cancer using cells engineered to produce tumor necrosis factor (TNF), a potent enzyme capable of rapidly dissolving bulging tumors in test animals, and which might have been a factor in Mr. DeAngelo's astounding medical hat trick.

A GLIMMERING PEARL

But the question of what had made Mr. DeAngelo different from other patients—of who he really *was*—is never answered, or even asked. Rosenberg's 1972 case report is maddeningly incurious. "No evidence of tumor or other masses could be found in the abdomen," he states simply. "No adenopathy could be palpated." Sieving through the medical annals of miracle, one is confronted with articles dry to the point of desiccation. If their subjects had psyches, relationships, or meaningful lives, the authors seem to be saying, these were of no more consequence than an oyster shell that accidentally produces within its dull gray housing an impossibly rare, glimmering pearl.

This has been an enduring frustration to investigators intrigued by the notion that there might be psychosocial factors conducive to spontaneous remission. However, as I and others have discovered, sometimes the simplest line of inquiry—*Would you mind telling me your story?*—leads beyond the mechanics of the human immune system toward the mysteries of the human soul; toward what one is tempted to call, for want of a better term, a psychology of the miraculous.

* * *

One such case is that of Mitchell May. When he was 21, May's destiny took a horrifying wrong turn. On his way to a bluegrass festival on a rain-slicked Alabama road, a car struck him head-on, reducing his van to a twisted wreck, collapsing his lung, and shattering his leg in 40 places. He was flown to UCLA in a full body cast, where a team of several dozen orthopedic, vascular, and plastic surgeons declared his leg unsalvageable.

"From just below the knee down to the ankle," remembers orthopedist Edgar Dawson, M.D., "there was just bare bone hanging out with no muscle or skin over it. The leg was grossly infected. It had to come off." But May stubbornly refused amputation, even when his brother, who said his leg "looked like a pride of lions had chewed on it until they had enough," was about to sign a court order allowing doctors to remove the dying appendage.

Desperate at the impasse, May's mother sought out a healer whose unorthodox methods included laying-on of hands, hypnosis, and prayer. Jack Gray was not the classic image of a healer, unless one's imagination ran to old-timers with impasto-thick New York accents in cheesy leisure suits. But Mitchell says this apparition, who drove a wheezing Pinto in from the Valley to stay by his side 12 hours a day, was seemingly able to bypass medical science completely.

"His hands would dance around me," recalls May. "He somehow managed to take me into very deep trance states, just using his voice." Within three days Mitchell's constant pain—the excruciating sensation of raw nerves exposed to air that had resisted the most powerful and addictive painkillers—was gone.

Over a period of months, with Jack "lending his energy," the two-inch gap in May's bone began to regenerate, the missing nerve and muscle tissue filled in, and his never-set fractures began to fuse. After years, against all medical expectation, he regained full use of his leg. Dr. Dawson, when asked to explain it all, says, "That's easy. It was a miracle."

But May, now a cheerful 42-year-old, claims his miracle was one of the human psyche. "Being literally dismembered somehow opened up a new world. It was as if by being taken apart, other energies could enter through the broken places. I was *forced* to discover the life of the soul, and I think *that* was most responsible for my healing."

May's description is reminiscent of the healing path described by shamans the world over: the plummet into helplessness and mortality, the awakening of a dormant treasure-source of power, and a phoenixlike ascent to wholeness. Writes anthropologist Joan Halifax about the "initiatory crisis" of the wounded healer: "The neophyte turns away from the secular life, either voluntarily, ritually, or spontaneously through sickness, and turns inward toward the unknown, the mysterium. This change of direction can be accomplished only through what Carl Jung has referred to as 'an obedience to awareness.'"

Nearly all the people I interviewed discovered their own version of this path —a journey that seemed most often to involve a sudden intensification of the inner life, replete with vivid dreams, psychological epiphanies, sometimes near-hallucinatory episodes and perceptual alterations.

One, a woman named Debby Ogg struggled to explain, "There's a science from the inside as well as the outside." Debby, whose spontaneous remission from lymphoma ("It wasn't spontaneous," she emends, "I worked my ass off for it.") was the subject of a made-for-TV movie, says that she experienced episodes of a "floating, timeless" state of mind that had reminded her of childhood, like when "the sign for the town of Worcester was only ten minutes from our house, but getting there seemed like a whole day's trip."

A SUBMERGED MEMORY

Many people described revisiting forgotten moments of childhood wholeness with unprecedented intensity. Peter Hettel, a Florida software engineer, was diagnosed with a deadly sarcoma in his sinus cavity. He had been offered a treatment so gruesome sounding that he refused. Instead, he drove to North Carolina to see an unorthodox therapist whose practice included "neurolinguistic programming." During his first session, Peter was suddenly plunged into a long-submerged memory.

"I was around six years old, living in the countryside. I'd woken up really early one morning, and there spread before me was a magical-looking field with dewdrops like diamonds, and a grazing deer with its breath smoking from the cold. What I remembered was this sense of newness, of infinite possibility. Suddenly I was in it again, just exactly. I felt like I was a different person, or a person I'd once been but had completely forgotten. I just burst out laughing."

Many ancient healing rituals seem to imply that the first turning point in the process of renewal is "becoming as a child again." Writes mythologist Joseph Campbell: "The first step of regeneration is a retreat from the desperations of the wasteland to the magic of childhood. All the life-potentialities that we never managed to bring to adult realization, those other portions of ourself, are there; such golden seeds do not die."

In the Greek Asklepian temple, the patient would be clothed in white linen and wrapped like a child in swaddling clothes. Interestingly, the late Australian psychiatrist Ainslee Meares apparently obtained several documented and dramatic spontaneous remissions teaching patients with advanced cancers a meditation technique aimed at producing psychological "regression . . . a return to that state of affairs prior to the onset of the cancer . . . before things went wrong. He postulated this return allowed the "self-righting" mechanisms of the body to again "come into play."

Vivid recall of childhood memories is a characteristic of people rated highly hypnotizable. Psychologists S. C. Wilson and T. X. Barber found that such people were as children more likely to indulge in make-believe and retain into adulthood an ability to immerse themselves in fantasy, to "live in" the images they create. One woman in Wilson and Barber's study described having to wrap herself in blankets in her well-heated living room while watching the Siberian winter scene in *Dr. Zhivago*.

Such so-called mind–body plasticity is also a hallmark of the placebo response, and may be a key component in self-

healing. Good placebo responders, says researcher Ian Wickramesekera, resemble good hypnotic subjects in their ability to shift out of "the critical, analytic mode of information processing. They will tend to be individuals who are prone to see conceptual or other relationships between events that seem randomly distributed to others. They will inhibit the interfering signals of doubt and skepticism."

It is intriguing to note how closely these descriptions tally with observations of the healers of the Africa's Kung Bushman tribe, who, Harvard anthropologist Richard Katz notes, have "easier access to a rich fantasy life and a primarily intuitive and emotional response, rather than a logical or rational one."

A RISING HEART

But Katz noticed another trait. The healers in the tribe, he says, seem to be more "emotionally labile [open to change]. They are said to be more *sga ku tsiu*; that is, their 'heart rises' more, they are more 'expressive' or 'passionate.' " During the healing dance ceremonies in which participants attempt to raise within their bodies the "boiling energy" called *num*, the healers' emotions seemed to be "readily available and capable of quickly changing their intensity and content."

I and other researchers have been struck by a similar emotional lability among self-healers. In contrast to some notions that the healing path winds through verdant swards of peace and love, many patients described the unexpected welling-up of hidden reservoirs of anger—"like a volcano," said a former rheumatoid arthritis patient—which they associated with their unexpected recoveries. Several studies of exceptional cancer patients have confirmed such people are not infrequently "hostile, compulsive, and demanding."

Dr. Hans Schilder, a researcher at the Helen Dowling Institute of Psychosocial Medicine in Rotterdam, Holland, has noted similar characteristics in the seven spontaneous remission cases he has studied. Schilder, who sports a mop of blond hair, looks scarcely older than 17, and is lanky almost to the point of elongation, is attempting to identify specific psychological changes that might precede healing—searching, in effect, for a Tumor Necrosis Factor of the Mind.

One of his cases, a woman with terminal breast cancer, her weight down to 90 pounds and near-comatose, had been moved to a hospice because her husband did not feel capable of caring for her in her final agonies. But realizing she had been relocated to a place to die, the woman suddenly became pugnaciously assertive. "From a neat and well-educated woman," says Schilder, "she changed into a woman who was cursing, singing dirty songs. She carried on like this for three weeks—although she still waited until people left the room to do it!" An internist was shocked to observe that her tumor was starting to regress. Ten years later, she remained in a good state of health—"still very tidy," says Schilder, "but now very earthy as well."

Japanese researcher Yujiro Ikemi, one of the pioneers in the study of spontaneous remission, also observed an increase in emotional expressivity and autonomous behavior. He describes the case of a 58-year-old farmer's wife who, after years of knuckling under to a harpy of a mother-in-law and a "bossy and self-centered husband," abruptly rebelled upon being diagnosed with terminal stomach cancer. As one token of her new assertiveness, lkemi notes, she insisted on joining a group that specialized in "the loud recitation of Chinese poems."

Although only one of Schilder's cases had a formal religious experience during their healings, Ikemi noted a particular quality of faith—the farmer's wife along with all four other cases in his initial study had, as he puts it, "completely committed themselves to the fate or the will of God."

But how integral is spiritual experience to the seeming occurrence of miracles? In his independent study of the reported healings at the shrine of Lourdes, psychologist Donald West observed that many cases were diseases known to normally undergo remission—tuberculosis, for example. Researcher Alexis Carrell concluded that most of the Lourdes cures that have been officially certified as *miracles* (a total of 65 out of 6,000 claimants and tens of millions of supplicants since 1884) seemed to occur through an enormous acceleration of the body's natural healing processes.

The Lourdes Medical Commission, however, insists that it bars cases of spontaneous remission when it deems these could have resulted from biological mechanisms that would require no spiritual intervention to explain them.

Until very recently, there seems to have been an odd collusion between conventional medicine and religion to make God a kind of catch basin of anomaly. "I can't explain why you got well," the doctor says to the patient who defies his prognosis. "The only word I can think of is 'miracle.'" James Gordon, M.D., a professor at Georgetown Medical School and director of the Center for Mind–Body Studies, notes that "science often ignores these cases because it is busy looking for statistical averages. This is not good science, just convenient science. Even if they hardly *ever* happen, these 'miracles' are the kinds of exceptions to the ruling paradigm that inevitably create new areas of study."

As Dr. Rosenberg wrote about the mystifying Mr. DeAngelo, "The single most important element of good science is to ask an important question." The Institute of Noetic Sciences' Caryle Hirshberg, Ph.D., a former Stanford biochemist, has become one of the leading inquirers into the subject of spontaneous remission. For the last eight years, beginning with a data base search on a donated computer and time spent "poring over big, dusty old volumes of the *British Medical Journal*," Hirshberg eventually gathered hundreds of cases into a massive book, *Spontaneous Remissions: An Annotated Bibliography*.

SIMPLY REMISSION

Her undertaking cannot help but spawn a few revolutionary questions. What percentage of *medical* cures, for example, may be instances of spontaneous healing mistakenly attributed to treatment? As Hirshberg writes, "Since remission happens with unknown frequency, it can convincingly be argued that some of both conventional and unconventional therapies' 'successes' are simply cases of remission and have nothing to do with the [therapies'] efficacy."

Could remissions be a more common phenomenon than we suspect? Says Patricia Norris of the Menninger Clinic, who's best known for her work with a nine-year-old boy who healed of a terminal brain tumor, after all treatment had failed, using only biofeedback and mental imagery, "It's completely natural

to heal. Spontaneous remission is too mystical-sounding; it's like the medieval term "spontaneous generation," when they didn't have enough science to see germs. Doctors think mind–body factors are a very minor part of curing cancer. But patients who heal say it's major. If our culture supported it, I think more people could get over cancer by bolstering their own immune systems."

In this, she edges further out on a theoretical limb than Hirshberg, who stressed at a recent conference, "We can't withhold treatment if statistics—at least, the ones available to us—tell us spontaneous remission is still only one chance in eighty thousand." She proposes "offering conscientious hope. We should ethically be able to say, 'Here are the survival statistics on your disease, here is the mortality rate, *and* five out of every three hundred or whatever have a spontaneous regression. You're just presenting the information."

But what *is* the information? Discussing the story of Dr. Rosenberg's Mr. DeAngelo, an alcoholic who polished off four quarts of bourbon a week, a doctor interrupted: "Did the guy quit drinking after they told him he had cancer?" Told no, he asked amid swelling laughter, "Well, what *kind* of whiskey did he drink?"

The lighthearted exchange belies its cut-to-the-chase significance. The mechanisms of spontaneous remission remain obscure. Mitchell May's orthopedist avers, "I have a lot of respect for the body's ability to heal itself—I literally take people half apart and put them back together again, and the human body comes through time after time." But in the case of his most famous patient, he says without hesitation, "We tried the ordinary and the extraordinary as far as medicine goes, from mind-altering medication right up to hypnosis and acupuncture. Nothing worked. Whatever turned the switch and made him heal, it did it much more rapidly than conventional explanations allow."

Perhaps, suggests Dr. Gordon of the Center for Mind–Body Studies, explanation isn't the only agenda. "Trying to systematize these phenomena may be the wrong way to go. Maybe for now we should concentrate more on how to create the conditions to help mobilize the amazing plasticity of the mind–body."

It is a strategy well known to shamans, whose elaborate, emotionally charged ritual ceremonies seem to create optimal conditions to arouse the inner capacity for healing. Journalist Rob Schultheiss, writing about his survival of a devastating climbing accident, suggested that "perhaps the powerful hidden self only appeared when the normal limited self was shocked or scarified or otherwise blown out of the way for an instant, clearing the boards." Perhaps it is the same hidden self the late Norman Cousins referred to when he surmised the existence of a "a healing system... a grand orchestration of all the body's systems in enabling human beings to meet a serious challenge."

But can the orchestra be conducted at will? Mitchell May, who eventually became an apprentice to healer Jack Gray, suggests that "dissecting a person's experience might not enable you to recreate it. It's like lightning." He pauses for a minute, looking for a better analogy. "Or like an amazingly delicious pot of soup, where there are all these ingredients plus something else, some art, that makes it *taste* so good."

Dr. Schilder, who believes it possible to create a psychology of healing, nonetheless reports the case of a woman who, returning to a stressful family situation, had a recurrence of a tumor after a year of apparent remission. "She tried to repeat a profound spiritual change that had occurred on a trip into the mountains, which she felt had started her spectacular recovery. But she found that she couldn't force that change to happen again.

"If you took these cases as literal instructions, you would have to somehow create a dramatic replay of a pivotal event —or an entire set of circumstances—in the person's life. It would certainly be a different sort of therapy than we're used to." In the meanwhile, it may be as one patient who had experienced a remission enigmatically put it: "You can't prescribe it, it can't be taught, and you *can* learn it."

What then can we draw from the archives of the miraculous? I find inspiration in the frequent evidence that, as the Arabic physician Ali Pul once wrote, "The medicine of the soul is the medicine of the body:" that what we do to live more wholeheartedly has innate healing power.

THE PSYCHOLOGICAL PIVOT

Dr. Schilder notes that spontaneous remitters "often gain access to something that is essential to them. Often the psychological pivot associated with healing is seemingly very small: For a patient who has been a strict, loyal housewife for 30 years, just taking a few minutes to sit in chair, stretch your legs, and let the kids run around and the hell with housekeeping can be a hell of a transformation." Schilder's story reminded me of the story of the Zen master who, asked if his practice of self-insight had enabled him to work miracles, replied, "My miracle is, I eat when I'm hungry, I sleep when I'm tired." Or of Rosa Parks, whose small act of authenticity on an Alabama bus mobilized the healing resources of the social body to defeat a seemingly invincible pathology.

"Spontaneous remitters," another physician told me, "almost invariably say they weren't shooting so much for a cure, but rather to live congruently at long last with their inner values." Rosa Parks just didn't feel like giving up her seat. Perhaps the most spectacular miracles begin with a single instance of self-listening, a few small acts of affirmation—with the tiniest mustard seed of faith in the deeper self. For some of those who walked the path of healing, disease seemed to have forced a moment that arrives for most of us all too infrequently, when life itself depended on becoming authoritatively, powerfully, even crazily, the person they were meant to be.

What most of the patients I interviewed wound up doing was the opposite of what sick people are usually expected to do: Rather than simply trying to "get back to normal," many had embarked, at the most harrowing of times, on a voyage of self-discovery. They had clung instinctively to the circumnavigator's faith that the only way home was forward, into the round, unknown world of the self. People who have been through illness's dark passage can occasionally give us a glimpse not only of what it is like to become whole, but what it is to be fully human.

NO
Ellen Switzer

BLAMING THE VICTIM

Are we psychologically responsible for our health—and illness? Experts point out that the cure to what ails us isn't always in our heads, our attitudes, or our ability to "visualize" it. Here, an unexpected take on the mind-over-medicine controversy.

Is cancer more likely to strike unhappy people than happy, well-adjusted ones? Can patients suffering from cancer or other life-threatening disease improve their chances of survival by learning to enjoy life more, thinking optimistically, giving or receiving "unconditional love," or learning to imagine sick cells being eaten away by healthy ones? Are heart attacks, peptic ulcers, inflammatory bowel disease, or arthritis consequences of having a certain personality type, and will changing that personality prevent or mitigate the course of such conditions?

Many surveys show that the vast majority of Americans will answer some or all of these questions with a resounding "yes." Too many of us have become convinced that there is scientific proof that our mental and emotional states or specific personality characteristics are the principal causes of *physical* illness, and that changes in attitude, outlook, and feelings can actually cure disease, not simply improve the quality of life for the patient.

The fact is that to date there is *no* scientific proof, either statistical or physiological, that any of these assumptions is true, according to *The New England Journal of Medicine*, one of the world's most prestigious medical publications. An editorial signed by Marcia Angell, M.D., the magazine's senior deputy editor, argues that many of our current beliefs are not only scientifically unjustified but damaging to a great many patients with serious disease. "The evidence for mental state as a cause and cure of today's scourges is not much better than it was for the afflictions of earlier centuries," she writes. "Most reports of such a connection are anecdotal. They usually deal with patients whose disease remitted after some form of positive thinking, and there is no attempt to determine the frequency of this occurrence and compare it with the frequency of remission without positive thinking. Other, more ambitious studies suffer from such serious flaws in design or analysis that bias is nearly inevitable."

Angell cites one frequently mentioned study that reports the death rate among those who have been recently widowed to be higher than among those still married: "Although the authors were cautious in their interpretation, others have been quick to ascribe the findings to grief, rather than to, say, a change in diet or other habits. Similarly, the known physiologic effects of stress on the adrenal glands are often over-interpreted so that it is a short leap to a view of stress as a cause of one disease or another."

But is there any harm in this belief apart from its lack of scientific substantiation? Angell believes that there definitely is. These assumptions may (and often do) lead lay persons and some physicians to blame the victim for (1) getting sick, and (2) not getting well: A patient gets cancer, it is assumed, because he or she is angry, is unable to give or to receive love, represses negative feelings, et cetera. Another is said to have had a heart attack because she is too driven, too obsessed with success to relax and smell the flowers. A third "needs" his illness to keep family members under control. And patients are said not to respond to treatment because they lack the will to live, are unable to exercise control over pain, or do not have the self-discipline to follow whatever mental therapy a "healer" has prescribed.

"The medical profession also participates in the tendency to hold the patient responsible for his progress," Angell adds. "In our desire to pay tribute to gallantry and grace in the face of hardship, we sometimes credit these qualities with cures, not realizing we may also be implying blame when there are reverses."

In the same issue of the *Journal* that contained this editorial, there was also a carefully researched study by Barrie R. Cassileth, Ph.D., and associates which concludes that there was no relationship between attitudes and survival or recurrence of cancer in 359 patients. According to Cassileth, the director of psychosocial programs at the University of Pennsylvania Cancer Center, in Philadelphia, the study is "the first methodologically sound investigation of the relationship between selected psychosocial factors and survival in advanced malignant disease." At the time the article was written, 75 percent of the patients with inoperable cancers had died, and 26 percent of those who had had cancers removed had had recurrences. Those who survived were "in no way different psychologically from those who died," Cassileth told a conference sponsored by the American Cancer Society in New York City last October. "Something about their own *biology* made them candidates for survival. The point is, their attitude is not what did it."

Jimmie Holland, M.D., the chief of psychiatric services at the Memorial Sloan-Kettering Cancer Center, in New York City, agrees with Cassileth and Angell. "The most common psychological problem I find among the cancer patients I see is a thoroughly understandable mixture of anxiety and depression," Holland says. "Some patients who have heard all about the mind-body connection in cancer blame themselves when they cannot have a positive, cheerful attitude all the time. Patients who get depressed should not be made to feel that they are responsible for getting sicker. Adding guilt to anxiety and depression obviously makes the patient feel worse and is, therefore, self-defeating."

Neither Cassileth nor Holland questions that in some ways the mind influences the body. Adrenaline is produced when someone is frightened; hypnotic suggestion can help to alleviate pain and induce relaxation; and placebos have been known to work—although they don't cure disease, they alleviate symptoms. Both doctors also agree that emotions and attitudes influence the way a person *behaves* in relation to health and illness. "We all know that someone who eats a high-fat diet, smokes three packs of cigarettes a day, and gets no exercise has a much higher chance of becoming seriously ill than someone who lives a healthier life," Holland says. "Someone who is so terrified of being sick that he or she refuses to seek medical help when symptoms appear is also apt to make a potentially dangerous situation worse. This is particularly true of cancer. But that kind of mind-body connection is very different from the belief that a person who is psychologically strong and vital will beat a life-threatening illness, when another person with a less optimistic outlook will not."

The blame-the-victim approach to serious illness is not exactly new. Historically, we have tended to believe that incurable illnesses of mysterious origin were somehow rooted in the personality or activities of the patient. In the Middle Ages, those who suffered from epilepsy or from various forms of mental illness were subjected, if they were lucky, to exorcism to banish evil spirits. Other, not-so-lucky ones were burned as witches.

Author Susan Sontag, who some years ago had surgery for breast cancer, describes the history of myths surrounding tuberculosis and cancer in her book *Illness as Metaphor* (Farrar, Straus & Giroux). In the nineteenth century tuberculosis was thought to be a disease of "excessive feeling," before science discovered that it was caused by a bacillus. Overly passionate persons, frequently artists, got the mysterious illness by "consuming" themselves physically and psychologically—indeed, it was often called "consumption."

In the nineteenth century, the tubercular look and personality became downright fashionable. "For snobs and parvenues and social climbers, TB was one index of being genteel, delicate, sensitive...," Sontag writes. "... The TB-influenced idea of the body was a new model for aristocratic looks...." Wan, hollow-chested young women and pallid young men vied with one another to capture the look of this incurable, really awful disease. "When I was young," wrote the French Romantic poet Théophile Gautier, "I could not have accepted as a lyrical poet anyone weighing more than ninety-nine pounds."

According to Sontag, cancer has never been romanticized in a similar way. The current mythology suggests that cancer is generated by "a steady repression of feelings.... In the earlier, more optimistic form of this fantasy, the repressed feelings were sexual; now, in a notable shift, the repression of *violent* feelings is imagined to cause cancer." Sontag points out that there are actually "cancerphobes," citing as an example Norman Mailer who "recently explained that had he not stabbed his wife... he would have gotten cancer and 'been dead in a few years himself.'" Unlike tuberculosis, which was seen as a metaphor for artistic sensitivity, cancer is often used as a metaphor for evil. These metaphors, or course, affect the way we think about people with disease.

Jan van Eys, M.D., Ph.D., the director of the division of pediatrics at the M. D. Anderson Hospital and Tumor Institute, in Houston, helped to write that institution's code of medical ethics. He has found that the mind-healing-the-body myths can be particularly damaging to sick children. "The parents desperately want the child to live, and they have allowed themselves to become convinced that it is in the youngster's power to make himself recover through some method of controlling his own mind," he says. "When the child, in spite of all their urging, does not improve, they often blame themselves, or even worse, they blame the child. A youngster, who is going through the kind of pain and suffering that terminal illness can produce, feels the withdrawal of parents' approval and love. This kind of situation is truly appalling, and every advocate of a direct mind-body connection, or any form of mental healing, should consider what he or she is doing to such an unfortunate family."

Scientists, of course, have known for several decades that some diseases, like asthma and high blood pressure, can be exacerbated by emotions, particularly stress and anxiety, and that neutralizing or changing negative feelings can have a beneficial effect on the course of the illness. Certainly Angell's editorial in the *Journal* is not directed at these practitioners.

Trying to change health-damaging behavior and teaching patients how to eliminate or at least to improve their management of stress is what Joan Borysenko, Ph.D., does at her Mind/Body Clinic at the New England Deaconess Hospital, in Boston. In her book, *Minding the Body, Mending the Mind* (Addison Wesley), she discusses how she helps patients suffering from migraines, allergies, high blood pressure, premenstrual tension, and other stress-related diseases by teaching them meditation and other relaxation techniques. "Recent major studies indicate that approximately 75 per-

cent of visits to the doctor are either for illnesses that will ultimately get better by themselves or for disorders related to anxiety or stress," she writes. "For these conditions, symptoms can be reduced or cured as the body's own natural healing balance is reinstated." Most scientists, including those who in the *Journal* attacked the mind-body connection, would approve of this kind of therapy, especially since Borysenko adds that "for many other chronic or potentially life-threatening disorders, symptoms may be lessened, but the progress of disease will lead inevitably toward death. Death, after all, . . . can be a powerful reminder to live life in a way that maximizes contentment, creativity, and love."

In other words, Borysenko does not assure her patients that positive thinking can cure cancer; at best, it can improve the quality of the patient's life. And she does not blame victims for their suffering.

Neither does Norman Cousins, Ph.D., whose popular book *Anatomy of an Illness as Perceived by the Patient* (Bantam) has been widely misrepresented and misunderstood. In his book, Cousins, formerly the editor of the *Saturday Review* and now an adjunct professor of medical humanities at the UCLA School of Medicine, relates how he used the power of positive emotions, especially laughter, to help himself recover from a disabling and exceedingly painful degenerative disease of the spinal tissue. Since this very popular book was published, however, he has given countless interviews to make it crystal clear that his message had been oversimplified and exaggerated. "I never meant to suggest that laughter is a substitute for competent medical attention," he said in an interview. "Positive attitude and medical science go hand in hand." He does not blame those patients who don't follow his precepts for not getting better or their personalities for having caused the sickness in the first place.

O. Carl Simonton, M.D., a California-based radiation oncologist who now counsels cancer patients, has written a much more disquieting book, *Getting Well Again* (Tarcher), which claims high survival rates for cancer patients practicing his visualization techniques along with medical treatment. Simonton suggests that patients concentrate on imagining, for example, that their white blood cells are fish swimming around in the body, devouring the "greyish cancer cells"— like Pac-Man. He also counsels patients to exercise, and to improve their diet and relationships in order to strengthen their will to live and thus to alter the course of their cancer. It is this book that Van Eys cites most frequently when he talks about parents putting pressure on their seriously ill children to "think themselves well."

In recent years, Simonton, like Cousins, has often said that his ideas may have been overstated by zealous followers. He told an interviewer, "I don't do anyone a service if I engender more depression and guilt. I know it happens, and I'm sorry. I'm glad that I did not know it would happen, or I never would have written the book." He emphasizes that "genuine belief" in his system is vital, and that "real enthusiasm" has to be the motivating factor. What he is describing, of course, is not a new cure to serious disease; it is what most scientists would describe as a placebo effect.

There are others who go much further than Borysenko, Cousins, or Simonton in insisting that patients can cure themselves of any disease by positive thinking and feeling. For instance, Bernie S. Siegel, M.D., a New Haven surgeon— whose book *Love, Medicine & Miracles: Lessons Learned about Self-Healing from a Surgeon's Experience with Exceptional Patients* (Harper & Row) was published in 1986 and has made *The New York Times*'s best-seller list—believes that "there are no incurable diseases, only incurable people." He even cites one patient, William Calderon, "who achieved the first documented recovery from [AIDS]." "By continuing at the job he loved, he refused to give in to the disease," Siegel writes. "Instead, he began meditating and using mental imagery to combat it. He worked to restore strained relationships with his family and achieved peace of mind by forgiving people he felt had hurt him.... Two years after the diagnosis, Calderon showed no sign of AIDS." One thing is seriously wrong with this case history, however: Calderon has died of an AIDS-related condition.

Illness is not just a metaphor to Siegel; it's a personality flaw. He quotes Elida Evans, a student of Carl Jung, who wrote in 1926, "Cancer is a symbol, as most illness is, of something going wrong in the patient's life, a warning to him to take another road." Siegel continues, "The typical cancer patient, let's say a man, experienced a lack of closeness to his parents during childhood, a lack of unconditional love that could have assured him of his intrinsic value and ability to overcome challenges.... Such a person tends to view himself as stupid, clumsy, weak, and inept at social games or sports, despite real achievements that are often the envy of classmates. At the same time, he may cherish a vision of the 'real me,' who is supremely gifted, destined to benefit the human race with vague but transcendent accomplishments...."

Not only the fact that the patient gets cancer, but the *site* of the cancer in the body is determined by personality and life events, according to Siegel. "Women whose children die young or who have unhappy love relationships are especially vulnerable to breast or cervical diseases," he writes. Testicular cancer in males, however, is not mentioned as a disease that is caused by negative emotions or events; only the primary and secondary sex organs of women seem to be affected by such factors.

According to Siegel, chronic rheumatoid arthritis (a disease of unknown cause for which there is no specific cure) also often originates in a personality disorder: "a *conscious* restriction of one's own achievement." Here, he cites his mother as an example: although frequently a vice president of organizations to which she belonged, she always refused to become president.

Other patients refuse to get well because they "need" their illness to control their families, Siegel claims. Gladys, for example, one of his least favorite cancer patients, refused to get well despite his best efforts. He had offered her a new "miraculous" injection, which, he assured her, would cure her at once. He made an appointment to give her the fictitious miracle drug, which she cancelled. She "needed" that illness, he says, to continue to tyrannize her unfortunate relations. It's possible, of course, that Gladys knew that no miracle drug existed and lost faith in a physician who was clearly trying to dupe her.

There is some preliminary research indicating that some mind states can minimally influence the immune system and the growth of cells. "We are looking at this research with great interest, but the changes are so tiny that they are medically insignificant," says Sloan-Kettering's Holland. "They certainly are not significant enough to influence the course of any disease. We hope to learn more... but to date there is simply not enough information on which to base even a workable theory, never mind a course of treatment."

Recently the American Cancer Society summed up what is known about the effects of emotion on cancer: "The American Cancer Society recognizes that a positive mental attitude, psychosocial techniques, and support are important for improving the quality of life for cancer patients. At the present time, available evidence does not support the theory that the use of techniques for reducing stress can change the risk of developing cancer, or duration of survival in humans. The Society recognizes the need for continued research in this area. However, the use of psychosocial interventions that claim to alter tumor growth or spread cannot be recommended at this time."

According to most scientists, including those in the mental-health professions, this statement reflects the extent of our knowledge about the mind-body connection and its relationship to serious disease. Mental and emotional exercises may help the patient feel better and thus improve the quality of life. But no one has proved that anyone with a life-threatening physical illness can get well simply by a change of mind and attitude. Many scientists believe that along that road lies a return to exorcism, anti-medical mumbo-jumbo, magical thinking, and witchcraft.

POSTSCRIPT

Can a Positive Mental Attitude Overcome Disease?

Significant research into the relationship between stress and health indicates that the more stress one encounters, the sicker one will be. Physiologist Suzanne Kobasa has even found that executives exposed to high levels of stress are more likely to become ill if they possess certain personality traits. She claims that "hardy" workers who are challenged by new ideas, are committed to their work, believe they make a difference in the world, and are in control of their lives stay healthy in spite of leading stressful lives. See "How Much Stress Can You Survive?" *American Health* (September 1984). Yale psychologist Judith Rodin also believes that a sense of control is important for individuals who wish to lose weight or to make their lives more productive. See "A Sense of Control," *Psychology Today* (December 1984). Dr. Bernard Siegel, writing in his bestseller *Love, Medicine and Miracles* (Harper & Row, 1986), claims that there are no "incurable diseases, only incurable people" and that illness is a personality flaw. In "Welcome to the Mind/Body Revolution," *Psychology Today* (July/August 1993), Marc Barasch further discusses how the mind and immune system influence each other. And journalist Susan Chollar, in "Mind Over Cancer," *American Health* (November 1994), claims that in treating cancer, "evidence grows that emotions can alter the course of the disease."

In *You Don't Have to Die: Unraveling the AIDS Myth* (Burton Goldberg Group, 1994), the chapter entitled "Mind-Body Medicine" discusses the body's innate healing capabilities and the role of self-responsibility in the healing process. The author, a long-term AIDS survivor, traveled the country interviewing other long-term survivors and found that the one thing they all shared was the belief that AIDS was survivable. They all also accepted the reality of their diagnosis but refused to see their condition as a death sentence.

Marcia Angell disagrees with the view that the mind controls the body. In "Disease as a Reflection of the Psyche," *The New England Journal of Medicine* (June 13, 1985), Angell argues that the cure to our illnesses is not always in our heads, our personalities, or our attitudes. B. R. Cassileth et al., in "Psychosocial Correlates of Survival in Advanced Malignant Disease," *The New England Journal of Medicine* (vol. 312, 1985), report that the results of a study of 359 cancer patients show no correlation between psychosocial factors and the progression of the illness. Research by R. B. Case et al., described in "Type A Behavior and Survival After Acute Myocardial Infarction," *The New England Journal of Medicine* (vol. 312, 1985), indicated no relationship between personality and heart attacks.

PART 3

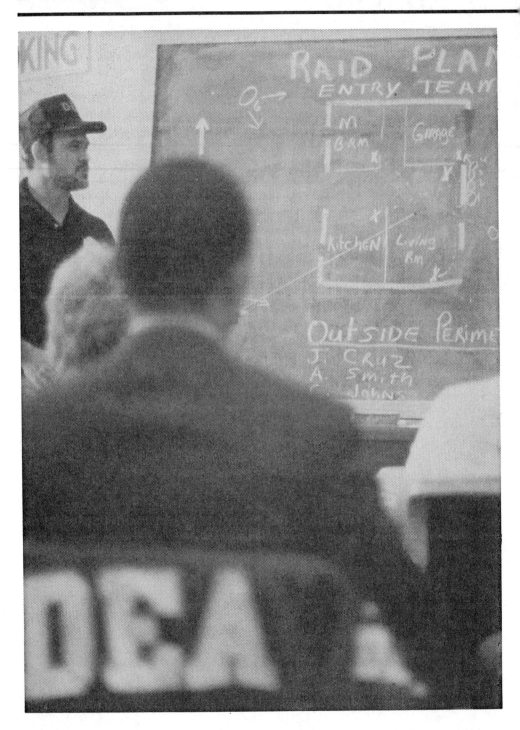

Substance Use and Abuse

While millions of Americans use and abuse drugs ranging from heroin and cocaine to alcohol and tobacco, experts continue to seek solutions for the related problems as well as the causes of addiction. The use of illegal drugs often leads to crime, while drinking and smoking are clearly associated with sickness and death. Smoking also has become an issue of personal rights as well as health—nonsmokers claim that secondhand smoke is a hazard to their well-being. The issues in this section deal with the complex concerns about drugs in our society.

- Is Secondhand Smoke a Proven Health Risk for Nonsmokers?

- Should Addiction to Drugs and Alcohol Be Considered a Disease Rather Than a Behavioral Problem?

- Should Drugs Be Legalized?

ISSUE 8

Is Secondhand Smoke a Proven Health Risk for Nonsmokers?

YES: Editors of *Consumer Reports,* from "Secondhand Smoke: Is It a Hazard?" *Consumer Reports* (January 1995)

NO: Jacob Sullum, from "Just How Bad Is Secondhand Smoke?" *National Review* (May 16, 1994)

ISSUE SUMMARY

YES: The editors of *Consumer Reports* argue that there is sound scientific data proving that the health of nonsmokers suffers when they are forced to breath tobacco smoke. They point out that many studies make a consistent case that secondhand smoke causes lung cancer and other illnesses.

NO: Editor and journalist Jacob Sullum argues that there is no evidence that secondhand smoking carries the dangers associated with actually smoking. He accuses the Environmental Protection Agency (EPA) of making inappropriate assumptions and manipulating data to arrive at a predetermined conclusion that is not accurate.

Smoking has become an established part of our culture. When cigarette manufacturing became a major industry at the turn of the century, the typical smoker was a middle-class working man. Beginning in the 1920s, however, cigarettes began to seem sophisticated and even fashionable, and women, too, started to smoke in increasing numbers. As advertising successfully penetrated the youth market and encouraged more and more young people to take up smoking, the number of smokers increased, and by 1964, 40 percent of the adult population smoked.

In 1964 the first major blow to smoking occurred: Then–surgeon general of the United States Luther L. Terry made his now-famous report positively linking smoking to lung cancer, heart disease, and other ailments. Other reports and stronger warnings on cigarette packs have contributed to the steady decline of smoking in the United States. Currently, approximately one-fourth of Americans continue to smoke.

Although the health effects of cigarette smoking are well known, until 1981 the risks associated with breathing others' smoke, or *secondhand smoke,* were not as clear. A Japanese study completed during that year showed that nonsmoking women who were married to smokers had a higher risk of lung cancer than those who were married to nonsmokers. This study indicated that breathing in the smoke from a family member's cigarettes on a daily basis is a significant risk factor for lung cancer. Since the publication of the Japanese study, secondhand smoke has been linked to numerous other diseases. Research suggests that not only are nonsmokers who are exposed to secondhand smoke—also called *environmental tobacco smoke* or *passive smoke* —at risk for lung cancer, they are also more susceptible to heart disease, asthma, and other upper respiratory diseases. The children of smokers are particularly vulnerable.

Based on the Japanese study and 30 other investigations, the EPA issued a report entitled *Respiratory Health Effects of Passive Smoking: Lung Cancer and Other Disorders* in the early 1990s. The report said, "Based on the weight of the available scientific evidence, the U.S. Environmental Protection Agency has concluded that the widespread exposure to environmental tobacco smoke in the United States presents a serious and substantial public health impact."

As a result of these health risks, nonsmokers' complaints about smokers, and the EPA report, most states now restrict smoking in public places. In addition, smoking is banned on most domestic airplane flights and in many workplaces. With the proliferation of clean indoor air regulations, smokers' freedom to light up in public is becoming more and more curtailed.

Although the nonsmoking majority may welcome these restrictions, there has been doubt cast as to the scientific validity of the research on secondhand smoke. John C. Luik, a senior associate of the Niagara Institute, claims that the substance of the EPA's report is flawed and that the agency only looked at studies involving smoking spouses and not workplace situations. Luik maintains that most of the studies involving secondhand smoke in the workplace have failed to find a statistically significant relationship between exposure to cigarette smoke and lung cancer among nonsmokers. Luik, in "Pandora's Box: The Dangers of Politically Corrupted Science for Democratic Public Policy," *Bostonia* (Winter 1993–1994), also argues that none of the studies on the health risks of nonsmoking spouses living with a smoker used by the EPA showed a strong relative risk for the nonsmokers.

In the following selections, the editors of *Consumer Reports* claim that numerous well-designed studies prove that exposure to others' smoke can cause lung cancer, heart disease, asthma, and bronchitis. The authors also assert that the tobacco companies are utilizing a small amount of scientific uncertainty along with a large amount of public relations to suggest that there is still a question as to whether or not passive smoking is harmful. Jacob Sullum argues that public policy restricting smoking in public places is based on unsound data. He claims that the risks of inhaling secondhand smoke are exaggerated and inaccurate.

YES

Editors of *Consumer Reports*

SECONDHAND SMOKE: IS IT A HAZARD?

In the 1950's and 60's, as scientists piled up a mountain of evidence on the life-threatening health consequences of smoking, the tobacco industry mounted a fierce and sophisticated campaign to keep doubt alive in the public mind.

The effort ultimately flopped; even scientists funded by tobacco-industry money today concede that smoking is bad for you. But it did succeed in putting off that day of reckoning when everyone acknowledged the hazard. That delay bought many years of robust sales.

The industry is at it again, only this time the target is secondhand smoke. A review of the record shows that tobacco companies are doing exactly what they did with "firsthand" smoke: They're using a little bit of scientific uncertainty and a lot of public relations to suggest there is still a serious debate about the health hazards of breathing smoke from other people's cigarettes.

At one time, such a controversy was real. When we reported on the subject 10 years ago, we described the evidence as "sparse and often conflicting." That's no longer true. A number of studies make a consistent case that secondhand smoke, like firsthand smoke, causes lung cancer. Many reputable groups that have inspected the evidence have reached this conclusion, including the U.S. Surgeon General's office, the National Research Council, the National Institute of Occupational Safety and Health, the International Agency for Research on Cancer, and the U.S. Occupational Safety and Health Administration (OSHA).

Other studies have found strong links between passive smoking and a host of other ills, such as asthma and bronchitis in children. Furthermore, evidence is accumulating that secondhand smoke contributes to the development of heart disease.

Early in 1993, the U.S. Environmental Protection Agency [EPA], after a painstaking and wide-ranging scientific review, declared secondhand smoke a known—not just "probable," or "possible"—human carcinogen. The EPA estimated that such smoke is responsible for several thousand cases of lung cancer in U.S. nonsmokers each year. Passive smoke joins a select company of only about a dozen other environmental pollutants in this risk category.

For the $48-billion U.S. tobacco industry, the EPA decision has been the worst setback since 1964, when the Surgeon General first declared that smoking causes cancer.

The EPA decision added momentum to widespread efforts to limit or ban smoking in public or at work. It gave employers a reason to fear workers' compensation claims based on exposure to workplace smoke. Businesses and organizations ranging from Taco Bell to the U.S. military have already banned or restricted smoking in their facilities. Seventy percent of the nation's shopping malls are now smoke-free.

Several states, including California, Maryland, Utah, Vermont, and Washington, have proposed or enacted strict controls on workplace smoking. As this report went to press, OSHA was considering nationwide rules that would, in effect, ban smoking on the job except in specially ventilated areas. Pending in the courts are at least two lawsuits brought against tobacco companies by relatives of nonsmokers who died of lung cancer after long exposure to secondhand smoke at work.

All those developments have helped to turn smoking from a public activity to a practice increasingly indulged in private. What's more they have helped persuade many smokers to cut back or quit. The smoking rate has dropped significantly, from one in three adults in 1980 to one in four today, cutting deeply into the tobacco industry's domestic market.

The industry is fighting back. It has sued in Federal court in an effort to overturn the EPA's decision. It has spent millions to block or roll back state and local public-smoking restrictions. Its public-relations firms are creating bogus "grass-roots" organizations as fronts for lobbying against smoking restrictions. (See "Public-Interest Pretenders," *Consumer Reports,* May 1994.)

In its most visible effort, a months-long national advertising campaign, the industry has attempted to spread doubt about the science behind the EPA decision and to recast the issue of secondhand smoke as one of individual rights versus an overzealous government agency.

THE EVIDENCE?

For years, researchers have accumulated information about the effects of the compounds in secondhand smoke. Cigarette smoke and tars condensed from it induce cancer in laboratory animals. The smoke causes genetic mutations in bacteria, another common test for carcinogenic potential. And several of its components are known or probable human carcinogens.

If scientists had only this animal and laboratory evidence to go on, secondhand smoke would still qualify as a "probable" or "possible" human carcinogen. But in addition, tobacco smoke is among a handful of substances—asbestos, vinyl chloride, and radon are others—for which abundant human evidence exists. That evidence comes from epidemiology, the study of disease patterns in human populations. It's the scientific field responsible for identifying all the know human carcinogens.

There are 33 published epidemiological studies of secondhand smoke, 13 of which were conducted in the U.S. Most used standard epidemiological technique: They looked at nonsmoking women who developed lung cancer, to see whether they were more likely to be married to smokers than were women who didn't get the disease. (Other researchers studied cancer rates in people exposed to smoke at work or from other family members; a few also studied husbands of women smokers.)

In all such studies, it is difficult to accurately measure every variable. Most of the smoking occurred decades ago, and the details can't be learned. Some women whose husbands didn't smoke might still have breathed smoke at work or with friends. And some wives of smokers might have been able to avoid their spouses' smoke. But both of those factors would tend to hide any true relationship between exposure and disease. So, if anything, the studies should underestimate the risk of secondhand smoke.

Nevertheless, 26 of the 33 studies indicated a link between secondhand smoke and lung cancer. Those studies estimated that people breathing secondhand smoke were 8 to 150 percent more likely to get lung cancer sometime later. Of the remaining seven studies, one found no connection with lung-cancer rates. Six suggested that people exposed to secondhand smoke had *lower* rates of lung cancer, although no one suggests passive smoking really reduces the risk.

Seven of the 26 positive studies included enough subjects, and found a sufficient effect, to attain "statistical significance"—meaning there was no more than a 5 percent probability that the results in those studies occurred by chance. In contrast, just one of the negative studies reached statistical significance.

STRENGTH IN NUMBERS

The nonsignificant studies can still be valuable when combined with all the rest for analysis. This technique, called meta-analysis, is commonly used with carefully designed clinical trials of drugs. But its use in epidemiology is controversial, since no two studies have identical designs and the analysts must make certain assumptions as they combine data. So, the result of a meta-analysis is supporting evidence but is not definitive by itself.

Six different meta-analyses have been carried out on the secondhand-smoke studies. Every one of them yielded a statistically significant increase in lung-cancer risk of approximately 20 to 40 percent. The EPA's study is the most recent of these meta-analyses. It found an increased risk of 19 percent among U.S. nonsmokers married to smokers.

More evidence for a link between cancer and secondhand smoke comes from 19 of the studies, which grouped subjects into exposure categories. In every one of those, women exposed to the most smoke for the most years had higher cancer risks that women exposed to less smoke. That dose-response relationship —an increase in risk with an increase in exposure—is an important indication of a true cause-effect relationship.

Evidence for a dose-response relationship got important support from the most recent secondhand-smoke study, published last summer by epidemiologist Elizabeth Fontham of Louisiana State University Medical Center. The largest such study ever done, it's also considered by experts in the field to be the best in design and execution. Fontham found increased risks of lung cancer with increasing exposure to secondhand smoke, whether it took place at home, at work, or in a social setting. A spouse's smoking alone produced an overall 30 percent increase in lung-cancer risk. Women with the greatest lifetime exposure—from smoking by parents, husbands, friends, and coworkers—had a 225 percent increase in risk. (That's much less than the hazard posed by active smoking, which confers a 1,100 to 2,400 percent increase in lung-cancer risk.)

For any given nonsmoker, the lifetime risk of getting lung cancer remains small —4 to 5 in 1,000 ordinarily, 6 to 7 in 1,000 if he or she has a smoking spouse. But exposure to secondhand smoke is so commonplace that, according to the EPA's calculations, it produces an extra 3000 lung-cancer deaths among adults in the U.S. each year.

That makes secondhand smoke the third-ranking known cause of lung cancer, after active smoking and indoor radon.

LUNG PROBLEMS

Despite all the attention given to lung cancer, it may not be the most significant health effect of secondhand smoke. Two others stand out as well—respiratory disorders in children and heart disease in adults.

The ill effects of smoke on children begin even before birth, since many of the components of smoke reach the developing fetus through the mother. Infants born to smoking mothers weigh less and have weaker lungs than unexposed newborns. Regardless of birth weight, babies born to smoking mothers are more likely to die in infancy than unexposed infants.

Whether from these prenatal effects or from secondhand exposure to smoke after birth, children reared around smoking parents have about twice as many respiratory infections—bronchitis and croup, for example—as the children of nonsmokers. After reviewing a number of studies, the EPA's risk analysis concluded that secondhand smoke causes an extra 150,000 to 300,000 respiratory infections a

year among the nation's 5.5 million children under the age of 18 months.

Asthma, the other major childhood respiratory ailment, also turns out to be about twice as common in children exposed to high levels of secondhand smoke. Wheezing from asthma and cough from bronchial irritation occur more frequently among children of smokers. And among children with asthma, living with smoking parents markedly worsens the disease. The EPA blames secondhand smoke for causing between 8,000 and 26,000 new cases of childhood asthma a year, and for aggravating the condition in about 200,000 children. "Children just should not be around people smoking," says Ross Brownson, professor of epidemiology at the St. Louis University School of Public Health.

HEART DISEASE

The epidemiological evidence on secondhand smoke and heart disease is not as abundant as that on lung cancer, and the experts are still debating the implications. But about a dozen studies exist, and they consistently show an elevated risk. Among nonsmokers who are exposed to their spouses' smoke, the chance of death from heart disease increases by about 30 percent. (The effects of active smoking on the heart were established some years ago. Smoking about doubles a person's chance of dying from a cardiovascular condition.)

Although the heart-disease evidence isn't as strong as that for lung cancer, a number of authorities have already declared secondhand smoke a risk factor for heart disease. They include the states of California and Maryland, OSHA, the American Heart Association, and the American College of Cardiology. They point not only to the epidemiological evidence, but to animal studies, which have shown that exposure to specific elements of secondhand smoke causes blood to clot more easily and damages arterial linings—two critical steps in the development of heart disease. In addition, human studies show that the carbon monoxide in secondhand smoke decreases the supply of oxygen reaching the heart muscle, which could cause serious problems for someone with coronary heart disease.

If exposure to secondhand smoke does increase the risk of heart disease by 30 percent, then it is causing an estimated 35,000 to 40,000 heart-disease deaths a year in the U.S.—about 10 times the number of lung-cancer deaths attributed to secondhand smoke. That would make the annual toll from secondhand smoke comparable to that from motor-vehicle accidents.

THE INDUSTRY'S CAMPAIGN

The tobacco industry foresaw the health debate over secondhand smoke—and the problems it would cause for cigarette makers. In 1978, a Roper poll commissioned by the Tobacco Institute, the industry's trade group, called growing public concern about secondhand smoke "the most dangerous development yet to the viability of the tobacco industry" and recommended "developing and widely publicizing clear-cut, credible medical evidence that passive smoking is not harmful."

In 1986, Imperial Tobacco Ltd., Canada's largest cigarette company, commissioned a secret study on how to combat the growing success of antismoking activists. The study documents, made public in the course of a lawsuit, lay out

in prescient detail the industry's current strategy on secondhand smoke:

"Passive smoking [should be] used as the focal point.... Of all the health issues surrounding smoking... the one which the tobacco industry has the most chance of winning [is] that the evidence proclaimed by the antigroup is flawed.... It is highly desirable to control the focus of the debate." The document goes on to urge "an attack on the credibility of evidence presented to date." The ideal advocate would be a medical professional, the report said, but "the challenge will be to find a sympathetic doctor who can be demonstrated to take a largely independent stance."

The recommended message on secondhand smoke: "Now that you have seen that all which has been said is not true, let's be adult and get down to the real business, a respect for each other's choices and space."

Whether or not U.S. tobacco companies ever saw the Canadian report, their current public-relations campaign is following its advice.

INFLUENCING SCIENCE

In its efforts to construct the sort of "credible medical evidence" its pollsters recommended, the tobacco industry has commissioned research from sympathetic scientists, sponsored scientific meetings carefully tailored to bring out their point of view, and published the results in the medical literature.

The research support comes through various channels: direct grants from companies or industry-funded research institutes—such as the Council for Tobacco Research and the Center for Indoor Air Research—and consulting contracts from tobacco companies, public-relations firms, and law firms. To get favorable research on the record, the industry has borrowed a technique from the pharmaceutical industry: sponsoring scientific symposia and seeing to it that their findings end up on medical library shelves.

Lisa Bero, a health policy analyst at the University of California, San Francisco, has documented the results of such symposia. She identified four symposia on passive smoking held between 1974 and 1990 that were paid for by the tobacco industry. She then compared the articles generated by the symposia with a random sample of articles on secondhand smoke that appeared in other scientific journals over the same period.

Only 4 percent of the articles from the industry-funded symposia said that passive smoking was unhealthful, compared with 65 percent of the other journal articles. Fully 72 percent of symposia reports argued that secondhand smoke wasn't harmful, compared with 20 percent of independent journal articles. (The balance of the articles were neutral.) The symposium reports did not undergo the standard scientific process of peer review, meaning they were not scrutinized by other experts in the field. Instead, they were published as non-peer-reviewed supplements to journals, or as freestanding books or monographs. Nevertheless, they can be found in the computerized databases of the medical literature. That makes them available for citation by others.

This careful construction of a citable scientific record came in handy when the tobacco industry set out to attack early drafts of the EPA's report on secondhand smoke. Bero found that two-thirds of comments critical of the report came from industry scientists, who drew heavily on industry-generated literature. The

Tobacco Institute's own submission, for instance, cited 32 papers from symposia, but only seven peer-reviewed articles.

As the industry has learned, however, research support doesn't guarantee that a scientist will go along with the company line. At least five members of an independent scientific advisory board that reviewed the EPA report had ties to industry research groups, either as advisers or grant recipients, including a scientist awarded a $1.2-million grant from Philip Morris [the largest cigarette manufacturer in the United States] during the review period. Yet the board unanimously agreed that passive smoking was a cancer risk.

PUBLIC PERSUASION

In a public-relations campaign, scientific articles don't mean much if only scientists read them. The industry is bringing its perspective to a much wider audience, with the help of a few journalists. This became clear when we studied industry-generated material on secondhand smoke and looked over newspaper and magazine articles sympathetic to the industry's position.

To read this material is to enter a house of mirrors that endlessly reflects the same set of opinions, voiced by the same few people, again and again. A person who saw nothing else could conclude that there were only four or five scientists in all of North America qualified to speak about secondhand smoke—all of them skeptical of its danger.

You can see how this works by tracing the public utterances of one of those scientists, Gary Huber, a lung specialist at the University of Texas. Shook, Hardy & Bacon, the tobacco industry's longtime law firm, pays Huber's university to support his group's compilation of research on lung disease. Despite this, he told us, his views are his own.

In 1991, Huber wrote an article for *Consumers' Research*—a small-circulation magazine not connected to *Consumer Reports*—in which he argued that the scientific evidence on the hazards of passive smoking is "shoddy and poorly conceived." He felt the epidemiological studies were too weak and the composition of secondhand smoke too poorly understood to reach a conclusion on any risk.

In early 1993, Huber was prominently quoted in an article in *Investor's Business Daily*. Writer Michael Fumento stated that "many in the scientific and medical community" dispute the EPA's opinion. All five scientists quoted to back up this viewpoint have received some type of industry support.

Both Huber's and Fumento's articles became, in turn, sources for a series of opinion pieces written by another journalist, Jacob Sullum. In *The Wall Street Journal* and *Forbes Media Critic*, Sullum built on Fumento's arguments and quoted three of the same scientists, including Huber. When we asked the Tobacco Institute for material on secondhand smoke, it sent us a packet that included Fumento's article.

R. J. Reynolds reprinted Sullum's *Wall Street Journal* article nationwide in a full-page ad. The ad's headline: "If We Said It, You Might Not Believe It." Philip Morris went even further, buying full-page ads in major national publications for six straight days to reprint Sullum's longer *Forbes Media Critic* article.

The effect: Huber's argument has undoubtedly now been seen by millions more people than ever read the original EPA report, never mind any of the

hundreds of scientific articles on the subject in medical journals.

The industry's strategy has been effective. John Pierce, a researcher at the University of California, San Diego, who specializes in tobacco issues, checked the calls made to a statewide smokers' hotline immediately after the Reynolds and Philip Morris ads started appearing in print. Although the hotline was intended to give support to smokers who wanted to quit, the calls coming in during that period were overwhelmingly accusatory. "We had a whole heap of people calling us, asking why we were misleading them," Pierce recalls. "There are all too many people willing to believe the industry when it says this thing's not really bad for you."

ATTACKING THE SCIENCE

The heart of the cigarette makers' campaign appears to be their attack on the scientific methods used to measure the risk of secondhand smoke. In its advertising, its public statements, and its lawsuit against the EPA, the industry argues that the agency "cherry-picked" data to reach a foregone conclusion and violated the rules of statistical analysis. That's a clever strategy; it takes advantage of the public's unfamiliarity with research methods and the common perception that one week's scientific report will be debunked the following week.

To evaluate the industry arguments, we consulted CU's own professional statisticians and also turned to Charles Hennekens and Julie Buring, epidemiologists at Harvard Medical School and coauthors of a leading edidemiology textbook. They have no ties to the tobacco industry, and their own research includes studying various causes of heart disease and cancer. Here's what they said about the criticisms.

Pooling Studies   The industry argues that the EPA had no business pooling smaller studies, many failing the "statistical significance" test, into one large collection of data. This is the meta-analysis technique we described above. "They've combined studies as different as night and day, which is not an accepted way to do a meta-analysis," says Walker Merryman, vice president of the Tobacco Institute.

In truth, the EPA made an effort to compare comparable studies. It sorted them by country or region, excluded the poorest-quality studies, and then pooled data only within each geographical group. The pooled results for Greece, Hong Kong, Japan, and the U.S. all showed statistically significant risk increases. The pooled results from Western Europe and China, though positive, didn't reach significance.

"Having a number of studies that show similar results but are not large enough individually to be statistically significant on their own is exactly the situation where meta-analysis is appropriate," Buring says.

The Significance Level   When they analyze their data, most researchers try to set their "statistical significance" hurdle at 5 percent. In everyday language, that means there is less than a 5 percent probability the results occurred by happenstance.

However, the tobacco industry argues that the EPA lowered its hurdle to 10 percent when it pooled the various studies. Jacob Sullum said it "in effect doubles the odds of being wrong." An industry scientific consultant called it a "confidence game."

But here too, the EPA played fair. It did set a 5 percent significance level. The agency used a standard statistical technique, called a one-tailed test, that allowed a 5 percent chance of wrongly concluding that secondhand smoke increases the risk of cancer. This technique, taught in every introductory statistics course, is appropriate when, as in this case, there is already independent evidence that a substance is harmful.

What's more, when Hennekens and Buring analyzed pooled data from the 11 U.S. studies on which the EPA relied most heavily, they found that the data do meet the even tougher standard the critics are demanding.

Confounding Factors   Since epidemiologists can't control everything that happens in the lives of their subjects, they have to be wary of confounding factors, possible alternative causes for the results. Relatively small risks, like that from secondhand smoke, are especially vulnerable to confounding.

The tobacco industry and its defenders have raised just such a possibility. "There are numerous, and in many cases unaccounted for, factors which makes the whole process exceedingly difficult," Merryman says. "Since we're dealing with an issue of such magnitude, I think it's proper to insist they be accounted for." The critics have usually focused on diet or socioeconomic status, both of which have been linked to the incidence of cancer. If people exposed to secondhand smoke were more likely to be poor or to have poor diets, data could be muddied.

In fact, the EPA considered possible confounding factors. Five of the studies it analyzed included information on diet. None of those five studies suggested that diet could account for the increased risk in people exposed to secondhand smoke.

The studies the EPA relied on didn't record socioeconomic status, but Fontham's newer study did—and found no link to risk. She also looked at diet and found that a diet high in fruits and vegetables did seem to protect people from lung cancer. But even after accounting for that, there was still a significant relationship between secondhand smoke and lung cancer.

Epidemiologists readily concede they can never account for all the factors that affect health. But since studies done in many countries with different cultures and habits all point to an elevated risk, confounding factors are not likely to be the explanation.

The 'Excluded' Studies   The industry has repeatedly implied that the EPA ignored two 1992 studies because they didn't support the agency's conclusions. In fact, both studies were published during the seven-month period after the EPA report was written but before the agency released it. And neither study suggests the EPA is wrong.

In one, University of South Florida researcher Heather Stockwell found that nonsmoking women married to smokers had a 60 percent higher risk of lung cancer than women married to nonsmokers. The most highly exposed group—women exposed for 40 years or more—had a 130 percent increase in risk. In the other study, Ross Brownson, then of the Missouri Department of Health, found no risk increase for all exposed women as a group—but the most highly exposed had a 30 percent increase.

Both the EPA and the industry have calculated, but not published, re-analyses that include all the new studies. The EPA says it still finds a statistically significant risk; R. J. Reynolds says it doesn't.

THE BOTTOM LINE

There's no question that all epidemiological studies have a built-in imprecision, Buring told us. "But when you see different investigators, using different definitions and study designs, all showing similar results, then you have to believe there's something going on."

The case against secondhand smoke has reached that point. Short of conducting an impossible experiment—deliberately exposing thousands of people to secondhand smoke for decades, to see what happens—this is about as good as the human evidence on secondhand smoke is likely to get.

When those results are combined with the laboratory studies, the abundant evidence that firsthand smoke causes cancer, and the evidence for a dose-response relationship, the health implications are clear—and the EPA's conclusion inescapable.

"If we didn't have the tobacco companies spending millions of dollars to confuse the facts, this issue would be an open-and-shut case," says Stanton Glantz, a longtime tobacco researcher at the University of California, San Francisco. "The fact is that passive smoking causes lung cancer."

Your personal risk? Since the amount of smoke inhaled appears related to the risk of disease, there probably is a minimal hazard from brief exposure. But steady doses of secondhand smoke at home or on the job aren't so benign.

A nonsmoker's individual risk of dying from lung cancer, normally small, is increased slightly by living or working for years among people who smoke heavily. And although the individual risk is relatively small, the numbers add up to an issue of public health. Thousands of people in the U.S. may be dying or made sick every year from other people's smoking.

James Repace and Alfred Lowrey, two statistical researchers who study the effects of secondhand smoke, have concluded that a lifetime increase in lung-cancer risk of 1 in 1,000 could be caused by long-term occupational exposure to air containing more than 6.8 micrograms of nicotine per cubic meter of air. (The nicotine itself doesn't cause lung disease but is a marker for smoke concentration.) Concentrations that heavy occur regularly in many homes and workplaces.

For its study, the EPA found 19 reports of measurements of nicotine levels in enclosed spaces where people smoked. Nicotine levels in homes of smokers had averages that ranged from study to study, between 2 and about 11 micrograms; in offices, the range of averages was about 1 to 13. Restaurants were even smokier, with averages between about 6 and 18 micrograms.

WHAT SHOULD BE DONE

If secondhand tobacco smoke were not connected to the profits of a powerful industry, we doubt there would be much argument about drastically restricting people's exposure to it.

The lifetime added risk of developing lung cancer from prolonged exposure to secondhand smoke is roughly 1 in 1,000—1,000 times greater than the one-in-a-million lifetime cancer risk considered unacceptable for many other environmental contaminants. Even in small doses, it can be an uncomfortable irritant, at the very least.

In response to the data, the tobacco industry has accelerated its campaign against public smoking restrictions. For instance, five companies together laid out nearly $8-million last year in an unsuccessful effort to persuade California voters to approve a smoking-control law that would have invalidated stronger state and local restrictions.

The 1994 elections greatly improved the industry's legislative prospects. Out as chairman of the House Subcommittee on Health and Environment is Democrat Henry Waxman of California. His hearings last year produced the widely seen image of tobacco-company chiefs swearing they didn't think cigarettes were addictive. His likely replacement is Republican Thomas Bliley. The major employer in Bliley's Virginia district is Philip Morris, and Bliley has already said, "I don't think we need any more legislation concerning tobacco."

We disagree. We believe nonsmokers have a right to breathe smoke-free air, and we have long favored restrictions on where people may smoke. The medical evidence makes it imperative to impose such limits. In particular, we support measures to keep smoke out of the workplace—not just offices and factories but also restaurants, stores, and public transportation, because of the risk to the millions of Americans who work there, too.

We support OSHA's efforts to limit workplace smoking to certain ventilated rooms. OSHA calculates that over the next 45 years a workplace smoking ban would eliminate between 5,500 and 32,500 lung-cancer deaths and 98,000 to 578,000 deaths from heart disease. (The variation comes from uncertainty about current levels of exposure to secondhand smoke.)

That makes control of smoke one of the great public-health bargains. Getting rid of workplace smoke requires posting signs, putting a few chairs and an ashtray outdoors, or putting an appropriate ventilation fan into a special smoking room —an improvement that OSHA estimates would cost $4,000 per building. In contrast, the bill for removing asbestos from a commercial building averages $300,000.

NO

Jacob Sullum

JUST HOW BAD IS
SECONDHAND SMOKE?

"Secondhand Smoke Kills." So says a billboard on Pico Boulevard in Los Angeles that I pass every day on the way to work. I'm still not convinced. But most Americans seem to be: a CNN / *Time* poll conducted in March found that 78 per cent believe secondhand smoke is "very" or "somewhat" harmful.

That idea was endorsed by the U.S. Environmental Protection Agency [EPA] last year, when it declared secondhand smoke "a known human lung carcinogen." Since then the EPA's report has helped justify smoking bans throughout the country: in cities such as Los Angeles and San Francisco (likely to be joined soon by New York); in Maryland, Vermont, and Washington state; and in government offices, including the Defense Department. On March 25, the Occupational Safety and Health Administration proposed a ban on smoking in workplaces, including bars and restaurants. A bill introduced by Representative Henry Waxman (D., Calif.) would go even further, banning smoking in almost every building except residences.

Most supporters of such measures probably believe that the EPA's report presents definitive scientific evidence that "secondhand smoke kills." But a closer look shows that the EPA manipulated data and finessed important points to arrive at a predetermined conclusion. The agency compromised science to support the political crusade against smoking.

The first line of defense for people who want to avoid scrutiny of the case against secondhand smoke (a/k/a environmental tobacco smoke, or ETS) is to argue by analogy. "We know that tobacco smoke causes disease and can kill you," says Scott Ballin, chairman of the Coalition on Smoking or Health. "It makes sense that a person who doesn't smoke cigarettes, who's sitting next to a smoker and inhaling the smoke, is also at some risk." The EPA offers a similar argument, devoting a chapter of its report on ETS to the evidence that smoking causes cancer.

Although superficially plausible, this analogy is misleading. A smoker breathes in hot, concentrated tobacco smoke and holds it in his lungs before exhaling. A nonsmoker in the vicinity, by contrast, breathes air that includes

From Jacob Sullum, "Just How Bad Is Secondhand Smoke?" *National Review* (May 16, 1994). Copyright © 1994 by National Review, Inc., 150 East 35th St., New York, NY 10016. Reprinted by permission.

minute quantities of residual chemicals from tobacco smoke. "ETS is so highly diluted that it is not even appropriate to call it smoke," says Gary Huber, a professor of medicine at the University of Texas Health Science Center, writing with two colleagues in the July 1991 *Consumers' Research.* Furthermore, since many of the compounds in tobacco smoke are unstable, it is not safe to assume even that a nonsmoker is exposed to the same chemicals as a smoker. Of 50 biologically active substances thought to be present in ETS, Huber and his colleagues report, only 14 have actually been detected.

Even if exposure to ETS were analogous to smoking, the doses involved are so small that it's not clear they would have any effect. Many chemicals that are hazardous or even fatal above a certain level are harmless (or beneficial) in smaller doses. James Enstrom, a professor of epidemiology at UCLA, estimates that someone exposed to ETS would be taking in the equivalent of a few cigarettes a year, perhaps one-hundredth of a cigarette a day. Yet studies of smoking have never looked at people who smoke that little; the lowest-exposure groups have been subjects who smoke up to five cigarettes a day.

THE EPA'S SMOKING GUN

So it's not reasonable to conclude that ETS must be dangerous because smoking is dangerous. You have to look at the research that deals specifically with ETS. The EPA's finding is based on 30 epidemiological studies that compared lung-cancer rates among nonsmokers (mainly women) who lived with smokers to lung-cancer rates among nonsmokers who lived with nonsmokers. None of the studies measured actual exposure to ETS; they simply assumed that people who lived with smokers were more exposed than people who didn't. In most of these studies, lung cancer was somewhat more common among the subject living with smokers, but in only 6 cases were the results statistically significant.

This is a crucial point. In any study that compares a group exposed to a suspected risk factor with a control group, the luck of the draw may result in a difference between the two groups that does not reflect a difference between the populations the groups are supposed to represent. Researchers do statistical tests to account for the possibility of such a fluke. By convention, epidemiologists call a result significant when the probability that it occurred purely by chance is 5 per cent or less. By this standard, 80 per cent of the studies discussed by the EPA did not find a statistically significant link between ETS and lung cancer.

But the EPA, which had always used the conventional definition of statistical significance in its risk assessments, adopted a different standard for the report on ETS. It considered a result significant if the probability that it occurred purely by chance was 10 per cent or less. This change essentially doubles the odds of being wrong. "The justification for this usage," according to the report itself, "is based on the *a priori* hypothesis ... that a positive association exists between exposure to ETS and lung cancer." Of course, the EPA was supposed to *test* that hypothesis, not simply assume that it is true.

Instead of presenting results from the epidemiological studies as they originally appeared, the EPA recalculated them using the less rigorous standard. As a report from the Congressional Research

Service drily notes, "it is unusual to return to a study after the fact, lower the required significance level, and declare its results to be supportive rather than unsupportive of the effect one's theory suggests should be present."

Even after the EPA massaged the data, the vast majority of the studies still did not show a significant association between ETS and lung cancer. Of the 11 U.S. studies, only 1 yielded a result that was significant according to the looser definition. (According to the usual definition, none of them did.) To bolster the evidence, the EPA did a "meta-analysis" of these studies. Dr. Enstrom notes that this technique was originally intended for clinical trials that assess the impact of a drug or procedure by randomly assigning subjects to treatment and control groups. By contrast, the data analyzed by the EPA came from retrospective case-control studies that "matched" people with lung cancer to people without lung cancer. Enstrom says using meta-analysis for such studies "is not a particularly meaningful exercise," because the studies are apt to differ in the way they define exposure, the confounding variables they take into account, the types of cancer they include, and so on.

In any event, the EPA's conclusion —that living with a smoker raises a woman's risk of getting lung cancer by 19 per cent—is justified only according to the definition of statistical significance adopted especially for these data. By the usual standard, even the meta-analysis does not support the claim that ETS causes lung cancer. Furthermore, the EPA excluded from its analysis a major U.S. study, published in the November 1992 *American Journal of Public Health*, that failed to find a significant link between ETS and lung cancer. Given the large size of the study, it could well have changed the outcome of the meta-analysis, so that the result would not have been significant even by the EPA's revised standard.

SMALL CLAIMS

Despite this "fancy statistical footwork," as a July 1992 article in *Science* described it, the EPA was able to claim only a weak association between ETS and lung cancer. With a risk increase as low as 19 per cent, it is difficult to rule out the possibility that other factors were at work. "At least 20 confounding variables have been identified as important to the development of lung cancer," write Huber et al. "No reported study comes anywhere close to controlling, or even mentioning, half of these."

Smokers tend to differ from nonsmokers in many ways—including diet, socioeconomic status, risk-taking behavior, and exercise—and it is likely that the spouses of smokers share these characteristics to some extent. "If wives of smokers share in poor health habits or other factors that could contribute to illness," the Congressional Research Service notes, "statistical associations found between disease and passive smoking could be incidental or misleading."

Misclassification could also account for some or all of the observed differences between wives of smokers and wives of nonsmokers. It's possible that some of the subjects thought to be nonsmokers were actually smokers or former smokers. Since spouses of smokers are more likely to be smokers themselves, such errors would have biased the results. The EPA adjusted the data to account for this effect, but it's impossible to say whether it fully compensated for misclassification.

These issues are especially important when the relationship between a suspected risk factor and a disease is weak. Based on the 11 U.S. studies, the EPA concluded that a woman who lives with a smoker is 1.19 times as likely to get lung cancer as a woman who lives with a nonsmoker. This ratio did not rise above 2.1 to 1 in any of the U.S. studies. In previous risk assessments, the EPA has seen such weak associations as cause for skepticism. When the agency examined the alleged connection between electromagnetic fields and cancer, for example, it said, "the association is not strong enough to constitute a proven causal relationship, largely because the relative risks in the published reports have seldom exceeded 3.0."

This concern did not prevent the EPA from reaching a firm conclusion about ETS, even though the agency recognized the limitations of the data. The head of the Scientific Advisory Board that reviewed the report conceded: "This is a classic case where the evidence is not all that strong."

The evidence is especially unimpressive when compared to the evidence that smoking causes lung cancer. In the latter case, there are thousands of studies, and virtually all of them have found a positive association, statistically significant in the vast majority of cases. And the associations are sizable: a typical female smoker is about 10 times as likely to get lung cancer as a female nonsmoker; for men the ratio is more like 20 to 1; and among heavy smokers, the figures are even higher. "The data on active smoking are so much stronger," Enstrom says. "That should be the focus of attention, not something which is so small and has the potential to be confounded by so many different things. I personally am baffled as to why people give it so much credibility."

PROTECTED FROM THEMSELVES

The explanation may be that the EPA's conclusion about ETS is useful in a way that the evidence about smoking is not. Although the share of adults who smoke has dropped from about 40 per cent to about 25 per cent since 1965, some 50 million Americans continue to smoke. And as Duke University economist W. Kip Viscusi shows in his recent book *Smoking: Making the Risky Decision*, this is not because they are ignorant about the health effects. Rather, they are willing to accept the risks in exchange for the benefits of smoking. From a "public-health" perspective, this is intolerable; no one should be allowed to make such a foolish decision. But the idea of protecting people from themselves still arouses considerable opposition in this country. Hence antismoking activists and public-health officials need a different excuse for restricting smoking: it endangers innocent bystanders.

When EPA Administrator Carol Browner testified in favor of Waxman's Smoke-Free Environment Act in February, she relied heavily on the ETS report. But the main benefit that she claimed for the bill was its expected impact on smokers. "The reduction in smoker mortality due to smokers who quit, cut back, or do not start is estimated to range from about 33,000 to 99,000 lives per year," she said. And six surgeons general, reported the *New York Times*, "echoed the theme that this simple measure could do more for the public health than any other bill in years."

If your main goal is improving "the public health," you may be inclined to shade the truth a bit if it helps to make smoking less acceptable and more inconvenient. Marc Lalonde, Canada's former minister of national health and welfare, offered a rationale for such a strategy in a highly influential 1974 report: "Science is full of 'ifs,' 'buts,' and 'maybes,' while messages designed to influence the public must be loud, clear, and unequivocal.... The scientific 'yes, but' is essential to research, but for modifying human behavior of the population it sometimes produces the 'uncertain sound.' This is all the excuse needed by many to cultivate and tolerate an environment and lifestyle that is hazardous to health."

Writing about the ETS controversy in *Toxicologic Pathology*, Yale University epidemiologist Alvan Feinstein quotes a colleague who appears to have been influenced by the Lalonde Doctrine: "Yes, it's rotten science, but it's in a worthy cause. It will help us get rid of cigarettes and become a smoke-free society."

This seems to be the attitude that the EPA brought to its risk assessment.

In June 1990 the agency released the first draft of *Environmental Tobacco Smoke: A Guide to Workplace Smoking Policies*, intended to advise employers to institute smoking restrictions. Yet this was three and a half years before the EPA officially determined that ETS was a health hazard. In a letter to Representative Thomas J. Bliley Jr., (R., Va.), then EPA Administrator William Reilly admitted that "beginning the development of an Agency risk assessment after the commencement of work on the draft policy guide gave the appearance of the very situation—i.e., policy leading science—that I am committed to avoid."

Reilly was so committed to avoiding this appearance that he decided not to release the final version of the policy guide, even though it was ready by December 1992. As he explained to the *Wall Street Journal*, putting out the guide along with the risk assessment would "look like we're trying to torque the science." But don't worry. Miss Browner, Mr. Reilly's successor, released the handy pamphlet last July.

POSTSCRIPT

Is Secondhand Smoke a Proven Health Risk for Nonsmokers?

The tobacco industry not only supports smokers' rights to smoke in public but also claims that passive smoking is not harmful. To justify the claim that passive smoking is harmless to health, industry representatives argue that the research is inconclusive and lacking in validity. The industry used similar tactics to try and persuade smokers that smoking had not been proven harmful to health after the surgeon general's proclamation that it had in 1964. The industry has more recently attacked research linking secondhand smoke with cancer, heart disease, and other health problems.

In addition to maintaining that secondhand smoke is not harmful, the tobacco industry holds that laws restricting smoking in public places violate smokers' civil rights; after all, smokers are taxpayers too. Also, smoking is a personal choice, and the industry contends that the government has no right to restrict when and where smokers may light up. Articles supporting this view include "Smoke and Mirrors," by Jacob Sullum, *Reason* (February 1991); "Zealots Against Science," *The American Spectator* (July 1990); "Coping With Smoking," by Tibor Machan, *Freeman* (April 1989); and "The Health Police Are Blowing Smoke," *Fortune* (April 25, 1988). Other writers also claim that proposed bans on tobacco advertising would be an example of unwanted government paternalism. See John Luik, "Tobacco Advertising Bans and the Dark Face of Government Paternalism," *International Journal of Advertising* (vol. 12, 1993). A recent article in the *Wall Street Journal* (April 15, 1994), p. A4, "Tobacco Executives Tell Panel Nicotine Is Not Addictive," typifies the tobacco industry's messages regarding the safety of active and passive smoking.

Because public smoking is an issue of both health and personal rights, it generates many arguments. Both nonsmokers and smokers claim that their rights are violated when one group's desires are allowed to prevail over the other's. In the battle over smoking, nonsmokers cite research showing that long-term exposure to passive smoke increases the risk of many illnesses, including heart disease and lung cancer. Researchers claim that passive tobacco smoke contains over 40 cancer-causing chemicals and is responsible for as many as 50,000 deaths each year. A recent study, "Environmental Tobacco Smoke and Lung Cancer in Nonsmoking Women: A Multicenter Study," *Journal of the American Medical Association* (June 8, 1994), confirms these findings: researchers found that nonsmoking women living with smoking spouses faced a 30 percent higher risk of developing lung cancer than nonsmoking women living with nonsmokers.

Numerous research studies have indicated that passive smoking is a health risk. The landmark investigation, which concluded that nonsmoking wives of smoking spouses have a higher risk of developing lung cancer, found that only a fraction of female lung cancer patients actually smoked cigarettes. It was concluded that the women who developed lung cancer were exposed to high levels of secondhand smoke from their husbands' cigarettes. See "Non-Smoking Wives of Heavy Smokers Have a Higher Risk of Lung Cancer: A Study from Japan," *British Medical Journal* (January 17, 1981). This classic study was followed by many others, all reaching the same conclusion: exposure to passive smoke is a risk for lung cancer and other smoking-related diseases. Further readings include "Passive Smoking and Lung Cancer," *The Lancet* (September 10, 1983); "Prevalence and Correlates of Passive Smoking," *American Journal of Public Health* (April 1983); "Cancer Risk in Adulthood from Early Life Exposure to Parents' Smoking," *American Journal of Public Health* (May 1985); "Passive Smoking May Cause Leukaemia," *New Scientist* (March 7, 1985); "Secondhand Smoke," *Newsweek* (June 11, 1990); "Passive Smoking, Active Risks," *American Health* (June 1990);"Urine Tests Confirm Fears About Passive Smoking," *New Scientist* (January 29, 1994); "Threat from Passive Smoking Is Upgraded," *Science News* (June 11, 1994); and "Passive Smoke and Lung Cancer," *American Health* (September 1994).

ISSUE 9

Should Addiction to Drugs and Alcohol Be Considered a Disease Rather Than a Behavioral Problem?

YES: George E. Vaillant, from "We Should Retain the Disease Concept of Alcoholism," *Harvard Medical School Mental Health Letter* (August 1990)

NO: Joann Ellison Rodgers, from "Addiction: A Whole New View," *Psychology Today* (September/October 1994)

ISSUE SUMMARY

YES: Physician George E. Vaillant maintains that alcoholism is genetically transmitted, so it should be treated as a disease and not as a behavioral problem or character flaw.

NO: Journalist Joann Ellison Rodgers argues that current ideas and policies regarding addiction to drugs and alcohol are outdated, particularly the theory that alcoholism and drug addiction are diseases.

There are many different theories as to why some individuals become addicted to alcohol or other drugs. Historically, drug and alcohol dependency has been viewed as either a disease or a moral failing. In more recent years, other theories of addiction have been developed, including behavioral, genetic, sociocultural, and psychological theories.

The view that drug addiction and alcoholism are moral failings maintains that abusing drugs is voluntary behavior that the user chooses to do. Users choose to overindulge in such a way that they create suffering for themselves and others. American history is marked by repeated and failed government efforts to control this abuse by eliminating drug and alcohol use with legal sanctions, such as the enactment of Prohibition in the late 1920s and the punishment of alcoholics and drug users via jail sentences and fines. However, there seem to be several contradictions to this behavioral model of addiction. Addiction may be a complex condition that is caused by multiple factors, including environment, biology, and others. It is not totally clear that addiction is voluntary behavior. And from a historical perspective, punishing alcoholics and drug addicts has been ineffective.

In the United States today, the primary theory for understanding the causes of addiction is the disease model rather than the moral model. The disease model is especially strong among the medical and alcohol treatment communities as well as self-help groups such as Alcoholics Anonymous and Narcotics Anonymous. The disease model implies that addiction is not the result of voluntary behavior, psychiatric problems, or lack of self-control; it is caused by biological factors. While there are somewhat different interpretations of the disease model, it generally refers to addiction as a disease with biological and genetic origins rather than voluntary and behavioral origins.

Many proponents of the disease model cite the claim that children of alcoholics are four times more likely to develop alcoholism than are children of nonalcoholics. In addition, they assert that some alcoholics have an enzyme abnormality related to alcohol activity that does not seem to exist in individuals who do not drink. These claims, which support genetics as the cause of alcoholism and other addictions, are largely based on a few studies that critics claim are flawed.

George Vaillant is a proponent of the disease model. He maintains that calling addiction a disease rather than a voluntary behavioral disorder is a useful device both to persuade the drug abuser to acknowledge the problem and to provide a ticket into the health care system.

Joann Ellison Rodgers does not believe that one theory can explain addiction. Addiction, she argues, is related to the individuals who use drugs and alcohol, their environment, and the drug itself.

YES
George E. Vaillant

WE SHOULD RETAIN THE DISEASE CONCEPT OF ALCOHOLISM

When I read expert discussions of why alcoholism is not a disease, I am reminded of the equally learned discussions by "the best and the brightest" of why the Viet Nam War was a good idea. These discussants had intelligence, advanced degrees, scholarship, prestige, literacy—every qualification but one. They lacked experience. None had spent much time in Viet Nam. Just so, the philosopher Herbert Fingarette, the psychoanalyst Thomas Szasz, the sociologist and theoretician Robin Room, and provocative, thoughtful psychologists like Stanton Peele and Nicholas Heather have every qualification but one for explaining why alcoholism is not a disease—they have never worked in an alcohol clinic. Why, I wonder, do experienced alcohol workers and recovering alcoholics, the thousands of competent common folk in the trenches, accept the view that alcoholism is a disease? Why is it mainly less competent people, the active alcoholics, who agree with Professor Fingarette that they are just "heavy drinkers"?

Let me summarize the evidence provided by the learned academics who have pointed out the folly of the medical model of alcoholism. First, alcohol abuse—unlike coughing from pneumonia, for example—is a habit under considerable volitional control. Second, there is compelling evidence that variations in alcohol consumption are distributed along a smooth continuum, although a medical model would suggest that in any individual, alcoholism is either present or absent. Third, when alcoholism is treated as a disease it can be used both by individuals and by society to explain away major underlying problems—poverty, mental deficiency, crime, and the like—which require our attention if efforts at prevention, treatment and understanding are to succeed. Fourth, to diagnose people as alcoholic is to label them in a way that can damage both self-esteem and public acceptance. Fifth, alcoholism

From George E. Vaillant, "We Should Retain the Disease Concept of Alcoholism," *Harvard Medical School Mental Health Letter* (August 1990). Copyright © 1990 by the President and Fellows of Harvard College. Reprinted by permission of the *Harvard Medical School Mental Health Letter*, 164 Longwood Avenue, Boston, MA 02115.

should not be considered a disease if it is regarded as merely a symptom of underlying personality or depression.

REFUTATION OF OBJECTIONS

Let me try to refute these objections one by one. First, it may be true that there is no known underlying biological defect in alcoholism. Rather, alcohol abuse is a multidetermined continuum of drinking behaviors whose causes are differently weighted for different people and include culture, habits, and genes. But the same can be said of high blood pressure and coronary heart disease. The incidence of hypertension varies with measurement procedures and psychological circumstances. It lies on a physiological continuum which defies precise definition. It has no known specific cause. It is powerfully affected by social factors; for example, it has become epidemic among young urban black males. The point of using the term 'disease' for alcoholism is simply to underscore that once a person has lost the capacity to control consistently how much and how often he or she drinks, continued use of alcohol can be both a necessary and a sufficient cause of a syndrome that produces millions of invalids and causes millions of deaths.

The second objection to the medical model of alcoholism is that only opinion separates the alcoholic from the heavy drinker. Supposedly one either has a disease or does not have it; diagnosis should depend on signs and symptoms, not value judgments. But consider the example of coronary heart disease. We regard it as a medical illness, although its causes are diverse and often poorly understood and there is no fixed point at which we can decide that coronary arteries become abnormal. So it is with alcoholism. Normal drinking merges imperceptibly with pathological drinking. Culture and idiosyncratic viewpoints will always determine where the line is drawn.

The third objection is that alcoholism is affected by so many situational and psychological factors that the drinking must often be viewed as reactive. Some people drink uncontrollably only after a serious loss or in certain specific situations, and some alcoholics return to normal drinking by an act of will. But these observations are equally true of hypertension, which often has an extremely important psychological component. Nevertheless, prospective studies show that alcohol dependence causes depression, anxiety, and poverty far more often than the other way around. In citing psychological problems as a cause of alcoholism, Fingarette reverses the position of cart and horse.

The fourth objection to calling alcoholism a disease is that it involves both labeling and a disparagement of free will. But in this case both labeling and the denial of free will are therapeutic. Some people believe that the label 'alcoholic' transforms a person into an outcast, akin to a leper. Well, should a doctor who knows that a person has leprosy keep the fact secret lest the patient be labeled a leper? Some people believe that if alcoholics are taught to regard alcoholism as a disease they will use this label as an excuse to drink or a reason why they should not be held responsible for their own recovery. It does not work out that way. Like people with high blood pressure, alcoholics who understand that they have a disease become more rather than less willing to take responsibility for self-care. That is why the self-help group, Alcoholics Anonymous, places such single-minded emphasis on the idea that alcoholism is a disease.

DIAGNOSIS HELPS

Once patients accept the diagnosis, they can be shown how to assume responsibility for their own care. Physicians stress the value of diagnosing hypertension early because it can provide a rational explanation for headaches and other symptoms that were hitherto regarded as neurotic or irrational. For years alcoholics themselves have labeled themselves 'wicked,' 'weak,' and 'reprehensible.' The offer of a medical explanation does not lead to irresponsibility, only to hope and improved morale.

The fifth argument against calling alcoholism a disease is the most compelling; it is said that uncontrolled maladaptive ingestion of alcohol is not a biological disorder but a disorder of behavior. Like compulsive fingernail biting, gambling, or child molesting, this form of deviant behavior can often be better classified by sociologists than by physiologists, and better treated by psychologists skilled in behavior therapy than by physicians with their medical armamentarium.

But unlike giving up gambling or fingernail biting, giving up alcohol abuse often requires skilled medical attention during acute withdrawal. Unlike gamblers and fingernail biters, most alcoholics develop secondary symptoms that do require medical care. Unlike child molesters, but like people with high blood pressure, alcoholics have a mortality rate two to four times as high as the average. In order to receive the medical treatment they require, alcoholics need a label that will allow them unprejudiced access to emergency rooms, detoxification clinics, and medical insurance.

The final argument for regarding alcoholism as a disease rather than a behavior disorder is that it often causes alcoholics to mistreat persons they love. Very few sustained human experiences involve as much abuse as the average close family member of an alcoholic must tolerate. Fingarette's "heavy drinking" model (which conveys a concept of misbehavior) only generates more denial in the already profoundly guilt-ridden alcoholic. Calling alcoholism a disease rather than a behavior disorder is a useful device both to persuade the alcoholic to acknowledge the problem and to provide a ticket for admission to the health care system. In short, in our attempts to understand and study alcoholism, we should employ the models of the social scientist and the learning theorist. But in order to treat alcoholics effectively we need to invoke the medical model.

Let me close with an anecdote. My research associate, reviewing the lives of 100 patients who had been hospitalized eight years previously for detoxification from alcohol, wrote to me that she mistrusted the diagnosis of alcoholism. To illustrate, she described one man who drank heavily for seven years after his initial detoxification. Although the alcohol clinic's staff agreed that his drinking was alcoholic, neither he nor his wife acknowledged that it was a problem. Finally he required a second detoxification, and the clinic staff claimed that they had been right.

"How can you call such behavior a disease," my associate wrote, "when you cannot decide if it represents a social problem [that is, requires a value judgment] or alcohol-dependent drinking?" Then she shifted her attention to the ninety-nine other tortured lives she had been reviewing. Oblivious of the contradiction, she concluded: "I don't think I ever fully realized before I did this follow-up what an absolutely devastating disease alcoholism is." I respectfully submit that if Professor Fingarette were to work in an alcohol clinic for two years, he would agree with the last half of my research associate's letter rather than the first half.

NO

Joann Ellison Rodgers

ADDICTION: A WHOLE NEW VIEW

Millions of Americans are apparently "hooked," not only on heroin, morphine, amphetamines, tranquilizers, and cocaine, but also nicotine, caffeine, sugar, steroids, work, theft, gambling, exercise, and even love and sex. The War on Drugs alone is older than the century. In the last four years, the United States spent $45 billion waging it, with no end in sight, despite every kind of addiction treatment from psychosurgery, psychoanalysis, psychedelics, and self-help to acupuncture, group confrontation, family therapy, hypnosis, meditation, education, and tough love.

There seems no end to our "dependencies," their bewildering intractability, the glib explanations for their causes and even more glib "solutions."

The news, however, is that brain, mind, and behavior specialists are rethinking the whole notion of addiction. With help from neuroscience, molecular biology, pharmacology, psychology, and genetics, they're challenging their own hard-core assumptions and popular "certainties" and finding surprisingly common characteristics among addictions.

They're using new imaging techniques to see how addiction looks and feels and where cravings "live" in the brain and mind. They're concluding that things are far from hopeless and they are rapidly replacing conjecture with facts.

For example, scientists have learned that every animal, from the ancient hagfish to reptiles, and rodents, and humans, share the same basic pleasure and "reward" circuits in the brain, circuits that all turn on when in contact with addictive substances or during pleasurable acts such as eating or orgasm. One conclusion from this evidence is that addictive behaviors are normal, a natural part of our "wiring." If they weren't, or if they were rare, nature would not have let the capacity to be addicted evolve, survive, and stick around in every living creature.

"Everyone engages in addictive behaviors to some extent because such things as eating, drinking, and sex are essential to survival and highly reinforcing," says G. Alan Marlatt, Ph.D., director of the Addictive Behaviors Research Center at the University of Washington. "We get immediate gratification from them and find them very hard to give up indeed. That's a pretty good definition of addiction."

"The inescapable fact is that nature gave us the ability to become hooked because the brain has clearly evolved a reward system, just as it has a pain system," says physiologist and pharmacologist Steven Childers, Ph.D., of Bowman Gray School of Medicine in North Carolina. "The fact that some things may accidentally or inadvertently trigger that system is somewhat beside the point.

"Our brains didn't develop opiate receptors to tempt us with heroin addiction. The coca plant didn't develop cocaine to produce what we call crack addicts. This plant doesn't care two hoots about our brain. But heroin and cocaine addiction certainly tell us a great deal about how brains work. And how they work is that if you taste or experience something that you like, that feels good, you're reinforced to do that again. Basic drives, for food, sex, and pleasure, activate reward centers in the brain. They're part of human nature."

NEW THINKING, OLD PROBLEM

What we now call "addictions," in this sense, Childers says, are cases of a good and useful phenomenon taken hostage, with terrible social and medical consequences. Moreover, that insight is leading to the identification of specific areas of the brain that link feelings and behavior to reward circuits. "In the case of addictive drugs, we know that areas of the brain involved in memory and learning and with the most ancient part of our brain, the emotional brain, are the most interesting. I'm very optimistic that

we will be able to develop new strategies for preventing and treating addictions."

The new concept of addiction is in sharp contrast to the conventional, frustrating, and some would say cynical view that everything causes addiction.

Ask 10 Americans what addiction is and what causes it and you might get at least 10 answers. Some will insist addiction is a failure of morality or a spiritual weakness, a sin and a crime by people who won't take responsibility for their behavior. If addicts want to self-destruct, let them. It's their fault; they choose to abuse.

For the teetotaler and politicians, it's a self-control problem; for sociologists, poverty; for educators, ignorance. Ask some psychiatrists or psychologists and you're told that personality traits, temperament, and "character" are at the root of addictive "personalities." Social-learning and cognitive-behavior theorists will tell you it's a case of conditioned response and intended or unintended reinforcement of inappropriate behaviors. The biologically oriented will say it's all in the genes and heredity; anthropologists that it's culturally determined. And Dan Quayle will blame it on the breakdown of family values.

The most popular "theory," however, is that addictive behaviors are diseases. In this view, an addict, like a cancer patient or a diabetic, either has it or does not have it. Popularized by Alcoholics Anonymous, the disease theory holds that addictions are irreversible, constitutional, and altogether abnormal and that the only appropriate treatment is total avoidance of the alcohol or other substance, lifelong abstinence, and constant vigilance.

ABSOLVING THE DISEASED

The problem with all of these theories and models is that they lead to control measures doomed to failure by mixing up the process of addiction with its impact. Worse, from the scientific standpoint, they don't hold up to the tests of observation, time, and consistent utility. They don't explain much and they don't account for a lot. For example:

• Not all drugs of abuse create dependence. LSD and other hallucinogens, caffeine, and tranquilizers are examples. Rats, for example, which can be easily addicted to heroin and cocaine just like humans, "just can't appreciate a psychedelic experience," notes Childers. "The same is true of marijuana and caffeine; it's hard to get animals to take them. People take these drugs for different reasons, not to feel pleasure."

At the same time, rats and other animals can become physically dependent on alcohol, but won't seek out alcohol even when they are in convulsions of withdrawal. Says Jack Henningfield, Ph.D., an addiction researcher at the National Institute of Drug Abuse [NIDA] in Baltimore, "we can get rats physically dependent on alcohol and even get them to go through DTs by withdrawing them. But we can't get them to crave alcohol naturally." Apparently, they have to learn, to be taught to want it. "Only when we give them the rat equivalent of smoke-filled rooms, soft jazz, and other rewards will they seek out alcohol."

• Some substances with clearly addictive properties are almost universally used and socially acceptable. Giving up coffee and colas containing caffeine can yield rapid heart beats, sweating, irritability, and headaches—markers of withdrawal.

• People can experience withdrawal syndromes with drugs that don't addict them or make them physically or psychologically dependent. Postsurgical morphine is always withdrawn gradually in the hospital, but most people who get morphine still undergo so-called white flu—flu-like symptoms after they leave the hospital. They are actually undergoing withdrawal symptoms, but they have not become dependent on or addicted to the morphine. There is also no evidence that terminal cancer patients in severe pain get "high" on heavy doses of morphine, although they do become dependent.

• Some drugs of abuse produce tolerance and some don't. Heroin addicts need more and more of it to avoid withdrawal symptoms. Cocaine produces no tolerance, yet most would say cocaine is far more addictive because craving accelerates to sometimes lethal doses. If permitted, lab rats will continue to take cocaine until they die.

• Some people, notably celebrities, check in regularly at the Betty Ford Center to overcome addiction to painkillers, alcohol, and barbiturates. Yet one of the most famous studies on Vietnam veterans shows that very few of those who returned addicted to heroin stayed addicted. Lots of planning went on for intensive treatment for them. But on follow-up back home, their rate of continuing addiction dropped to levels no different than those of the general population, despite their exposure to lots of drugs, stress, high-risk environments, youth, and other risk factors that predicted a serious addiction epidemic. They had no trouble for the most part leaving their addictions behind in the jungles, while in the U.S., relapses are legendary and widespread.

For decades, we've sent heroin addicts to Lexington, Kentucky, for treatment in an isolated treatment facility; the idea was to remove them for long periods from their conducive environments. Almost all got "clean" and stayed that way, but when released, still sought out their old haunts and relapsed. Yet the majority of people living in drug-infested cultures never get addicted.

• The children of alcoholics have a much higher risk of alcohol abuse than children of nonalcoholics. Some studies show that alcoholics have an enzyme abnormality related to alcohol activity that doesn't seem to exist in people who've never had a drink. Yet some people who are classic alcoholics can and do learn to drink moderately and safely. Others quit even when they know they can drink moderately.

DEBUNKING THE DOMINO THEORY

"I began to understand the bankruptcy of many addiction theories when a lot of my predictions about alcoholism and treatment for it were dead wrong," says William R. Miller, Ph.D. A professor of psychology and psychiatry and director of the Center on Alcoholism, Substance Abuse, and Addictions at the University of New Mexico, his controversial studies of "controlled drinking" in the early 1970s were among the first to clash with the "disease" theory of addictions.

"I developed a reasonably successful program that taught alcoholics how to drink moderately. Lots of them eventually totally quit and became abstainers. I would never have predicted that. The prevalent theories were that they would either eventually relapse and lose control of their drinking or that they would

quit because moderation did not work. We knew from blood and urine tests that they were able to moderate but quit anyhow. The old domino theory that one drink equals a drunk proved, for some, to be baloney. We know with cigarette smoking and alcohol and other addictive behaviors that moderation, tapering, and 'warm turkey' can be very effective." Miller blames mostly the persistent strength of the addiction-as-disease concept on the peculiarly American experience with alcohol and Prohibition.

"During Prohibition, alcohol was marked as completely dangerous and the message was that no one could use it safely. At the end of Prohibition, we had a problem: a cognitive dissonance. Clearly many people could use it safely, so we needed a new model to make drinking permissible again. That led to the idea that only 'some' people can't handle it, those who have a disease called alcoholism."

Everyone likes this model, Miller says. People with alcohol problems like it because they get special status as victims of a disease and get treatment. Nonalcoholics like it because they can tell themselves they don't need to worry if they don't have the "disease." The treatment industry loves it because there's money to be made, and the liquor industry loves it because under this theory, it's not alcohol that's the problem but the alcoholic.

"What's really bizarre," says Miller, "is that the alcohol beverage industry spends a lot of money to help teach us about the disease model. It's the inverse of the temperance movement, which many now laugh at, but which saw alcohol more realistically as a dangerous drug. It is."

Today, Miller notes, heroin and cocaine are looked upon the way the temperance movement once looked on alcohol. "Ironically, too," he says, "we are treating nicotine and gluttony the way we once treated alcohol. It's easy to see how the disease model and all other single-cause theories of addiction can lead to blind alleys and bad treatments in which therapists adopt every fad and reach into a bulging bag of tricks for whatever is in hand or intuitively meets the immediate moment. But what we wind up with are three myths about alcoholism and other addictions: that nothing works, that one particular approach is superior to all others, and that everything works about equally well. That's nonsense."

NO EASY TARGETS

The most likely truth about addiction is that it's not a single, basic mechanism, but several problems we label 'addiction,'" says Michael F. Cataldo, Ph.D., chief of behavioral psychology at Johns Hopkins Medical Institutes. "No one thing explains addiction," echoes Miller. "There are things about individuals, about the environment in which they live, and about the substances involved that must be factored in." Experts today prefer the term "addictive behaviors," rather than addiction, to underscore their belief that while everyone has the capacity for addiction, it's what people do that should drive treatment.

So while all addictions display common properties, the proportions of those factors vary widely. And certainly not all addictions have the same effect on the quality of our lives or capacity to be dangerous. Everyday bad habits, compulsions, dependencies, and cravings clearly have something in common with heroin and cocaine addiction, in terms of their mechanisms and triggers. But what about people who are Type A personalities; who eat chocolate every day; who, like Microsoft's Bill Gates, focus almost pathologically on work; who feel compelled to expose themselves in public, seek thrills like race-car driving and fire fighting, or obsess constantly over hand washing, hair twirling, or playing video games. They have—from the standpoint of what their behavior actually means to themselves and others—very little in common with heroin and crack addicts.

Or consider two of the more fascinating candidates for addiction—sex and love. Anthropologist Helen Fisher, Ph.D., of the American Museum of Natural History, suggests that the initial rush of arousal and romantic, erotic love, the "chemistry" that hooks a couple to each other, produces effects in the brain parallel to what happens when a brain is exposed to morphine or amphetamines.

In the case of love, the reactions involve chemicals such as endorphins, the brain's own opiates, and oxytocin and vasopressin, naturally occurring hormones linked to male and female bonding. After a while, though, this effect diminishes as the brain's receptor sites for these chemicals become overloaded and thus desensitized. Tolerance occurs; attachment wanes and sets up the mind for separation, so that the "addicted" man or woman is ready to pursue the high elsewhere. In this scenario, divorce or adultery becomes the equivalent of drug-seeking behavior, addicts craving for the high. According to Fisher, the fact that most people stay married is "a triumph of culture over nature," much the way, perhaps, nonaddiction is.

Experts generally agree on the most common characteristics of addictions that trouble society:

- The substance or activity that triggers them must initially cause feelings of pleasure and changes in emotion or mood.
- The body develops a physical tolerance to the substance or activity so that addicts must take ever-larger amounts to get the same effects.
- Removal of the drug or activity causes painful withdrawal symptoms.
- Quite apart from physical tolerance, addiction involves physical and psychological dependence associated with craving that is independent of the need to avoid the pain of withdrawal.
- Addiction always causes changes in the brain and mind. These include physiological changes, chemical changes, anatomical changes, and behavioral changes.
- Addiction requires a prior experience with a substance or behavior. The first contact with the substance or activity is an initiation that may or may not lead to addiction, but must occur in order to set in motion the effects in the brain that are likely to encourage a person to try that experience again.
- Addictions cause repeated behavioral problems, take a lot of a person's time and energy, are openly sanctioned by the community, and are marked by a gradual obsession with the drug or behavior.
- Addictions develop their own motivations. For addicts, their tolerance and dependence in and of themselves become reinforcing and rewarding, independent of their actual use of the drug or the "high" they may get. "One way of understanding this," says Cataldo, "is to analyze what is happening behaviorally in withdrawal. Given that withdrawal is so punishing, why do addicts let themselves go through it

more than once? One answer is that the withdrawal, when combined with relapse and returning to the use of the substance, itself may be 'rewarding.'"

HAIR OF THE DOG

The withdrawal and relapse cycle suggests that like any behavior, the addict "gets something out of" the pain of withdrawal—attention, perhaps, or help. But in any case, enough so that he not only is willing to do it again, but also may seek out the cycle the way he once sought out the drug.

In gambling addictions and certain eating disorders, particularly, says Toni Farrenkopf, Ph.D., a Seattle psychologist, the "rush" for the addict often comes from pursuit of the activity after "getting clean and clear" for a while, along with eluding police, spouses, parents, bill collectors, and employers.

"We know this is the case with animals we can train to do something, even if they never get a positive reward out of it," Cataldo says. The "reward" is escape from or absence of an electric shock or punishment, even if it's only occasional escape or unpredictable escape. The cocaine addict may be addicted to the pursuit of cocaine and stealing to get money to buy the drug; using coke may be secondary to the reward of not getting caught and the "high" of pursuing the drug life-style.

If addictions have characteristics in common, so do addicts, the experts say.

They have particular vulnerabilities or susceptibilities, opportunity to have contact with the substance or activity that will addict them, and a risk of relapse no matter how successfully they are treated. They tend to be risk takers and thrill seekers and expect to have a positive reaction to their substance of abuse before they use it.

Addicts have distinct preferences for one substance over another and for how they use the substance of abuse. They have problems with self-regulation and impulse control, tend to use drugs as a substitute for coping strategies in dealing with both stress and their everyday lives in general, and don't seek "escape" so much as a way to manage their lives. Finally, addicts tend to have higher-than-normal capacity for such drugs. Alcoholics, for example, often can drink friends "under the table" and appear somewhat normal, even drive (not safely) on doses of alcohol that would put most people to sleep or kill them.

The biological, psychological, and social processes by which addictions occur also have common pathways, but with complicated loops and detours. All addictions appear now to have roots in genetic susceptibilities and biological traits. But like all human and animal behaviors, including eating, sleeping, and learning, addictive behavior takes a lot of handling. The end product is a bit like Mozart's talent: If he'd never come in contact with a piano or with music, it's unlikely he would have expressed his musical gifts.

Floyd E. Bloom, M.D., chairman of neuropharmacology at the Scripps Clinical and Research Foundation in La Jolla, California, once gave a talk called "The Bane of Pain Is Mainly in the Brain." His point was that both pain and pain relief occur in the brain, triggered by the release, control, uptake, and quantity of assorted brain chemicals and other natural substances. The same might be said for addiction. Regardless of the source of addiction, the effects are "mainly in the brain," physically, chemically, and psychologically affecting emotions and energy levels.

The new view of addiction ties together biology, chemistry, behavior, and emotions in the brain. Among others, Edythe London, Ph.D., chief of neuroimaging and the drug-action section of NIDA, has conducted experiments demonstrating that such links are in fact formed and offering some clues as to how that happens.

In her work, the first of its kind funded by the Office of National Drug Control Policy, she is using positron emission tomographic (PET) scans to figure out how drugs and behaviors produce the rewards that create addicts and keep them addicted even when the euphoria ends, the tolerance builds, and the withdrawals occur. She is homing in on areas of the brain where craving lives both neurochemically and psychologically.

PET scans measure the brain's uptake of glucose, the principal source of energy used by the brain to function, and locate areas of the brain affected by various experiences. By tagging glucose molecules with radioactive and other "tracers," scientists like London can watch the brain react to stimuli such as drugs, noise, stress, and work.

In early studies, she and her colleagues gave addictive drugs under carefully controlled conditions to addicts and gauged their mood and feelings while monitoring the rate of glucose use. "The surprising thing we found is that *all* drugs of abuse—even those that differ radically in structure such as morphine and cocaine—do the same thing. They reduce use of glucose in the brain, so providing a way to observe which areas of the brain are involved in specific psychological effects. The amount of glucose used in certain parts of the brain's cortex, moreover, was closely related to how good people felt, regardless of where any drug binds.

London says this common pathway of reduced brain metabolism should not really have surprised her. "If you think about it, it makes sense," she says, "because glucose is an index of brain activity and brain activity in any given area is a function of not only what drugs are binding right there, but of nerve connections feeding into that area. The final picture of drug action usually looks quite different than the pattern of where a drug binds. That's because the brain is a highly interconnected organ. Clearly, if a drug acts on dopamine-neurotransmitter systems in part of the limbic brain initially, it's easy to see that there would be wider distribution through the brain's networks and that the impact of the drug could be very diffuse and varied."

So far, London and others have seen this reduction in glucose use with morphine, cocaine, nicotine, buprenorphine (a treatment for opiate addicts), amphetamine, benzodiazepine, barbiturates, and alcohol. "All drugs of abuse do this."

From these studies, London moved on to experiments designed to show that an addict's brain is permanently different from what it was before and after the initial exposure. "I wanted to know where craving lived in the brain," she says.

Her first idea was wrong. "I thought that drug addicts had the same kind of situation as people with obsessive-compulsive disorder (OCD) in terms of where the brain was affected," she says, "because all OCD victims, like drug abusers, had a lack of impulse control. Studies had shown that they had disorders of the orbital frontal cortex, the part of the brain near the temple, and that's where I went looking."

She conducted experiments in which she gave a lot of drug-related cues—but not drugs—to cocaine addicts. These cues included videotapes showing crack houses, mounds of white powder, $10 bills, and people "high." "We thought that would make them crave the drug and we'd be able to see glucose use diminish in the orbital frontal cortex."

The bad news was that the orbital frontal cortex showed nothing. The good news was that they got a "pretty dramatic effect" in two other areas of the brain, the amygdala and the hippocampus.

The hippocampus is a bundle of fibers linked to learning and short-term memory and carries signals in and around the limbic system, forming electrochemical junctions for the emotional seat of the brain. The amygdala, located in the lower arc of the limbic system, is the seat of "fight or flight" reactions, and impairment or injury can lead to profound behavior changes. There is also evidence that the amygdala has a role in recalling pleasant or painful consequences of experiences and damage to this may flatten or remove some of this recall.

London hasn't entirely abandoned her notion that the orbital frontal cortex also is involved in addicts' recall of their drug experience and the onset of craving. Recent research suggests this part of the brain may be the anatomical location of "source memory," the place that helps people remember when and where and how a memory was formed, or whether it is a "real" memory at all.

London says she is convinced that addiction takes place in stages and requires not only initiation to a substance or to an activity that brings great pleasure, physiologically and/or psychologically, but also creation of nondrug "incentives" to keep using the drug and craving it. The incentives include the creation of memories—via the creation of neural pathways—of the pleasure and good mood and the excitement of getting the drug, preparing it, or sharing it with others.

"What we're talking about is like conditioning," says London. "Over time, events that happen concurrently with the euphoria begin to contribute to the drug experience and are involved in a sensitization process. They too probably produce a biochemical effect in the brain and become very important in the addiction process."

* * *

If that happens, it goes a long way to explaining why relapse rates are so high, even for addicts who are "detoxified" and off drugs for long periods. Even when people clean up their act and stay clean for some time, they are still very vulnerable and this may have something to do not only with receptor sites and neurotransmitters, but also with biochemical processes that produce long-term, stored memories of the drug experience. Says London: "In my view, biochemical and psychological memories act in the same way. What we're talking about is learning at the molecular level—and the reason that addicts, long after they are free of a drug, can experience intense craving when presented with stimuli—even photographs or sounds—that remind them of the drug experience."

If there is a hitch in this new picture of addiction it is that it is far from simple. It is also politically incorrect, unlikely to make the "Just Say No" and "law and order" crowd very happy. But it is putting solid foundations under prevention and treatment programs and promising entirely new strategies to combat drug abuse. The implications of this new view of addiction are in fact profound for treatment, prevention, and public policy.

L. H. R. Drew, an Australian addiction expert, notes that "if the idea prevails that drug use—and more particularly drug addiction—is a special type of behavior which is highly contagious, irreversible, inevitably leads to disease, and is due to the special seductive properties of certain drugs, then our approach to reducing drug problems is not going to change. If, however, the ideas prevail that drug use is more similar than different to other behaviors and that there is little that is special about drug addiction compared with other addictions that are universally experienced, then the drug hysteria may abate and a rational approach to policies to reduce drug problems may be possible. It must be known that people get into trouble with drugs in the same way that they do with many other things... particularly behaviors giving short-term rewards."

In the new view of addiction, says Childers, people vary in their ability to manage problems and pleasures, "but we must recognize that we all share the same circuits of pleasure, rewards, and pain. Anyone who takes cocaine will enjoy it; anyone who has sex will enjoy it. There is nothing abnormal about getting high on cocaine. Everyone will. There is a natural basis of addiction and we need to get away from the concept that only bad or weak or diseased people have problems with addiction. Telling someone to 'just say no' is like telling someone to just say no to eating and drinking and sex. We must begin to see how very human and very hard this is. But it is far from hopeless."

POSTSCRIPT

Should Addiction to Drugs and Alcohol Be Considered a Disease Rather Than a Behavioral Problem?

One of the most valuable aspects of the disease model is that it removes alcohol and drugs from the moral realm. It proposes that addiction sufferers should be treated and helped, rather than scorned and punished. Though the moral model of addiction has by no means disappeared in the United States, today more resources are directed toward rehabilitation than punishment. Increasingly, it is being recognized and understood that fines and imprisonment do little to curb alcohol and drug abuse in society.

Another strength of the disease model is its simplicity. It is straightforward and relatively easy to teach to recovering addicts. They, in turn, are often comfortable with the concept that what they have is a disease, rather than moral degeneration. And finally, the disease model provides the substance abuser with a mechanism for coping with any shame or guilt resulting from past misdeeds. The disease model teaches that problem behaviors are *symptoms*, not causes, of the disease process and that the user is not to blame. Further readings supporting the disease model include *Twelve Steps and Twelve Traditions* (Alcoholics Anonymous World Services, 1981); *Alcoholism: The Genetic Inheritance* by Kathleen W. FitzGerald (Doubleday, 1988); and "Alcoholics Anonymous and Behavior Therapy: Can Habits Be Treated as Diseases?" *Journal of Consulting and Clinical Psychology* (December 1994).

The role of genetics in alcoholism is discussed in "Prisoners of Pleasure?" *New Scientist* (October 1, 1994); "Why Some Children of Alcoholics Become Alcoholics Themselves," *Adolescence* (Spring 1994); and "Alcoholism and Your Genes," *Edell Health Letter* (September 1993).

Critics argue that the disease model either underemphasizes or ignores the impact of environmental forces, learned behaviors, and many other factors of alcohol and drug abuse. Furthermore, most treatment programs in the United States are based on the disease model, and most are considered to be generally ineffective when judged by their high relapse rates. A detailed, critical evaluation of the disease model can be found in Herbert Fingarette's *Heavy Drinking: The Myth of Alcoholism as a Disease* (University of California Press, 1988). In "The Disease Concept of Alcoholism: Its Impact on Women's Treatment," *Journal of Substance Abuse and Treatment* (March 1994), the negative outcome of using the disease model with women alcoholics is discussed. According to the authors, this model validates feelings of powerlessness and helplessness of women in dependent and subordinate roles.

ISSUE 10

Should Drugs Be Legalized?

YES: Joseph P. Kane, from "The Challenge of Legalizing Drugs," *America* (August 8, 1992)

NO: Gerald W. Lynch and Roberta Blotner, from "Legalizing Drugs Is Not the Solution," *America* (February 13, 1993)

ISSUE SUMMARY

YES: Theologian Joseph P. Kane asserts that legalizing drugs will help prevent crime and violence associated with the illegality of these substances.

NO: Gerald W. Lynch, president of the John Jay College of Criminal Justice, and Roberta Blotner, director of the City University of New York's substance abuse prevention programs, claim that legalizing drugs would actually increase violent crime as well as drug usage and addiction.

At one time there were no laws regulating the use or sale of drugs and alcohol. Rather than legislation, their use was regulated by religious teaching and social custom. As society grew more complex and more heterogenous, the need for more formal regulation of drug sales, production, and use developed.

Attempts at regulating patent medications through legislation began in the early 1900s. In 1920 Congress, under pressure from temperance organizations, passed the Eighteenth Amendment prohibiting the manufacture and sale of all alcoholic beverages. From 1920 until 1933, the demand for alcohol was met by members of organized crime, who either manufactured it illicitly or smuggled it into the United States. The government's inability to enforce the law and increasing violence finally led to the repeal of Prohibition in 1933.

Many years later, in the 1960s, drug usage again began to worry many Americans. Heroin abuse had become epidemic in urban areas, and many middle-class young adults began to experiment with marijuana and LSD by the end of the decade. Cocaine also became popular—first among the middle class; later among inner-city residents. Today, crack houses, babies born with drug addictions, and drug-related crimes and shootings are the images of a new epidemic of drug abuse.

This new epidemic encouraged President Ronald Reagan to begin a drug education program in the 1980s, characterized by a "Just Say No" campaign. In 1989 President George Bush declared a "war on drugs" and appointed former education secretary William J. Bennett—who resigned a year later—to the post of "drug czar." Although Bennett declared a victory, drug usage continues to be of concern to most Americans. In a 1989 poll, a majority of Americans cited drugs as the nation's greatest threat.

The way to end these drug-related problems, some experts maintain, is to follow the example of the repeal of Prohibition—legalize drugs. Proponents of legalization believe that if laws prohibiting the sale, manufacture, and use of drugs were repealed, there would be a significant reduction in the enormous profits earned by major drug suppliers. This, in turn, would reduce the violent crimes related to drug dealing.

Opponents of drug legalization believe that repealing drug laws is not the answer to crime and other drug-related problems. Drug usage would probably rise, as did the use of alcohol following the repeal of Prohibition; alcohol consumption rose 350 percent after 1933. With more users, there would doubtlessly be an increase in crime, drug-addicted babies, and other social ills.

In the following selections, Joseph P. Kane maintains that illegal drugs net astronomical profits for which people are willing to kill. Reasonable prices for drugs controlled by the government, he believes, would eliminate the associated crimes. Kane further argues that if drugs were legalized, then addicts would not be treated as criminals but as ill people in need of help. Gerald W. Lynch and Roberta Blotner argue that legalizing drugs would not only increase their usage but also increase violent crime.

YES

Joseph P. Kane

THE CHALLENGE OF LEGALIZING DRUGS

Why are many responsible people proposing that the manufacture and distribution of drugs should be legally regulated just as alcohol is? Has legalization effectively controlled alcohol use? Alcohol consumption, we know, actually increased with the repeal of Prohibition. Given the devastating harm that addictive drugs cause, and the heartache, broken homes and carnage on U.S. highways caused by alcohol, why would intelligent and well-intentioned people like Milton Friedman and many other conservatives want to legalize drugs? In this article, I want to examine attitudes toward drug users, evaluate some positive and harmful effects of present drug policies and discuss what America needs to deal effectively with drugs. Finally, I will argue, legalizing drugs is only part of the solution.

HOW PROHIBITION FOSTERS CRIME AND ABUSE

How does legalization affect drug users and addicts? America's history with addictive drugs suggests that policy for drug users is more effectively developed by a Surgeon General than by an Attorney General. During Prohibition, society often abused moonshiners and drunks. When a drunkard violated the law, we often saw only a criminal and forgot the person. Prohibition surely did not create the proper attitudes within America to treat alcoholism effectively. Today, however, precisely because alcohol consumption is legal, alcoholics can be treated compassionately as sick people. The same result would obtain, I suggest, if we legalized addictive drugs.

Even if legalization could increase opportunities for compassionate treatment toward users/abusers, would not legalizing drugs increase crime? I doubt it. In fact, present drug policies actually foster crime in four ways.

First, because the price of illegal drugs is very high, poor addicts rob and burglarize. Wealthy users/abusers can afford not to steal. As a prison chaplain, I do not see addicted movie stars, sports figures or Wall Street brokers, because their money buys expensive drugs without the need to steal and obtains drug therapy without months of waiting. Pricing drugs reasonably by legalization would virtually eliminate the crimes that terrify us. How many Americans rob or kill, I ask you, for a six-pack of beer?

Second, illegal drugs net astronomical profits for which people are willing to kill. Drug-related homicide rates are soaring, and innocent bystanders are caught in the cross fire. The same thing happened during the Prohibition era. "The Untouchables" and similar film portrayals of the roaring 20's depict the ruthless violence among alcohol pushers that afflicted mainstream society. Today's slaughter mirrors those Prohibition homicide rates, which dropped immediately upon repeal. Homicides did not rise to the same rates until 1979. Such figures invite reflection on lessons painfully learned during Prohibition.

Third, present drug policies foster crime by overwhelming our criminal justice system with drug arrests. Police resources, courts and prisons are mired in drug arrests and consequently unable to deal effectively with other serious threats to our safety.

Fourth, by subjecting addicts to imprisonment instead of offering therapy, we further debase and alienate them. Such treatment confirms their belief that they are bad people and makes awareness of their sickness and possible treatment less probable. Ex-convicts return to our streets as angry and desperate addicts more likely to rob for a fix.

ABUSING THE POOR

Besides fostering crime, present drug policies abuse our society in many ways. Illegal drugs foster irresponsible attitudes about work. On my block, for example, kids who work in supermarkets or McDonald's are considered "chumps."

Who would work for $120 a week when they can earn $300 *per evening?* This fast money buys fancy clothing and may even earn respect at home for young dealers paying their families' bills. A local Boy Scout leader surprised me by insisting that drug legalization is the only way to save his friends from the lucrative and dangerous drug world. These illegal dealers are not evil. They say, "Good evening, Father," and I respond warmly with the same respect that I give to bartenders.

Our war on drugs, furthermore, teaches that some people are "better dead than drugged." Heroin users/abusers are dying from AIDS, and still we refuse to legalize the dispensation of clean syringe needles to them. In effect, our drug policies deliberately endanger any person who wants to use a drug that may be lethal, just as "hooch" and "moonshine" endangered another generation—because these drugs are produced by outlaws.

Then, by not providing adequate detoxification and therapy programs, we systematically abuse addicted people who want to stop their drug use. New York City incarcerates one drug user/abuser at a cost of more than $150 per day—whereas therapy programs that actually deal with the problem of addiction cost half that. Drug-war money hires police, Federal agents, judges, court personnel, prison contractors, correctional officers and parole officers—and for all practical purposes ignores the needs of people who use/abuse drugs. Addicts without money face at least a four-month waiting period for therapy. Without access to drug programs upon request, they cannot break the bonds of addiction.

Indeed, the so-called drug war grievously abuses minorities with grossly higher rates of incarceration. New York City, for example, warehouses about 20,000 prisoners on any given day; over 14,000 are incarcerated for drug-related crimes. They are the city's poor and over 90 percent are young blacks and Hispanics. Percentages vary throughout the country, but statistics clearly indicate that America disproportionately imprisons minorities with the highest incarceration rate in the world. Illegal drugs are sold to these prisoners even in maximum security prisons—with much higher profits for illegal distributors. What does this say about stopping drugs at our borders?

In addition, America's drug war abuses poor people in other countries. Can we honestly expect Peruvians to grow their nation's food when coca increases their earnings astronomically? All the violence over drug turf that we experience in the United States has become a tragic reality in some very poor areas of South America. Our Government's use of military operations against the coca industry exposes nothing so much as the futility of drug policies that must battle uphill against the power of sheer economics. Worse yet, desperately poor foreigners become "mules." They swallow balloon bags of cocaine or conceal drug packages in terrifying attempts to pass through U.S. Customs and earn $3,000. After they are arrested, our justice system destroys them. "Three years to life" is the usual minimum sentence that I hear; often they receive eight years to life. Unfortunately, selling lucrative illegal drugs is also a sore temptation for many poor Americans when their legal income is inadequate for basic needs.

CHANGING ATTITUDES

Merely legalizing dangerous drugs, of course, does not solve drug problems. Our attitudes toward even legal drugs must change. As educated, middle-class Americans cut down on drinking and stop smoking cigarettes, tobacco and liquor companies focus their advertising upon third-world people within and outside the United States. This was recently dramatized by a clergyman in Harlem. He and some parishioners whitewashed billboards advertising alcohol and cigarettes. The pastor's message was clear: "Don't seduce my people with death-dealing drugs." In effect, they were protesting against America's tendency to lose interest in issues that do not affect mainstream people—and our lack of commitment to those who are least able to protect themselves from exploitative advertising.

In order to deal effectively with additive drugs, our perceptions need to include the broader and disturbing reality of America's use and abuse of medicinal drugs. Many average Americans use such drugs irresponsibly. Bathroom medicine chests of the 1930's contained aspirin, band-aids, cotton, mercurochrome, peroxide; open a medicine chest today and you discover a whole pharmacy. Indigestion must be relieved so that we can return immediately to eating irresponsibly. Bloodshot eyes, nasal congestion, insomnia, heartburn or headaches—all require drugs. Unfortunately, we and our doctors often turn to drugs before determining whether a change of behavior might be more appropriate. This "quick-fix" mentality, I say, provides the context for America's abuse of more menacing drugs.

There has always been, is now and will always be abuse/addition. Some who seek escape from too much pressure or too little meaning in their lives will become alcoholics, addicted gamblers or "crack heads." But the normal way to limit the damage is to ban 100 percent alcohol, to crack down on loan sharks and to legalize lotteries—and we could do the same with cocaine. Unless we see drug users/abusers in this context, we will remain unable to respond to them humanely and effectively. The law is misused if it aspires to make saints.

In addition, we need to realize, first, that seductive advertising for alcohol and nicotine, although legal, is immoral and should become a serious issue for everyone. Given America's present concern for the danger of cocaine, heroin and marijuana, we have a unique opportunity to restrict all dishonest advertising that irresponsibly tempts people to use any addictive substances. We can enact regulations that foster responsible advertising and distribution of tobacco or alcohol. Such controls will be appropriate, as well, for advertising and distributing other dangerous drugs that Americans seek for a buzz even at the risk of addiction.

Second, Americans need to learn more about the sickness called addition. Drug-rehabilitation centers show us proven methods for treating drug addicts and helping their families. The highly effective 12-step programs for various addictions are based on spiritual healing, which is diametrically opposed to our present drug laws based on *coercion and violence that can never heal.*

Despite the adamant rejection of legalization by many ex-addicts and drug-program personnel, we need to face the fact that today's drug policies incarcerate and debase people just for using drugs, whereas addicts need drug programs. Is there not something dishonest about drug policies in which lower-class drug users, labeled criminals, go to prison while middle-class addicts, labeled alcoholics, go to therapy?

EFFECTIVE POLICY

The legalization of hard drugs does not mean that we don't need law enforcement to help protect us from dangerous drug users. Everyone who wants to operate cars, trains and buses should be monitored for alcohol or other drug consumption that would impede his or her performance. We also require protection from abusive drug and alcohol users who constitute a menace to other citizens. But why arrest people just for using addictive drugs?

What we need instead are "statutory abuse" laws similar to statutory rape laws that protect minors. Anyone arrested for selling drugs to a minor would have no excuse based on ignorance of the purchaser's age. Seller beware!

We also need to empower young people to deal responsibly with seductive invitations to drug use. Adults can help to protect children by showing them the fantasy and intent of captivating commercials. Responsible concern for honest advertising entails more than minuscule skull-and-bones warnings on cigarette packs. Laws do not remove our obligation to educate others about the danger surrounding us—and laws that lull America into complacency are no substitute for that education.

Mothers Against Drunk Drivers (MADD) provides a good model. Instead of lobbying to restore Prohibition, this group educates us about the danger of mixing alcohol and driving. The mothers lobby for the enforcement of strict laws against driving while under the influence of a drug, and thus they show us that education and intelligent law enforcement—not prohibition—are the effective approaches to addictive and potentially dangerous drugs.

Education about drugs is essential; otherwise, drugs—legal or not—will remain a grave problem. The elementary and middle schools in the town of Islip, N. Y., recently published a booklet of students' articles and drawings to educate youngsters about the dangers of drugs. The approach showed concern for alcohol and tobacco use and abuse. There was no mention of jails. Powerful drugs were treated as substances dangerous to one's health and well-being. The message was positive: We are concerned for you. Love yourself and treat yourself well. This should be America's attitude to *all drug users*.

LEGALIZATION: PART OF A FIRST STEP

Legalizing addictive drugs would probably increase their use. At least we know that the repeal of alcohol prohibition had that effect. So, how can we responsibly legalize them? For the same reasons that we keep alcohol legal! Just as we do not choose to return to Prohibition because we do not want gang wars, a growing disrespect for law, astronomical illegal profits, corrupted law enforcement personnel or the sickness and even deaths from impure substances, so we do not want our loved ones—whether addicts or social users who want a buzz from a drug or a drink—to become involved with outlaws.

A responsible approach to addictive drugs requires control of production with safe dosages, accountable advertising and restricted distribution through state-managed "drug stores." Distribution centers should offer drug education, counseling and treatment referrals to adequately funded programs. This responsible tone is absent in today's liquor stores, off-track betting parlors and gambling casinos. Offering these addictive drugs and activities in a responsible manner might show the way for using them in a saner manner. Our present policies are unable to fulfill these requirements.

What could we expect from a new drug policy that promoted respect, education and therapy? Drug dealers would be licensed and supervised in a market controlled by laws—not, as now, by outlaws. Eliminating inflated prices would reduce the crimes perpetrated by people desperate for a fix. Law enforcement personnel would be freed to protect us from crime. The release of Drug War prisoners convicted of drug use, possession and sales would save vast sums of money. Taxes on all legalized drugs should fund the education and treatment programs that a responsible society would create as a sane response to addictive drugs.

Changing present drug laws makes sense. Americans wisely rejected the prohibition of alcohol and we are not considering it for tobacco because we realize the waste of money involved. Instead of prisons for people who use or abuse drugs, the United States needs legal control, education and therapy programs.

NO

Gerald W. Lynch and
Roberta Blotner

LEGALIZING DRUGS IS
NOT THE SOLUTION

In "The Challenge of Legalizing Drugs" (*America*, Aug. 8, 1992), Joseph P. Kane, S. J., presents a compelling description of the devastation wreaked on our society by drug abuse, but draws some troubling conclusions supporting the legalization of drugs. Father Kane argues that illegal drugs promote the proliferation of crime because of the huge profits associated with their import and sales. Violence and murder have increased dramatically as dealers and gangs compete for turf and drug profits. Youngsters are attracted to selling drugs in order to earn more money than they could ever hope to earn in legitimate jobs. Addicts steal to pay for their drugs. The criminal justice system is overwhelmed by the increasing number of drug arrests.

He further argues that because drugs are illegal, addicts are treated as criminals rather than as sick people in need of help. Addicts are often arrested and processed through the criminal justice system rather than offered legitimate rehabilitation or treatment. Finally, he states that illegal drugs exploit the poor, whose struggle to survive makes drug dealing a sometimes necessary alternative.

The solution to the problem, he concludes, is to legalize drugs while at the same time 1) changing attitudes within our society about drugs; 2) changing laws and public policy; 3) and providing drug education and treatment to all those who want it. While Father Kane's description of the toll drugs are taking on our society and our citizens is poignant, the solution to this problem is not legalization.

Legalizing drugs will almost certainly increase their use. This has been well documented in a number of studies. J. F. Mosher points out that alcohol usage and rates of liver disease declined significantly during Prohibition ("Drug Availability in a Public Health Perspective" in *Youth and Drugs: Society's Mixed Messages* [1990]). Moreover, following repeal of the 18th Amendment, the number of drinkers in the United States increased by 60 percent.

The most widely abused drugs in our society are tobacco, alcohol and prescription drugs—the legal drugs and those which are most widely available.

A recent report issued by the Federal Government states that approximately 57 million people in this country are addicted to cigarettes, 18 million are addicted to alcohol and 10 million are abusing psychotherapeutic drugs. By comparison, crack, heroin and hallucinogens each accounts for one million addicts. Further, the report states that every day in this country 1,000 people die of smoking-related illnesses, 550 die of alcohol-related accidents and diseases, while 20 die of drug overdoses and drug-related homicides. In addition, the annual costs of health care and lost productivity to employers are estimated at $600 billion for alcoholism and $60 billion for tobacco-related ailments. For all illegal drugs, however, the comparable cost is an estimated $40 billion (see "Making America Drug Free: A New Vision of What Works," *Carnegie Quarterly* [Summer 1992]). These data clearly demonstrate that the drugs which are most available are the most abused, the most dangerous and the most costly.

* * *

As the number of people using drugs increases, babies born to addicted mothers will increase as well. According to a report issued by the New York City Public Schools in 1991, during the preceding 10 years babies born to substance-abusing mothers increased 3,000 percent. It is estimated that each year approximately 10,000 babies are born exposed to drugs. With greater availability of drugs, it is inevitable that more babies will be born to substance-abusing mothers. According to guidelines offered by the Children Prenatally Exposed to Drugs Program of the Los Angeles Unified School District, the following are among the characteristics of the child prenatally exposed to drugs: neurological problems, affective disorders, poor concentration, delayed language development, impaired social skills, difficulty in play. The extent to which children of addicted fathers may be impaired is not yet known. Legalizing drugs will surely compound the tragedy to our society of these most innocent victims.

* * *

Drug legalization would not eliminate crime. Although crimes associated with obtaining drugs might decrease with legalization, other crimes, especially violent crimes, would increase. As many as 80 percent of violent crimes involve alcohol and drugs. A number of studies have demonstrated the relationship between drugs and homicides, automobile deaths, child abuse and sexual abuse. It is estimated that drugs and alcohol are involved in 50 percent to 75 percent of cases of suicidal behavior. According to recent pharmacological research, certain drugs, especially cocaine, have the tendency to elicit violent behavior because of changes that take place in the neurotransmitter systems of the brain.

Many experts think that unless there were free access to unlimited quantities of drugs, there would be a black market even after legalization. Drugs, even if legal, would still cost money. Since many addicts cannot maintain jobs, they would continue to engage in stealing and prostitution to pay for drugs and would continue to subject their families and friends to abuse.

Experiments with the decriminalization of drugs have failed. A case in point is Zurich, Switzerland. There the city set aside a park, the Platzpitz, in which drugs were decriminalized and were available with no legal consequences. Health care was made accessible and clean syringes were supplied. It was hoped that there would be a reduction in crime, better health care for addicts and containment of the problem to a defined area of the city. The experiment failed dramatically.

As reported in *The New York Times* on Feb. 11, 1992, and London's *Financial Times* on Jan. 4, 1992, Zurich's drug-related crime and violence actually increased. Drug users and dealers converged on the Swiss city from other countries throughout Europe. The health-care system was overwhelmed as drug users had to be resuscitated. As drug dealers began to compete for business, the cost of drugs decreased. One addict was quoted as saying, "Too many kids were getting hooked too easily." The Platzpitz, a garden spot in the center of Zurich, was devastated. Statues were marred with graffiti. The ground was littered with used syringes and soaked with urine. Citizens avoided the area and the city finally ended its experiment. The park was closed and surrounded by a high fence to keep out the drug addicts and dealers. Plans are now being implemented to renovate the park and restore its original beauty. Zurich has served as a real-life experiment that proves the failure of decriminalization.

We believe that we must change public attitudes toward drugs and focus on prevention and treatment, but we must also maintain the laws making drugs illegal. A goal of prevention is to create an environment that rejects drug use and dealing. Effective prevention involves a comprehensive approach that includes the following components: education, including information about drugs; helping children understand the pressures from friends, family and school that may promote the use of drugs; social-competency skills to assist them in resisting the temptations of drugs; making available intervention (counseling, treatment) to those who have begun to use drugs; promoting positive alternatives to drug use; providing training to those who relate to children and influencing social policies (see *An Assessment of Substance Abuse Prevention*, New York State Division of Substance Abuse Services, October 1989).

Effective prevention efforts also attempt to promote negative attitudes toward drug use by communicating clear, consistent anti-substance-abuse messages through the mass media, within communities and in educational settings. A final important prevention strategy is to enforce stringently the laws against illegal drugs in order to control their availability.

* * *

When community prevention efforts are coupled with strong and decisive national leadership, the chances for change are greatly enhanced. Perhaps the most dramatic examples of the effectiveness of these partnerships are the anti-drunk driving and anti-smoking campaigns. These campaigns grew out of public intolerance of problems that not only plagued their communities, but decimated their children. Volunteers, community activists, parents and youth groups organized, developed community prevention strategies and applied unrelenting pressure on public officials, the private sector and the media. These activists were influential in shifting public attitudes. At the same time, Federal as well as state and local officials passed laws and changed public policies to regulate smoking in public areas, limit advertising and increase drunk-driving penalties. The result has been fewer traffic fatalities and a decrease in the social acceptability of drunk driving and smoking.

A study conducted by the New York State Division of Substance Abuse Services in 1990 found that during the preceding 12 years marijuana, cocaine and alcohol use had declined among school-age children. National data show similar trends. Studies of high school seniors conducted over the past decade have shown a dramatic decline in drug use as well. Legalizing drugs now would only send a confused message that could be interpreted as implying that the Government condones their use.

While legalization may appear to be a realistic solution to a very difficult problem, it would be a tremendous mistake. With legalization would come an increase in availability of drugs and an increase in the problems associated with their abuse: the suffering of addicts and their loved ones; the death and loss of thousands of innocent lives; great costs to society, to the health-care system, to employers, and, above all, social, economic and emotional costs to our children.

Instead of legalizing drugs, we must devote massive resources to education and treatment. We must communicate the clear and consistent message that drugs are destructive and will not be tolerated. We must so change public policy and attitudes that every addict who wants treatment can receive it. We must continue to use our resources to enforce the laws against drugs in order to keep drugs out of our communities. Rather than giving up the fight and legalizing drugs, it is crucial that we redouble our efforts to solve the problem.

POSTSCRIPT

Should Drugs Be Legalized?

Prohibition is generally considered to have been a failure in curbing alcohol use, and today, many see the current drug laws as being similarly ineffective in halting the work of drug dealers or diminishing the number of drug users. But the debate continues over whether or not drugs should be legalized: If drugs were legal, dealers would be out of business, thus reducing drug-related crime. Legalization would not, however, necessarily reduce the usage or abuse of drugs. An overview of the debate can be found in *The Drug Legalization Debate* by James A. Inciardi (Sage Publications, 1991).

A third route, decriminalization, is another option. Under this plan, certain less dangerous drugs, such as marijuana, would be neither strictly legal nor illegal. There would be no penalty for personal use or possession, although there would continue to be criminal penalties for sale for profit and distribution to minors.

This third category appeals to journalist Robert Hough, who argues that marijuana should be decriminalized in "Reefer Sadness," *Toronto Globe and Mail* (November 9, 1991). Also in support of decriminalization are attorney Peter Riga, "The Drug War Is a Crime: Let's Try Decriminalization," *Commonweal* (July 16, 1993), and physician Marcia Angell, "Alcohol and Other Drugs: Toward a More Rational and Consistent Policy," *The New England Journal of Medicine* (August 25, 1994). D. Keith Mano, in *National Review* (May 14, 1990), argues that marijuana has genuine medicinal purposes and is, as a recreational drug, considerably less harmful than alcohol. Brian Hecht, in "Out of Joint," *The New Republic* (July 15, 1991), also asserts that marijuana should be legalized for medicinal purposes. Eric Scholsser, in "Reefer Madness," *The Atlantic Monthly* (August 1994), argues that there are far too many people in jail for marijuana offenses.

In early 1992 the Drug Enforcement Administration published a document claiming that the government was justified in its continued prohibition of marijuana for medicinal purposes. The report indicated that too many questions surrounded the effectiveness of medicinal marijuana. See "Agency Says Marijuana Is Not Proven Medicine," *The New York Times* (March 19, 1992).

Additional views of the drug legalization issue can be found among the following selections: "Discontinuous Change and the War on Drugs" and "The Moral Culture of Drug Prohibition," *The Humanist* (September/October 1994); "A Content Analysis of the Drug Legalization Debate," *Journal of Drug Issues* (Fall 1993); "The Legalization Debate," *Federal Probation* (March 1993); and "How to Win the War on Drugs," *The New Republic* (May 21, 1990).

PART 4

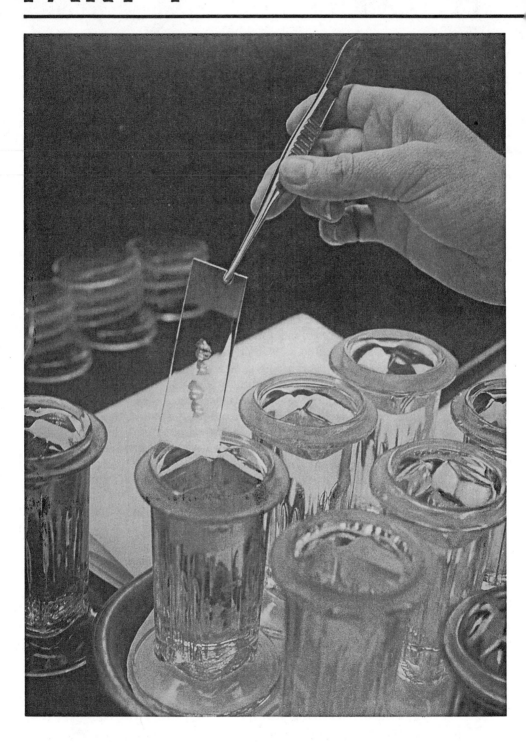

Sexuality and Gender Issues

Few issues can promote greater controversy than those concerning sexuality and gender. Recent generations of Americans have thrown out "traditional" sexual roles and values, which has resulted in a significant increase in the number of babies born out of wedlock, the spread of sexually transmitted diseases, and the decriminalization and proliferation of abortion. This section debates the morality of abortion, the gender gap in health care, and the extent to which non-drug-abusing heterosexuals are at risk for AIDS.

- Can Abortion Be a Morally Acceptable Choice?

- Does Health Care Delivery and Research Benefit Men at the Expense of Women?

- Is AIDS a Major Threat to the Heterosexual, Non-Drug-Abusing Population?

ISSUE 11

Can Abortion Be a Morally Acceptable Choice?

YES: Mary Gordon, from "A Moral Choice," *The Atlantic Monthly* (April 1990)

NO: Jason DeParle, from "Beyond the Legal Right: Why Liberals and Feminists Don't Like to Talk About the Morality of Abortion," *The Washington Monthly* (April 1989)

ISSUE SUMMARY

YES: Author Mary Gordon believes that abortion is an acceptable means to end an unwanted pregnancy and that women who have abortions are neither selfish nor immoral.

NO: Editor Jason DeParle argues that liberals and feminists refuse to acknowledge that the 3 out of 10 pregnancies that currently end in abortion raise many moral questions.

Few issues have created as much controversy and resulted in as much opposition as has the topic of abortion. Those involved in the abortion debate not only have firm beliefs, but each side has a self-designated label—pro-life and pro-choice—that clearly reflects what they believe to be the basic issues. The supporters of a woman's right to choose an abortion see individual choice as central to the debate. They believe that if a woman cannot choose to end an unwanted pregnancy, a condition that affects her body and possibly her whole life, then she has lost one of her most basic human rights. The pro-choice people feel that although the fetus is a potential human being, its life cannot be placed on the same level as that of the woman. On the other side, supporters of the pro-life movement argue that the fetus *is* a human being and that it has the same right to life as the mother. They believe that abortion is not only immoral but murder.

Although abortion appears to be a modern issue, it has a very long history. In the past, women in both urbanized and tribal societies have used a variety of dangerous methods to end unwanted pregnancies. Women sometimes consumed toxic chemicals, or various tools were inserted into the uterus in hopes of expelling its contents. Modern technology has simplified the procedure and has made it considerably safer. Before abortion was legalized in the United States, approximately 20 percent of all deaths from childbirth or pregnancy were caused by botched illegal abortions.

In 1973 the U.S. Supreme Court's decision of *Roe v. Wade* determined that an abortion in the first three months (trimester) of pregnancy is a decision between a woman and her physician and is protected by a right to privacy. During the second trimester, the Court ruled, an abortion could be performed on the basis of health risks. During the final trimester, an abortion could be performed only to preserve the mother's life.

Since 1973 abortion has become one of the most controversial issues in America. The National Right to Life Committee, one of the major abortion foes, currently has over 11 million members, who have become increasingly militant. In the summer of 1991, a major battle between pro-life and pro-choice forces took place in Wichita, Kansas. A similar demonstration followed during the spring of 1992 in Buffalo, New York, and others are planned. Largely as a result of these and other efforts, legislators have introduced various proposals to reduce, and eliminate, abortion rights in the United States.

Despite opposition from the right-to-life groups, abortion remains safe and legal in the United States today. However, what continues to kindle the debate are these questions: Does an abortion involve killing what may be a human being? Is abortion moral? Does the fetus have a right to life, liberty, and the pursuit of happiness, as guaranteed by the U.S. Constitution? Or do women have a right to a safe means of terminating an unwanted pregnancy?

In the following selections, Mary Gordon writes that abortion is neither immoral nor selfish. Because abortions usually take place when the embryo is merely a clump of cells and not a developed fetus, Gordon argues, abortion is not immoral, and she maintains that a woman's life is more important than that of a *potential* human. Jason DeParle argues that there is nothing more vulnerable than the unborn. DeParle cannot understand how liberalism can "hope to regain the glory of standing for morality and humanity while finding nothing inhumane or immoral in the extermination of so much life."

YES

Mary Gordon

A MORAL CHOICE

I am having lunch with six women. What is unusual is that four of them are in their seventies, two of them widowed, the other two living with husbands beside whom they've lived for decades. All of them have had children. Had they been men, they would have published books and hung their paintings on the walls of important galleries. But they are women of a certain generation, and their lives were shaped around their families and personal relations. They are women you go to for help and support. We begin talking about the latest legislative act that makes abortion more difficult for poor women to obtain. An extraordinary thing happens. Each of them talks about the illegal abortions she had during her young womanhood. Not one of them was spared the experience. Any of them could have died on the table of whatever person (not a doctor in any case) she was forced to approach, in secrecy and in terror, to end a pregnancy that she felt would blight her life.

I mention this incident for two reasons: first as a reminder that all kinds of women have always had abortions; second because it is essential that we remember that an abortion is performed on a living woman who has a life in which a terminated pregnancy is only a small part. Morally speaking, the decision to have an abortion doesn't take place in a vacuum. It is connected to other choices that a woman makes in the course of an adult life.

Anti-choice propagandists paint pictures of women who choose to have abortions as types of moral callousness, selfishness, or irresponsibility. The woman choosing to abort is the dressed-for-success yuppie who gets rid of her baby so that she won't miss her Caribbean vacation or her chance for promotion. Or she is the feckless, promiscuous ghetto teenager who couldn't bring herself to just say no to sex. A third, purportedly kinder, gentler picture has recently begun to be drawn. The woman in the abortion clinic is there because she is misinformed about the nature of the world. She is having an abortion because society does not provide for mothers and their children, and she mistakenly thinks that another mouth to feed will be the ruin of her family, not understanding that the temporary truth of family unhappiness doesn't stack up beside the eternal verity that abortion is murder. Or she is the dupe of her husband or boyfriend, who talks her into having an abortion because

From Mary Gordon, "A Moral Choice," *The Atlantic Monthly* (April 1990). Copyright © 1990 by Mary Gordon. Reprinted by permission of Sterling Lord Literistic, Inc.

a child will be a drag on his life-style. None of these pictures created by the anti-choice movement assumes that the decision to have an abortion is made responsibly, in the context of a morally lived life, by a free and responsible moral agent.

THE ONTOLOGY* OF THE FETUS

How would a woman who habitually makes choices in moral terms come to the decision to have an abortion? The moral discussion of abortion centers on the issue of whether or not abortion is an act of murder. At first glance it would seem that the answer should follow directly upon two questions: Is the fetus human? and Is it alive? It would be absurd to deny that a fetus is alive or that it is human. What would our other options be—to say that it is inanimate or belongs to another species? But we habitually use the terms "human" and "live" to refer to parts of our body—"human hair," for example, or "live red-blood cells"—and we are clear in our understanding that the nature of these objects does not rank equally with an entire personal existence. It then seems important to consider whether the fetus, this alive human thing, is a *person*, to whom the term "murder" could sensibly be applied. How would anyone come to a decision about something so impalpable as personhood? Philosophers have struggled with the issue of personhood, but in language that is so abstract that it is unhelpful to ordinary people making decisions in the course of their lives. It might be more productive to begin thinking about the status of the fetus by examining the language and customs that

*[*Ontology* refers to the nature of being or existing. —Ed.]

surround it. This approach will encourage us to focus on the choosing, acting woman, rather than the act of abortion— as if the act were performed by abstract forces without bodies, histories, attachments.

This focus on the acting woman is useful because a pregnant woman has an identifiable, consistent ontology, and a fetus takes on different ontological identities over time. But common sense, experience, and linguistic usage point clearly to the fact that we habitually consider, for example, a seven-week-old fetus to be different from a seven-month-old one. We can tell this by the way we respond to the involuntary loss of one as against the other. We have different language for the experience of the involuntary expulsion of the fetus from the womb depending upon the point of gestation at which the experience occurs. If it occurs early in the pregnancy, we call it a miscarriage; if late, we call it a stillbirth.

We would have an extreme reaction to the reversal of those terms. If a woman referred to a miscarriage at seven weeks as a stillbirth, we would be alarmed. It would shock our sense of propriety; it would make us uneasy; we would find it disturbing, misplaced—as we do when a bag lady sits down in a restaurant and starts shouting, or an octogenarian arrives at our door in a sailor suit. In short, we would suspect that the speaker was mad. Similarly, if a doctor or a nurse referred to the loss of a seven-month-old fetus as a miscarriage, we would be shocked by that person's insensitivity: could she or he not understand that a fetus that age is not what it was months before?

Our ritual and religious practices underscore the fact that we make distinctions among fetuses. If a woman took the bloody matter—indistinguishable from a heavy period—of an early miscarriage and insisted upon putting it in a tiny coffin and marking its grave, we would have serious concerns about her mental health. By the same token, we would feel squeamish about flushing a seven-month-old fetus down the toilet—something we would quite normally do with an early miscarriage. There are no prayers for the matter of a miscarriage, nor do we feel there should be. Even a Catholic priest would not baptize the issue of an early miscarriage.

The difficulties stem, of course, from the odd situation of a fetus's ontology: a complicated, differentiated, and nuanced response is required when we are dealing with an entity that changes over time. Yet we are in the habit of making distinctions like this. At one point we know that a child is no longer a child but an adult. That this question is vexed and problematic is clear from our difficulty in determining who is a juvenile offender and who is an adult criminal and at what age sexual intercourse ceases to be known as statutory rape. So at what point, if any, do we on the pro-choice side say that the developing fetus is a person, with rights equal to its mother's?

The anti-choice people have one advantage over us; their monolithic position gives them unity on this question. For myself, I am made uneasy by third-trimester abortions, which take place when the fetus could live outside the mother's body, but I also know that these are extremely rare and often performed on very young girls who have had difficulty comprehending the realities of pregnancy. It seems to me that the question of late abortions should be decided case by case, and that fixation

on this issue is a deflection from what is most important: keeping early abortions, which are in the majority by far, safe and legal. I am also politically realistic enough to suspect that bills restricting late abortions are not good-faith attempts to make distinctions about the nature of fetal life. They are, rather, the cynical embodiments of the hope among anti-choice partisans that technology will be on their side and that medical science's ability to create situations in which younger fetuses are viable outside their mothers' bodies will increase dramatically in the next few years. Ironically, medical science will probably make the issue of abortion a minor one in the near future. The RU-486 pill, which can induce abortion early on, exists, and whether or not it is legally available (it is not on the market here, because of pressure from anti-choice groups), women will begin to obtain it. If abortion can occur through chemical rather than physical means, in the privacy of one's home, most people not directly involved will lose interest in it. As abortion is transformed from a public into a private issue, it will cease to be perceived as political; it will be called personal instead.

AN EQUIVOCAL GOOD

But because abortion will always deal with what it is to create and sustain life, it will always be a moral issue. And whether we like it or not, our moral thinking about abortion is rooted in the shifting soil of perception. In an age in which much of our perception is manipulated by media that specialize in the sound bite and the photo op, the anti-choice partisans have a twofold advantage over us on the pro-choice side. The pro-choice moral position is more complex, and the experience we defend is physically repellent to contemplate. None of us in the pro-choice movement would suggest that abortion is not a regrettable occurrence. Anti-choice proponents can offer pastel photographs of babies in buntings, their eyes peaceful in the camera's gaze. In answer, we can't offer the material of an early abortion, bloody, amorphous in a paper cup, to prove that what has just been removed from the woman's body is not a child, not in the same category of being as the adorable bundle in an adoptive mother's arms. It is not a pleasure to look at the physical evidence of abortion, and most of us don't get the opportunity to do so.

The theologian Daniel Maguire, uncomfortable with the fact that most theological arguments about the nature of abortion are made by men who have never been anywhere near an actual abortion, decided to visit a clinic and observe abortions being performed. He didn't find the experience easy, but he knew that before he could in good conscience make a moral judgment on abortion, he needed to experience through his senses what an aborted fetus is like: he needed to look at and touch the controversial entity. He held in his hand the bloody fetal stuff; the eight-week-old fetus fit in the palm of his hand, and it certainly bore no resemblance to either of his two children when he had held them moments after their birth. He knew at that point what women who have experienced early abortions and miscarriages know: that some event occurred, possibly even a dramatic one, but it was not the death of a child.

Because issues of pregnancy and birth are both physical and metaphorical, we must constantly step back and forth between ways of perceiving the world. When we speak of gestation, we are often talking in terms of potential, about events and objects to which we attach our hopes, fears, dreams, and ideals. A mother can speak to the fetus in her uterus and name it; she and her mate may decorate a nursery according to their vision of the good life; they may choose for an embryo a college, a profession, a dwelling. But those of us who are trying to think morally about pregnancy and birth must remember that these feelings are our own projections onto what is in reality an inappropriate object. However charmed we may be by an expectant father's buying a little football for something inside his wife's belly, we shouldn't make public policy based on such actions, nor should we force others to live their lives conforming to our fantasies.

As a society, we are making decisions that pit the complicated future of a complex adult against the fate of a mass of cells lacking cortical development. The moral pressure should be on distinguishing the true from the false, the real suffering of living persons from our individual and often idiosyncratic dreams and fears. We must make decisions on abortion based on an understanding of how people really do live. We must be able to say that poverty is worse than not being poor, that having dignified and meaningful work is better than working in conditions of degradation, that raising a child one loves and has desired is better than raising a child in resentment and rage, that it is better for a twelve-year-old not to endure the trauma of having a child when she is herself a child.

When we put these ideas against the ideas of "child" or "baby," we seem to be making a horrifying choice of life-style over life. But in fact we are telling the truth of what it means to bear a child, and what the experience of abortion really is.

This is extremely difficult, for the object of the discussion is hidden, changing, potential. We make our decisions on the basis of approximate and inadequate language, often on the basis of fantasies and fears. It will always be crucial to try to separate genuine moral concern from phobia, punitiveness, superstition, anxiety, a desperate search for certainty in an uncertain world.

One of the certainties that is removed if we accept the consequences of the pro-choice position is the belief that the birth of a child is an unequivocal good. In real life we act knowing that the birth of a child is not always a good thing: people are sometimes depressed, angry, rejecting, at the birth of a child. But this is a difficult truth to tell; we don't like to say it, and one of the fears preyed on by anti-choice proponents is that if we cannot look at the birth of a child as an unequivocal good, then there is nothing to look toward. The desire for security of the imagination, for typological fixity, particularly in the area of "the good," is an understandable desire. It must seem to some anti-choice people that we on the pro-choice side are not only murdering innocent children but also murdering hope. Those of us who have experienced the birth of a desired child and felt the joy of that moment can be tempted into believing that it was the physical experience of the birth itself that was the joy. But it is crucial to remember that the birth of a child itself is a neutral occurrence emotionally: the charge it takes on is invested in it by the people experiencing or observing it.

THE FEAR OF SEXUAL AUTONOMY

These uncertainties can lead to another set of fears, not only about abortion but about its implications. Many anti-choice people fear that to support abortion is to cast one's lot with the cold and technological rather than with the warm and natural, to head down the slippery slope toward a brave new world where handicapped children are left on mountains to starve and the old are put out in the snow. But if we look at the history of abortion, we don't see the embodiment of what the anti-choice proponents fear. On the contrary, excepting the grotesque counterexample of the People's Republic of China (which practices forced abortion), there seems to be a real link between repressive anti-abortion stances and repressive governments. Abortion was banned in Fascist Italy and Nazi Germany; it is illegal in South Africa and in Chile. It is paid for by the governments of Denmark, England, and the Netherlands, which have national health and welfare systems that foster the health and well-being of mothers, children, the old, and the handicapped.

Advocates of outlawing abortion often refer to women seeking abortion as self-indulgent and materialistic. In fact these accusations mask a discomfort with female sexuality, sexual pleasure, and sexual autonomy. It is possible for a woman to have a sexual life unriddled by fear only if she can be confident that she need not pay for a failure of technology or judgment (and who among us has never once been swept away in the heat of a sexual moment?) by taking upon herself the crushing burden of unchosen motherhood.

It is no accident, therefore, that the increased appeal of measures to restrict maternal conduct during pregnancy—and a new focus on the physical autonomy of the pregnant woman—have come into public discourse at precisely the time when women are achieving un-precedented levels of economic and po-litical autonomy. What has surprised me is that some of this new anti-autonomy talk comes to us from the left. An ex-ample of this new discourse is an ar-ticle by Christopher Hitchens that ap-peared in *The Nation* last April, in which the author asserts his discomfort with abortion. Hitchens's tone is impeccably British: arch, light, we're men of the left.

> Anyone who has ever seen a sonogram or has spent even an hour with a textbook on embryology knows that the emotions are not the deciding factor. In order to terminate a pregnancy, you have to still a heartbeat, switch off a developing brain, and whatever the method, break some bones and rupture some organs. As to whether this involves pain on the "Silent Scream" scale, I have no idea. The "right to life" leadership, again, has cheapened everything it touches. ["Silent Scream" refers to Dr. Bernard Nathanson's widely debated antiabortion film *The Silent Scream*, in which an abortion on a 12-week-old fetus is shown from inside the uterus.—Ed.]

"It is a pity," Hitchens goes on to say, "that... the majority of feminists and their allies have stuck to the dead ground of 'Me Decade' possessive individualism, an ideology that has more in common than it admits with the prehistoric right, which it claims to oppose but has in fact encouraged." Hitchens proposes, as an alternative, a program of social reform that would make contraception free and support a national adoption service. In his opinion, it would seem, women have abortions for only two reasons: because they are selfish or because they are poor. If the state will take care of the economic problems and the bureaucratic messiness around adoption, it remains only for the possessive individualists to get their act together and walk with their babies into the communal utopia of the future. Hitchens would allow victims of rape or incest to have free abortions, on the grounds that since they didn't choose to have sex, the women should not be forced to have the babies. This would seem to put the issue of volition in a wrong and telling place. To Hitchens's mind, it would appear, if a woman chooses to have sex, she can't choose whether or not to have a baby. The implications of this are clear. If a woman is consciously and volitionally sexual, she should be prepared to take her medicine. And what medicine must the consciously sexual male take? Does Hitchens really believe, or want us to believe, that every male who has unintentionally impregnated a woman will be involved in the lifelong responsibility for the upbringing of the engendered child? Can he honestly say that he has observed this behavior—or, indeed, would want to see it observed—in the world in which he lives?

REAL CHOICES

It is essential for a moral decision about abortion to be made in an atmosphere of open, critical thinking. We on the pro-choice side must accept that there are in-deed anti-choice activists who take their position in good faith. I believe, however, that they are people for whom childbirth is an emotionally overladen topic, peo-ple who are susceptible to unclear think-ing because of their unrealistic hopes and fears. It is important for us in the pro-choice movement to be open in dis-cussing those areas involving abortion which are nebulous and unclear. But we must not forget that there are some things that we know to be undeniably true.

There are some undeniable bad consequences of a woman's being forced to bear a child against her will. First is the trauma of going through a pregnancy and giving birth to a child who is not desired, a trauma more long-lasting than that experienced by some (only some) women who experience an early abortion. The grief of giving up a child at its birth—and at nine months it is a child whom one has felt move inside one's body—is underestimated both by anti-choice partisans and by those for whom access to adoptable children is important. This grief should not be forced on any woman—or, indeed, encouraged by public policy.

We must be realistic about the impact on society of millions of unwanted children in an overpopulated world. Most of the time, human beings have sex not because they want to make babies. Yet throughout history sex has resulted in unwanted pregnancies. And women have always aborted. One thing that is not hidden, mysterious, or debatable is that making abortion illegal will result in the deaths of women, as it has always done. Is our historical memory so short that none of us remember aunts, sisters, friends, or mothers who were killed or rendered sterile by septic abortions? Does no one in the anti-choice movement remember stories or actual experiences of midnight drives to filthy rooms from which aborted women were sent out, bleeding, to their fate? Can anyone genuinely say that it would be a moral good for us as a society to return to those conditions?

Thinking about abortion, then, forces us to take moral positions as adults who understand the complexities of the world and the realities of human suffering, to make decisions based on how people actually live and choose, and not on our fears, prejudices, and anxieties about sex and society, life and death.

NO

Jason DeParle

BEYOND THE LEGAL RIGHT: WHY LIBERALS AND FEMINISTS DON'T LIKE TO TALK ABOUT THE MORALITY OF ABORTION

It's hard to hold these two images—the dismembered body of the fetus and the enveloping body of the mother, each begging the allegiance of our conscience—in mind at the same time. One of the biggest problems with the abortion debate is how rarely we do it, at least in public discourse. While contentious issues naturally produce one-dimensional positions, the remarkable thing about abortion is that many otherwise sensitive, nuanced thinkers hold them. To one side, visions only of women in crisis, terrified and imperilled by an invasive growth; to the other, only legions of innocent children, chased by the steely needle.

The inhumanity that issues from baronies within the right-to-life movement is well known: the craziness of a crusade against birth control; the view of women as second-class citizens; even the descent into bomb-throwing madness. The insistence that an unborn child must always be saved, no matter the cost, isn't compassion but a compassionate mask, and it obscures a face of cruelty.

But what ought to be equally if not more disturbing to feminists, liberals, and others on the Left is the extent to which prominent prochoice intellectuals mirror that dishonesty and denial. One-and-a-half million abortions each year is not the moral equivalent of the Holocaust, precisely because of the way in which fetuses *are* distinguishable: growing inside women, they can wreck the lives of mothers and of others, including her children, who depend upon her. But the fact that three of 10 pregnancies end in abortion poses moral questions that much of the Left, especially abortion's most vocal defenders, refuses to acknowledge. This lowering of intellectual standards offers a useful way of looking at the reflexes of liberals in general, and also reveals much about the passions—many of them just—that underpin contemporary feminism.

From Jason DeParle, "Beyond the Legal Right: Why Liberals and Feminists Don't Like to Talk About the Morality of Abortion," *The Washington Monthly* (April 1989). Copyright © 1989 by The Washington Monthly Company, 1611 Connecticut Avenue, NW, Washington, DC 20009, (202) 462-0128. Reprinted by permission.

WHAT THE SUCTION MACHINE SUCKS

The declaration of a legal right to an abortion doesn't end the discussion of what our attitude toward it should be, it merely begins it.... [M]any of the prochoice movement's writers and intellectuals would have us believe that the early fetus (and 90 percent of abortions take place in the first three months) is nothing more than a dewy piece of tissue, to be excised without regret. To speak of abortion as a moral dilemma, [Barbara Ehrenreich, prolific writer and contemporary feminist and socialist] has written, is to use "a mealy-mouthed vocabulary of evasion," to be compromised by a "strange and cabalistic question."

Yet everything we know—not just from science and religion but from experience, intuition, and compassion—suggests otherwise. A pregnant woman, even talking to her doctor, doesn't call the growth inside her an embryo or fetus. She calls it a *baby*. And she is admonished, by fellow feminists among others, to hold it in trust: Don't drink. Don't smoke. Eat well, counsels the feminist manual, *Our Bodies, Ourselves:* "think of it as eating for three—you, your baby, and the placenta...." Is it protoplasm that she's feeding? Or is it protoplasm only if she's feeding it to the forceps?

Grant for a moment that it is; agree that what the suction machine sucks is nothing more than tissue. Why then the feminist fuss over abortions for purposes of sex selection? If a couple wants a boy and nature hands them the makings of a girl, why not abort and start again? All that matters—no?—is "choice."

It wasn't sex selection but nuclear power that got a feminist named Juli Loesch rethinking her own contradictory views of fetuses. As an organizer attempting to stop the construction of Three Mile Island, she had schooled herself on what leaked radiation can do to prenatal development. At a meeting one day, she says, a group of women issued an unexpected challenge: "if you're so concerned about what Plutonium 239 might do to the child's arm bud you should go see what a suction machine does to his whole body."

In fact, we need neither *The Silent Scream* [Dr. Bernard Nathanson's antiabortion film, which was widely publicized and debated in the United States during the mid-1980s and which showed, from inside a uterus, an abortion being performed on a 12-week-old fetus] nor a degree in fetal physiology to tell us what we already know: that abortion is the eradication of human life and should be avoided whenever possible. Should it be legal? Yes, since the alternatives are worse. Is it moral? Perhaps, depending on what's at stake. Fetal life exists along a continuum; our obligations to it grow as it grows, but they must be weighed against other demands.

The number of liberals, feminists, and other defenders of abortion eager to simplify the moral questions is, at the very least, deeply ironic. One of the animating spirits of liberalism and other factions on the Left, and proudly so, is the concern for the most vulnerable. But what could be more vulnerable than the unborn? And how can liberalism hope to regain the glory of standing for humanity and morality while finding nothing inhumane or immoral in the extermination of so much life?

The problem with much prochoice thinking is suggested by the movement's chief slogan, "a woman's right to control her body," which fails to acknowledge that the great moral and biological conundrum is precisely that another body is involved. Slogans are slogans, not dissertations; but this one is revealing in that it mirrors so much of the prochoice tendency to ignore the conflict in an unwanted pregnancy between two competing interests, mother and embryo, and insist that only one is worthy of consideration. Daniel Callahan, a moral philosopher, has written of the need, upon securing the right to a legal abortion, to preserve the "moral tension" implicit in an unwanted pregnancy. This is something that too few members of the prochoice movement are willing to do.

One fine example of preserving the moral tension appeared several years ago in a *Harper's* piece by Sallie Tisdale, an abortion clinic nurse with a grudging acceptance of her work. First the mothers: "A twenty-one-year-old woman, unemployed, uneducated, without family, in the fifth month of her fifth pregnancy. A forty-two-year-old mother of teenagers, shocked by her condition, refusing to tell her husband. A twenty-three-year-old mother of two having her seventh abortion, and many women in their thirties having their first.... Oh, the ignorance.... Some swear they have not had sex, many do not know what a uterus is, how sperm and egg meet, how sex makes babies.... They come so young, snapping gum, sockless and sneakered, and their shakily applied eyeliner smears when they cry.... I cannot imagine them as mothers."

Then the fetus: "I am speaking in a matter-of-fact voice about 'the tissue' and 'the contents' when the woman suddenly catches my eye and asks, 'How big is the baby now?'.... I gauge, and sometimes lie a little, weaseling around its infantile features until its clinging power slackens. But when I look in the basin, among the curdlike blood clots, I see an elfin thorax, attenuated, its pencilline ribs all in parallel rows with tiny knobs of spine rounding upwards. A translucent arm and hand swim beside.... I have fetus dreams, we all do here: dreams of abortions one after the other; of buckets of blood splashed on the walls; trees full of crawling fetuses...."

It's not surprising that the defenders of abortion don't like pictures of fetuses; General Westmoreland didn't like the cameras in Vietnam either. Fetuses aren't babies, and the photos don't end the discussion. But they make it a more sober one, as it should be. Fetuses aren't just *their* image but our image too, anyone's image who is going to confront abortion.

If the prochoice movement doesn't like the way *The Silent Scream* depicts the fetus, turn to an early edition of *Our Bodies, Ourselves*. Describing an abortion at 16 weeks by means of saline injection, the feminist handbook explains: "Contractions will start some hours later. Generally they will be as strong as those of a full-term pregnancy.... The longest and most difficult part will be the labor. The breathing techniques taught in the childbirth section of this book might help make the contractions more bearable. After eight to fifteen hours of labor, the fetus is expelled in a bedpan in the patient's bed."

HEIL MARY

When Suzannah Lessard wrote about abortion in *The Washington Monthly* in 1972 ("Aborting a Fetus: the Legal Right, the Personal Choice"), a year before *Roe v. Wade*, she described what she called a "reaction formation along ideological lines... of the new feminist movement" as it related to abortion. This was a time when Gloria Steinem was insisting that a fetus was nothing more than "mass of dependent protoplasm" and aborting it the moral equivalent of a tonsillectomy. "I think a lot of women need to go fanatically ideological for a while because they can't in any other way overthrow the insidious sense of themselves as inferior," Lessard wrote, "nor otherwise live with the rage that comes to the surface when they realize how they have been psychically mauled." This is an observation about the psychology of oppression that could be applied to any number of righteous rebellions; the path to autonomy tends to pass, by necessity perhaps, through stages of angry defiance. "But I don't think that state of mind—hopefully temporary—is the strength of the movement," Lessard wrote. "It has very little to do with working out a new, undamaging way of living as women."

But to judge by much contemporary prochoice writing, the mere-protoplasm camp still thrives. Certainly, there are exceptions, Mario Cuomo's 1984 speech at Notre Dame perhaps being the most famous: "A fetus is different from an appendix or set of tonsils. At the very least... the full potential of human life is indisputably there. That—to my less subtle mind—by itself should demand respect, caution, indeed... reverence.... [But] I concluded that the approach of a constitutional amendment is not the best way for us to seek to deal with abortion." And others on the Left have gone even further: Nat Hentoff, who supports a legal ban, has written a number of attacks on abortion in the *Village Voice*; Mary Meehan, a former antiwar activist, published an article in *The Progressive* that

attacked the magazine's own editorial stance in favor of legal abortion.

But these are the exceptions. Pick up the past 10 years of *The Nation, Mother Jones,* or *Ms.* Read liberals and feminists on the op-ed pages of *The Washington Post* or *The New York Times*—you're likely to find more concern about the snail darter than the 1.6 million fetuses aborted each year....

LIBERAL PRECINCTS

... [T]he point is clear: questioning abortion—not only the legal right but also the moral choice—is often viewed, even by otherwise sensitive and thoughtful activists, as a betrayal of the highest order. (Except, at times, for Catholics, whose antiabortion views are usually dismissed as a quaint if unfortunate quirk of faith.)

A great irony about this public demonstration of zeal is that there may be more ambivalence on the Left than is usually acknowledged. When *The Progressive* published Mary Meehan's prolife piece in 1980, it drew more mail than any article save the famous guide to the workings of the H-bomb. About half were predictable: "your knees buckle at the mere thought of taking a forthright stand for women's rights," "prolife is only a code word representing the neo-fascist absolutist thinking." Etc, etc.

But the others: "I support most of the positions of the women's movement, but I part company with those who insist on abortion as a 'right of women to control their own bodies.' There's a lot more than just one body that is being controlled here." "I have no religious objection to abortion, but I do oppose it from a humanitarian point of view." "I was awfully glad to see a liberal publication printing an antiabortion article."

Why aren't there more voices like these heard in liberal precincts? The answers come in two general sets, one pertaining to liberal and progressive values generally and the other connected more specifically to the passions of contemporary feminism.

Right or wrong, abortion helps further values that liberals and progressives generally hold in esteem. Among them is public health. Even those with qualms about abortion tend to back the legal right, if for no other reason than to stem the mutilation that a return to back alleys would surely entail. There's also an equity-between-the-classes argument: if abortion is banned all women may experience trouble getting one, but the poor will have the most trouble of all. For others, there are always planes to Sweden.

Beyond questions of abortion's legality, the Left tends to hold values that encourage the acceptance of abortion's morality too. There's the civil liberties perspective, which argues that the state should "stay out of the bedroom." There's a population control argument; without abortion, wrote one *Progressive* reader, "there will be a more intense scramble for food and all the world's natural resources." There's a help-the-poor strand of thinking; what, liberals constantly ask, about the welfare mother who can't afford another child? And there's a fairness-in-the-marketplace argument, which maintains that without absolute control of their fertility, women cannot compete with men: if two Arnold & Porter associates conceive a child at a Christmas party tryst, bringing it into the world, whether she keeps it or not, will penalize her career much more than his.

These principles—a thirst for fairness between genders and classes, for civil liberties, for economic opportunity—are honorable ones. And they speak well of those who hold them as caring not only for life itself but also for its quality.

Careful, though. Quality-of-life arguments sometimes stop focusing on quality and start frowning on life. Concerns about population control have their place; but whether abortion is a fit means of seeking it raises questions that go well beyond environmental impact studies. One of the most troubling prochoice arguments is the what-kind-of-life-will-the-child-have line. Yes, poverty may appropriately enter the moral calculus if an additional child will truly tumble the family into chaos and despair, and those situations exist. (And there is little cruelty purer than child abuse, which afflicts unwanted children of all classes.) But liberal talk about the quality of life can quickly devolve into a form of cardboard compassion that assumes life for the poor doesn't mean much anyway. That sentiment says to an unborn child of poverty: life is tough, so you should die. Compassionate, that....

THE CHRISTMAS PARTY TRYST

While the values of the Left in general provide one set of explanations for the contours of the abortion debate, the specific passions and experiences of feminists provide another. These concerns don't, finally, answer the question of what our personal, as opposed to legal, obligations toward fetal life need to be. But they do underline the history of injustice that women have inherited.

In rough outline, one persuasive feminist argument for keeping abortion *legal* —an argument I accept—goes something like this: Without the option of abortion, women cannot be as free as men. Not just socially and economically but psychologically as well. And not just those with unwanted pregnancies. As Ellen Willis of the [*Village*] *Voice* has put it, "Criminalizing abortion doesn't just harm individual women with unwanted pregnancies, it affects all women's sense of themselves. Without control of our fertility we can never envision ourselves as free, for our biology makes us constantly vulnerable." Vulnerable to failed birth control. To rape or other coercive sex. Or simply to passion. Vulnerable in a way that men are not. And in a society that rightly prizes liberty as much as ours, it's unacceptable for one half of its members to be less free, at an essential level, than the other. Therefore the legal right.

Of course, having the legal right to do something doesn't tell us whether it's a desirable thing to do. Women have the legal right to smoke and drink heavily during pregnancy, but few of us would hesitate to dissuade them from doing so. Why don't more feminists take the same view toward abortion—defending the right, but urging women to incline against it whenever possible? The feminist defenders of abortion I spoke with reacted to that proposal with a litany of past and present injustices against women—economic, social, political, and cultural, all of them quite real. "You can sit around all day talking about what's the morally right thing to do—rights and sacrifices and the sanctity of life and all that—but I don't think it can be divorced from women's lives in this society," [poet and critic Katha] Pollitt said.

Leaving aside for a moment the wrenching emotional issues, one obvious burden is economics. Having a child—even one put up for adoption—costs not only trauma but time and money, and takes them from women, not men. The financial burden is one reason why poor women are more likely to have abortions than others.

But the same inequity is true among professional women. To return to the Arnold & Porter Christmas party tryst, what would happen if the female associate does the right thing by prolife standards and decides to have the child? At $65,000 a year, she can certainly afford to do it, and her insurance is probably blue chip. But in the eyes of some senior partners, the luster of her earlier promise begins to fade. They may be reluctant to keep her on certain accounts, for fear of offending the clients. What's more, even if the clients understand, she'll be missing at least six to eight weeks of work—just, as fate would have it, when she's needed in court on an important case. The long-term penalties may be overestimated—good employees are in short demand in most professions; it's the marginal who will suffer the most—but the fears are nonetheless real. What's more, the burden is unequally shared. Her trystee suffers no such repercussions. The clients love him, he shines in court, and his future seems assured. Unfair? Yes, extremely.

These inequities are one reason why the right-to-life movement has the obligation, often shirked, to support measures that would make it easier for women of all incomes to go through pregnancy —health care, maternity leave, parental leave, day care, protections against employment discrimination. But even if all these things were provided—as they should be—it's unlikely that the strength of feminist feeling on abortion would recede. Economic opportunity is an important facet of the abortion debate, but it's not, finally at its core. Of all the women I spoke with, the one I most expected to forward an economic argument was Barbara Ehrenreich—since she is co-chair of Democratic Socialists of America—but she never mentioned it. When I finally asked her about it she said that no amount of money or servants would change the essential moral equation, which centers, in her mind, on female autonomy. "The moral issue has to do with female personhood," she said.

CRUEL CHOICES

What surprised me in my talks with the female defenders of abortion, was how many of them seemed to view the abortion debate as some sort of referendum by which society judged women's deepest levels of self. Words like *guilt* and *sin, punishment* and *shame* kept issuing forth. They did so both about abortion and about sex in general. "The whole debate is more about the value of women's lives and the respect we have for women than it is about the act of abortion itself," said Kate Michelman, the head of the National Abortion Rights Action League.

A few days before my scheduled meeting with Michelman, I got a phone call from her press secretary. "We hear a nasty rumor," she said, "that you're writing something that says abortion is immoral." I mentioned the rumor when I sat down to speak with Michelman, who quickly told me about the very difficult circumstances surrounding her own abortion. Her first husband had walked out on her and her three small children when she was destitute, ill, and pregnant. She had to make a difficult moral judgment, she said, weighing her responsibilities to her family against those to the fetus. Then, this being 1970, she couldn't even make the decision herself but had to obtain the consent of a panel of doctors and then, to further the pain, get her ex-husband's signature. Call me immoral, she seemed to say, in an I-dare-you way.

But it seemed to me that Michelman's decision, like those, certainly, of a great number of women, had involved a thoughtful handling of difficult questions —as she herself was underlining. "Sure the fetus has interests, absolutely," she said, as do other things, like a woman's commitments to her family and her health. It was only when I began asking why those leading the prochoice movement didn't discuss these moral tensions more often that her reasoning turned curious and defensive.

"The ethical questions are being raised," she said. "And if [a woman] makes a decision [to have an abortion] then she's made the right decision."

I asked her how she knew. With 1.6 million abortions a year, there seems to be a lot of room for error.

Merely asking the question, she said, implied that women had abortions for frivolous reasons. "To even raise the question of when it's immoral," she said, "is to say that women can't make moral decisions."

In considering the way a legacy of injustice fuels the adamance over abortion, it is helpful to consider three generations of women: those who preceded the feminist movement of the late sixties and early seventies; those who soldiered in it; and those who inherited its gains. Each has faced the tyranny of a man's world in a way that primes passions about abortion, but each has done so in a different way.

Women who became sexually active outside of marriage in the days of blanket abortion bans faced a world prepared to hand them the cruelest choice: the life-wrecking stigma of pregnancy out-of-wedlock or the back alley; a "ruined" life or a potentially lethal trip through a netherworld. Men, meanwhile, made the decisions that crafted that world while escaping the brunt of its cruelty. That *was* an unjust life, and the triumph over it is among feminism's proudest achievements....

ACCEPTING FEMALE SEXUALITY

... [W]hat's interesting about the observations of male irresponsibility [in casual sexual relationships], as it relates to abortion, is that both sides cite it. Prolife feminists, like Juli Loesch, argue that the acceptance of abortion actually *encourages* exploitation. The "hit and run" artist can pony up $200, send a woman off to a clinic, and imagine himself to have done the gallant thing. "The idea is that a man can use a woman, vacuum her out, and she's ready to be used again," Loesch says."It's like a rent-a-car or something." (In such scenarios, Loesch argues, abortion has the same blame-the-victim effect that the Left is typically quick to condemn, with the victimized mother perpetrating the injustice through violence against the fetus.)

When I asked Katha Pollitt about this, she dismissed it with the argument that men will be just as irresponsible with or without abortion, and that the only difference will be the burden left to women. To some extent she's right: irresponsible sexual behavior—by men and women both—will no doubt continue under any imaginable scenario. Then again, it's not unreasonable to suspect that casual attitudes about abortion, particularly among men, could increase precisely the kind

of "stallion" behavior that Pollitt rightly protests. And abortion can become a tool of male coercion in other ways as well. "He said that if I didn't have an abortion, the relationship would be over," a friend recently explained. Many women have experienced the same.

Of course, feminist emotion toward abortion isn't just a reaction to male sexuality but also an assertion that women's own sexual drive is equally legitimate. Feminists argue that antiabortion arguments reflect a larger cultural ambivalence, if not outright hostility, toward female sexuality. This is where words like *guilt* and *shame* and *punishment* continue to arise. I recently sat down with Katha Pollitt for a long conversation about abortion. She cited the many ways in which women (and the children antiabortionists want them to raise) are injured by society: poor health care, poor housing, economic discrimination, male abuse. We talked also about power, politics, religion, and the other forces that play into the abortion debate, like the unflagging responsibilities that come with parenthood. (She is a new, and proud, mother.) But when I asked her which, of the many justifications for abortion, she felt most deeply—what, in her mind, was the real core of the issue—her answer surprised me. "Deep down," she said, "what I believe is that children should not be a punishment for having sex."

Ellen Willis of the *Voice* advances a similar argument. Opposition to abortion, she's written, is cut of the same cloth as the more general "virginity fetishism, sexual guilt and panic and disgrace" foisted on women by a repressive society. The woman's fight for abortion without qualm, she says, is part of the fight for the "acceptance of the erotic impulse, and one's own erotic impulses, as fundamentally benign and necessary for human happiness."

Pollitt agreed. "The notion of female sexuality being expressed is something people have deeply contradictory feelings about," Pollitt said....

BIOLOGY AND DESTINY

What the argument for abortion-without-qualm comes down to is this: the fetus doesn't exist unless we want it to. But the whole crisis over abortion is that we know precisely the opposite to be true. It's there physically, feminists say, but not morally. But how could it be one without the other—there to nurture one day (remember, plenty of fresh vegetables, we're eating for three: you, baby, and placenta), but free to dismember the next? Qualm-less advocates argue that all that finally matters is whether the woman, for whatever reason, desires to bring it into the world. Yet the fetus is already there, no matter what we plan or desire. Forces may conspire against a woman and leave her *unable* to bring it into the world, or unable to do so without a great deal of harm to herself and others. That is, *other* moral obligations may overrule. But it is suspicious in the extreme to argue—as the qualmlessness position does—that our moral obligations are nothing more than what we want them to be, a wish-it-away view of the world. Inconveniently fetuses exist, quite outside our fluctuating emotions and desires.

Finally, Ellen Willis's argument that by giving fetuses any moral status at all we reduce women to vessels breaks down because women *are* vessels. They're not *just* vessels. They're much more than vessels. But the attempt to reconcile the just desire for full female autonomy with

our moral obligations toward fetuses by insisting that we have none attempts to wish away a very real collision; it refuses to acknowledge a (so far) inalterable conflict buried in biology. Willis argues this is precisely the oppressive "biology equals destiny" argument that feminism has fought to overturn. Biology doesn't equal destiny; but it does affect destiny, and it leaves us with the extremely difficult fact that women, for any number of reasons, get burdened with unwanted pregnancies to which there are no easy moral solutions. Something important is lost—female autonomy or fetal life—in either event.

There are two highly imperfect ways of dealing with this conflict. The first is abstinence (since birth control fails). But not much chance of that. The second is adoption—another imperfect solution. The first argument against it is that there aren't enough parents to go around, particularly for minority and handicapped children. Ironically those quickest to point this out tend to be those for whom putting up a child for adoption really is a plausible option —white professionals. George Bush's "adoption not abortion" line brought quick ridicule by Pollitt in *The Nation* and Ehrenreich in *Mother Jones*. He's wrong to suggest it as a panacea— babies would quickly outstrip parents, as Pollitt insists—but right to encourage its wider use. The real challenge for liberals and progressives would be to turn the thought back toward Bush, and demand the governmental support, in health care and other ways, needed to get through pregnancy, and needed to raise a child.

The second argument against adoption focuses not on demand but supply: nine months of illness culminating in a "physiological crisis which is occasionally fatal and almost always excruciatingly painful," as Ehrenreich has written.... "It's almost unimaginable to me to think about giving up the baby," said Ehrenreich. "Talk about misery. Talk about 20 years of grief and ambivalence." The grief is real—particularly for people of conscience, like Ehrenreich. (And people of conscience are the targets of moral suasion in the first place.) But where does that argument lead? That in order to spare a child the risks of an adoptive life, we offer the kindness of a suction machine?

"A VERY SCARY TIME"

A few years ago, I was sharing an apartment with a friend who became pregnant just before breaking up with her fiance. Like many men... he just walked away, dealing with the dilemma through denial. My friend dealt with it with a lot of courage. I called her recently to see how the experience seemed in retrospect, and perhaps she should provide the coda, since her view complicates both Ehrenreich's position and my own. Though she said that putting her child up for adoption was "the right thing," she said she "would never, ever, pressure someone to go through the same thing."

It surprised me to hear her say that abortion "crossed my mind several thousand times," since that was the one option she had seemed to rule out from the start. When she realized she was pregnant, she said, she went riding her bicycle into potholes "trying to jar something loose. It was very, very easy for me to think of the sperm and the egg as having just joined. It was like a piece of mucous to me." She decided against abortion after about a week, "a very lonely, very scary time."

"At some point, I realized I was old enough, and mature enough, that I could do it [have the baby]," she said, but she emphasized that this calculus could have been altered easily by any number of factors—including less support from family and friends, a less understanding employer, or the lack of medical care. She spent months in counseling trying to decide whether to raise the child or put it up for adoption, and the decision to give the baby away "was the most difficult thing I've ever had to do." Since the baby was healthy and white the adoption market was on her side—"I could have dictated that I wanted two Finnish socialists," she said—and her certainty that the new parents would not only love the child but pass on certain shared values was an essential thing to know.

"When I think about her," she said, "just the miracle of being able to have brought her into this life, even if she's not here with me right now, she's with people who love her. It's a miracle."

"When she left to go to her adoptive parents, it was the most devastating and wonderful thing," she said. "I kept thinking this is my child, and I love her."

"It always kept coming back to that—I love her."

POSTSCRIPT

Can Abortion Be a Morally Acceptable Choice?

The abortion issue continues to be complex and polarizing. In June 1983, in a series of decisions, the Supreme Court reaffirmed its support of abortion rights. Similar decisions in 1986 also confirmed the Court's support. However, the Court has become more conservative and pro-life in recent years. With pressure and support from pro-life groups throughout the country, *Roe v. Wade* may continue to come before the Supreme Court for reconsideration. While the majority of Americans favor a woman's right to an abortion, the vocal and well-organized pro-life groups have been successful in keeping the abortion issue in the media and in the political arena.

Nancy Meyers, the media director of the National Right to Life Committee, asserts that abortion is never justified and that it is a violation of human rights in "Abortion is Morally Wrong," *The World and I* (1989), as does William F. Buckley in "Abortion: The Debate," *National Review* (December 1989). Writing in the *Humanist* (January/February 1991), Faye Wattleton, the president of Planned Parenthood Federation of America, argues that women's reproductive rights are inviolable and that no government, court, or politician should ever interfere with these rights.

Many people believe that if abortion becomes illegal again, dangerous self-induced and back-alley abortions would reappear. But whether or not legalized abortion has improved women's health is still the subject of controversy. In her book *The Choices We Made* (Random House, 1991), Angela Bonavoglia claims that *Roe v. Wade* made abortion both safe and legal and that legal abortion saves women's lives. She notes that of the 1.6 million legal abortions performed each year in the United States, only 6 women die from the procedure. In contrast, in Mexico, where abortion is not legal, 140,000 women die annually from the procedure.

David C. Reardon, in *Aborted Women: Silent No More* (Loyola University Press, 1987), counters that the legalization of abortion has not improved the health of women. While the number of deaths from legal abortions is low, Reardon claims, the infection and bleeding rates are high. He believes that, overall, the health risks associated with abortion have increased due to the sheer numbers of women having abortions.

The following selections debate the moral concerns surrounding abortion: "Life Terms," *New Republic* (July 15, 1991); "A Basic Human Right," *Ms* (August 1989); and "Abortion: The Politics—What the People Really Say," *National Review* (December 22, 1989).

ISSUE 12

Does Health Care Delivery and Research Benefit Men at the Expense of Women?

YES: Leslie Laurence and Beth Weinhouse, from *Outrageous Practices: The Alarming Truth About How Medicine Mistreats Women* (Fawcett Columbine, 1994)

NO: Andrew G. Kadar, from "The Sex-Bias Myth in Medicine," *The Atlantic Monthly* (August 1994)

ISSUE SUMMARY

YES: Health and medical reporters Leslie Laurence and Beth Weinhouse claim that women have been excluded from most research on new drugs, medical treatments, and surgical techniques that are routinely offered to men.

NO: Physician Andrew G. Kadar argues that women actually receive more medical care and benefit more from medical research than do men, which explains why women generally live longer than men.

In 1989 Harvard University reported that taking an aspirin tablet every other day could prevent heart disease based on a study involving 22,000 male physicians. The findings were generalized to include both men and women, and the final reports claimed that aspirin, which helps prevent blood clotting, would be useful to all adults. Dr. Suzanne Oparil, president of the American Heart Association, however, believes that aspirin might not be beneficial to women because they have generally faster rates of blood clotting than men.

Why weren't women included in the Harvard aspirin study or in other research that might help prevent their premature deaths or disabilities? The answer goes back to 1975, when the National Commission for the Protection of Human Subjects of Biomedical and Behavioral Research issued guidelines limiting research on pregnant women. This ban on using women stemmed from fears following the thalidomide crisis in the late 1950s. Thalidomide, a sedative and antinausea drug that was used to help treat morning sickness during early pregnancy, was responsible for many children being born with deformities after their mothers used the drug while they were pregnant. Two years after this incident the Food and Drug Administration (FDA) published recommendations that all women of "childbearing potential" be excluded from early phases of drug trials to avoid any damage to fetuses.

By the mid-1980s many women began to question the FDA-mandated exclusion of women from drug trials. In 1985 the National Institutes of Health

(NIH) issued a statement urging researchers to include women in their studies. In 1990 it was reported, however, that women were still not included in major federally funded clinical studies and that the NIH was not enforcing its policy of including women.

Things began to change, beginning with the 1991 launching of the *Women's Health Initiative*, a 14-year study of women's health. And in 1993 the FDA lifted its ban on using women in drug trials. Although there has been obvious progress, claims are still being made that women and men are not treated equally regarding medical care and research. Many argue that women are being shortchanged with regard to research on heart disease and AIDS and that they are also twice as likely *not* to be tested for lung cancer as men, even though lung cancer is the leading cancer killer of women.

A relatively recent concern pertains to AIDS and HIV-related conditions. In particular, AIDS research has a proportionately higher number of men participating in drug and other scientific trials. Additionally, though AIDS is a major killer of women, especially in urban areas, the official definition of AIDS has until recently excluded HIV-related conditions that were specific to females. What is known about HIV and AIDS seems to have been acquired from research on men only.

Despite concerns that health care and research in the United States benefit men at the expense of women, there is ample evidence to the contrary: Department of Health and Human Services studies show that women see their physicians more frequently, have more surgery, and are admitted to hospitals more often than men. Currently, two out of three medical dollars are spent by women. A 1981 study conducted at the University of California at San Diego reviewed over 40,000 patient office visits and found that the health care men and women received was similar over two-thirds of the time. When the care differed, it was women who were given more lab tests, drug prescriptions, and return appointments.

Women have also benefitted from medical research involving high-tech procedures. Laparoscopic surgery and ultrasound are two advanced techniques that were first developed for use on women's bodies (these procedures were later adapted for men). Women's diseases have also been the recipient of research dollars. Breast cancer, the second leading cancer killer of women, has received more funding than any other tumor research. In 1993 the National Cancer Institute spent over $213 million dollars on breast cancer and $51 million dollars on prostate cancer. Although one-third more women die of breast cancer than men of prostate cancer, research into breast cancer received more than four times the funding of prostate cancer research.

In the following selections, Leslie Laurence and Beth Weinhouse argue that women have been short-changed with regard to health care and medical research. Andrew G. Kadar disagrees, claiming that though it is often believed that women do not get the same consideration in medical care and research as men, the truth appears to be exactly the opposite.

YES

Leslie Laurence and
Beth Weinhouse

OUTRAGEOUS PRACTICES: THE ALARMING TRUTH ABOUT HOW MEDICINE MISTREATS WOMEN

There is unfortunately a clear path from the ignorant attitudes about women's bodies prevalent in the last century to the ignorant attitudes that exist today. A century ago physicians removed women's ovaries to treat a variety of unrelated complaints. They believed women's reproductive organs were responsible for almost everything that can and did go wrong with the human body. How much has changed? Recent medical students say that, during anatomy lectures on the female reproductive system, lecturers take pains to describe the female reproductive system as inefficient, badly designed, and prone to problems....

We may be horrified by the "ovariotomies" and "clitoridectomies" of the nineteenth century, but what of the hundreds of thousands of unnecessary hysterectomies being performed today?...

Nearly 550,000 hysterectomies are performed in the United States each year, making hysterectomy one of the most common operations of all. Yet the vast majority of these operations are elective, not lifesaving. When the American College of Obstetricians and Gynecologists recently announced its wish for ob-gyns to become the primary-care physicians for postmenopausal women, one woman doctor retorted, "If they want to do that, they're going to have to leave some organs in first."

How far have we really come from the days when women were told their psychological symptoms were due to physical problems and their reproductive organs were removed as a cure? Today women are frequently told that their very real physical symptoms—chest pains, menstrual problems, endometriosis, gastrointestinal pain—are psychological, and are handed a prescription for antidepressants or tranquilizers.

The medical textbooks of the 1800s may seem laughably ignorant today, but as recently as the 1970s physicians were being taught that morning sickness was caused by a woman's resentment at being a mother, PMS [premenstrual syndrome] was also a psychological disorder, and menopause represented the end of a woman's usefulness in life. And the doctors who were trained with those textbooks are still practicing medicine.

Instead of putting today's inequities in perspective, the examples of past abuses of women serve only to show that we haven't come as far as we thought....

THE RESEARCH GAP

In June 1990, American women got a rude shock. For all the complaints women leveled against the health care system —most having to do with insensitive male doctors and dissatisfaction with gynecological and obstetric care—the majority of women still assumed that at least they were included in America's state-of-the-art medical research. But they were wrong. For at least the past several decades women in this country had been systematically excluded from the vast majority of research to develop new drugs, medical treatments, and surgical techniques.

It was on June 18, 1990, that the government's General Accounting Office (GAO) released its report of an audit of the National Institutes of Health (NIH). The audit found that although NIH had formulated a policy in 1986 for including women as research subjects, little had been done to implement or monitor that policy. In fact, most researchers applying for NIH grants were not even aware that they were supposed to include women, since the NIH grant-application book contained no mention of the policy. Because the 1986 policy urged rather than required attention to gender bias, most institutes, and most researchers, had simply decided to ignore it altogether or pay it only slight heed: "It used to be

enough for a researcher to say, 'Women and minorities will not be excluded from this study,'" explains one woman in NIH's Division of Research Grants. But not excluding women is very different from actively recruiting and including them....

The GAO found that women were being underrepresented in studies of diseases affecting both men and women. In the fifty applications reviewed, one-fifth made no mention of gender and over one-third said the subjects would include both sexes, but did not give percentages. Some all-male studies gave no rationale for their exclusivity. "The [NIH] may win the Nobel Prize, but I'd like to see them get the *Good Housekeeping* seal of approval," said Congresswoman Barbara Mikulski (D-Md.), voicing her hopes that the behemoth medical institution could be made more woman-friendly.

As if medical research were some kind of exclusive male club, some of the biggest and most important medical studies of recent years had failed to enroll a single woman:

• The Baltimore Longitudinal Study, one of the largest studies to examine the natural process of aging, began in 1958 and included no women for its first twenty years because, according to Gene Cohen, then deputy director of the National Institute on Aging (NIA), the facility in which the study was conducted had only one toilet. The study's 1984 report, entitled "Normal Human Aging," contained no data on women. (Currently 40 percent of the participants in this study are women... although 60 percent of the population over age sixty-five is female.)
• The by-now-infamous Physicians' Health Study, which concluded in 1988

that taking an aspirin a day might reduce the risk of heart disease, included 22,000 men and no women.

- The 1982 Multiple Risk Factor Intervention Trial, known as Mr. Fit, a long-term study of lifestyle factors related to cholesterol and heart disease, included 13,000 men and no women. To this day no definitive answer exists on whether dietary change and exercise can benefit women in preventing heart disease.

- A Harvard School of Public Health study investigating the possible link between caffeine consumption and heart disease involved over 45,000 men and no women.

- Perhaps most unbelievably, a pilot project at Rockefeller University to study how obesity affected breast and uterine cancer was conducted solely on men. Said Congresswoman Olympia Snowe (R-Me.) upon hearing of this study, "Somehow, I find it hard to believe that the male-dominated medical community would tolerate a study of prostate cancer that used only women as research subjects."...

Protection or Paternalism?

The objection to women's participation in health research that is most difficult to counter is the concern over exposing a fetus to a drug or treatment that might be dangerous, or at least has not been proven safe. Recent history makes it impossible to dismiss these fears. In the 1950s the drug thalidomide, given to European women to combat nausea during pregnancy, caused thousands of children to be born with severe deformities. In this country the drug diethylstilbestrol (DES) was widely prescribed to pregnant women during the 1940s and 1950s to prevent miscarriage, but has led to gynecological cancers and other medical problems in the offspring of the women who took it.

But in their effort to expose the fetus to "zero risk," scientists have shied away from including not just pregnant women in their studies, but any woman who could potentially become pregnant.

Translated into research practice, that meant that no woman between the ages of fifteen and fifty could participate in the earliest stages of new drug research unless she had been surgically sterilized or had a hysterectomy. (And since many studies have an upper age limit of sixty-five, that leaves a narrow window of opportunity for women to participate.) Exceptions were made only in the case of extremely severe or life-threatening illnesses.

While policies to protect unborn children seem to make sense on first reading, upon closer examination they represent protectionism run amok. An increasing number of studies are showing that exposure to chemicals and environmental toxins can affect *sperm*, yet no one is suggesting that men be excluded from research in order to protect their unborn children. When Proscar, a drug used to treat enlarged prostate glands, was found to cause birth defects in the offspring of male animals given the drug, men in the drug trials simply had to sign a consent form saying they would use condoms. Women weren't given the option of using contraception during the trial. By grouping together all women between the ages of fifteen and fifty as potentially pregnant, researchers were implying that women have no control over their reproductive lives....

WOMEN'S HEARTS: THE DEADLY DIFFERENCE

Kathy O'Brien (not her real name), a forty-two-year-old smoker, had been experiencing chest pains on and off for about a year. Her father and two of her uncles had died of heart attacks when young. She went to a clinic in the rural area of northwest New Jersey where she lived, and there the local doctors told her she probably had gallstones. When the pain got worse, she went back to the clinic, where they told her she'd have to have a sonogram of her gallbladder. She left without having it done. Instead Kathy went home, collapsed from chest pain, and nearly died. She had suffered a massive heart attack and gone into cardiac arrest. Technically dead, she had to be defibrillated with electrical shocks on the way to the hospital. The following day she was transferred to a larger, teaching hospital, where doctors did an angiogram and found a blockage in a major blood vessel. After bypass surgery she recovered well. But why, wondered the cardiologists at the larger hospital, didn't anyone recognize heart disease in a heavy smoker with chest pain and a serious family history of death from heart attack?

Though it has been the leading cause of death in American women since 1908, heart disease is one of the best-kept secrets of women's health. It wasn't until 1964 that the American Heart Association [AHA] sponsored its first conference on women and heart disease....

The real topic of this conference wasn't women and heart disease, however. It was how women could take care of their *husbands'* hearts. "Hearts and Husbands: The First Women's Conference on Coronary Heart Disease" explained to women the important role they played in keeping their spouses healthy. "The conference was a symposium on how to take care of your *man:* how to feed him and make sure he didn't get heart disease, and how to take care of him if he did," explains Mary Ann Malloy, M.D., a cardiologist at Loyola University Medical Center in Chicago, and head of the AHA's local Women and Heart Disease committee. The conference organizers prepared an educational pamphlet called "Eight Questions Wives Ask." There was no discussion at all of ways for women to recognize their own symptoms or to prevent the disease that was killing more of them than any other, no mention of how women could look after their own heart health. And no one objected, including women, because, for the medical profession and the public, heart disease was an exclusively male problem.

Both physicians and the public still harbor the misconception that women do not suffer from heart disease. Yet many more women die from cardiovascular disease—478,000 in 1993—than from all forms of cancer combined, which are responsible for 237,000 deaths. Although women seem to fear breast cancer more, only one in eight women will develop it (and not all of them will die of it), while one in two will develop cardiovascular disease. And for those who persist in thinking of heart disease as a male province, in 1992 (the most recent statistics available), more women than men died of cardiovascular disease. Among women, 46 percent of all deaths are due to cardiovascular disease; in men it's 40 percent. Because heart disease tends to be an illness of older, postmenopausal women, the incidence of heart disease, and the number of deaths, have been rising as women's life expectancies have increased. "Women didn't die of heart disease when the median age of death was the fifties or sixties," says Nanette K. Wenger, M.D., professor of medicine (cardiology) at Emory University School of Medicine in Atlanta.

Yet despite these ominous numbers, the vast majority of research into coronary artery disease, the type of heart disease that causes most heart attacks, has been done on middle-aged men. "We're very much in an infancy in terms of understanding heart disease in women," says Irma L. Mebane-Sims, Ph.D., an epidemiologist at the National Heart, Lung and Blood Institute. Compared with men's hearts, women's hearts are still largely a mystery....

"IT'S ALL IN YOUR HEAD": MISUNDERSTANDING WOMEN'S COMPLAINTS

Just as the physical diseases of women are poorly understood, so, too, are a panoply of psychosomatic disorders, extremely controversial diagnoses in which emotional distresses are transferred into physical symptoms for which people then seek treatment. Somatization, as this process is known, has existed for centuries and is, to this day, remarkably common: Some 80 percent of healthy adults are believed to have psychogenic symptoms in any given week—for instance a stomachache that coincides with an important deadline or a headache that comes on after a fight with the boss....

Such a dynamic has a great bearing on women: they make up the majority of people suffering from such psychosomatic disorders as chronic fatigue syndrome, fibromyalgia, irritable bowel syndrome, and chronic pelvic pain (which

can also be the result of an organic disorder such as endometriosis). The hidden scandal is that there is no shortage of doctors who will treat women's psychogenic complaints as if they're organic in origin, often leading to a chamber of medical horrors, including an array of unnecessary surgeries instead of the treatment women may really need: help in understanding the emotional reasons for their disease.

Of course women are willing participants in their mistreatment. Resisting psychological consultation, they embark on a medical odyssey, dragging their strange array of symptoms from specialist to specialist until they find someone who will give them the one thing they desperately need: a diagnosis. "These are very beleaguered patients," says Nortin Hadler, M.D., a North Carolina rheumatologist with a particular interest in somatization. "The worst thing to happen to any patient is not to be believed. You can't get better if you can't prove you're ill."

The corollary is that, because women suffer from psychosomatic illness disproportionately and express their medical problems in a more open and emotional style compared with men, their complaints frequently *aren't* listened to—even when they're directly related to an organic disease. "The perception among many physicians is that women tend to complain a lot, so you shouldn't pay too much attention to them," says Donna Stewart, head of women's health at Toronto Hospital, a teaching hospital affiliated with the University of Toronto. As a result, many of women's *legitimate* physical ailments are not attended to, sometimes with serious consequences....

WOMEN AND DOCTORS: A TROUBLED RELATIONSHIP

Most women who visit physicians aren't aware of the lack of research into women's health, the difficulties in diagnosing women with cardiac disease, or the discrimination against women in medical school. What they *are* aware of is dissatisfaction with their physicians and with their health care in general. They base these opinions on what goes on in the doctor's office and the respect—or lack of it—they receive there. "The usual experience for a woman going to a gynecologist includes humiliation, depersonalization, even pain, and too seldom does she come away with her needs having been met," asserts gynecologist John M. Smith, M.D., author of *Women and Doctors*. And gynecologists are certainly not the only physicians guilty of this mistreatment.

Marianne J. Legato, M.D., associate director of the Center for Women's Health at Columbia–Presbyterian Medical Center, has toured the country talking with women about their experiences as patients. "The general mood is anger," she says. Women complained to her that their physicians were insensitive, uninterested, rushed, arrogant, and uncommunicative. Because women's health care is fragmented, with women seeing a gynecologist for reproductive health, an internist for a general physical, and other specialists for more specific problems, one woman told her she felt "like a salami, with a slice in every doctor's office in town."

None of this surprises Dr. Legato, who says that medicine is a mirror of the rest of society and its values. "Women, the old, the poor, children, and minority groups as a whole who haven't achieved economic power are taken less seriously and held in less regard ... which kind of leaves the emphasis on white males."

Many physicians interact with their women patients based on a view of the female sex that was already archaic decades ago. "If she's premenopausal, she is dismissed as suffering from PMS; if she's postmenopausal, then she obviously needs hormone replacement therapy; if she's a homemaker, she has too much time on her hands; if she's a business executive, then the pressure of her job is too much for her. She just can't win," writes Isadore Rosenfeld, M.D.

Medical school textbooks from only two decades ago portray women not much differently from the "walking wombs" that physicians treated in the 1800s. In this century gynecologists embraced the idea that hormones were the long-suspected link between the uterus and the brain. This theory led them to believe that a pelvic exam could help diagnose mental problems. Conditions such as painful or irregular periods, excessive morning sickness or labor pain, and infertility became indications that a woman was battling her femininity. One 1947 obstetrics textbook, still on a practicing physician's shelf, introduces a chapter on such pregnancy problems as heartburn, nausea and vomiting, constipation, backache, varicose veins, and hemorrhoids with the sentence "Women with satisfactory self-control and more than average intelligence have fewer complaints than do other women."

Things still hadn't improved by the 1970s. A 1973 study of how women were portrayed in gynecology textbooks found that most textbooks were more concerned with the well-being of a woman's husband than with the woman herself. Wrote the authors, "Women are consistently described as anatomically destined to reproduce, nurture, and keep their husbands happy." A popular 1971 ob-gyn textbook portrayed women as helpless, childlike creatures who couldn't survive sex, pregnancy, delivery, or child raising without their doctors and added, "The traits that compose the core of the female personality are feminine narcissism, masochism, and passivity."

While current textbooks seem generally more sensitive and realistic, the physicians who trained on the older books are still in practice. When *JAMA*, a leading medical journal, ran an article in 1991 about gender disparities in medical care, they received a letter from a physician in Ohio who wrote that perhaps women's "overanxiousness" about their health and their greater use of health services "may be due to temperamental differences in gender-mediated clinical features of depression, which are manifested by women's less active, more ruminative responses that are linked to dysfunction of the right frontal cortex in which the metabolic rate is higher in females." In other words women are more anxious about their health because they are somehow brain-damaged. With doctors like this, no wonder women are unhappy.

Women as Patients
Surveys show that women are more dissatisfied with their physicians than men are. And the dissatisfaction is not necessarily due to the quality of the medical care women receive, but to the lack of communication and respect they perceive in the encounter. In a 1993 Commonwealth Fund survey of twenty-five hundred women and a thousand men on the subject of women's health, women reported greater communication problems with their physicians, and were more likely to change doctors because of their dissatisfaction. One out of four women said she had been "talked down to" or treated like a child by a physician. Nearly one out of five women had been told that a reported medical condition was "all in your head."

The perception nationwide is that doctors and patients just don't understand each other. A study of one thousand complaints from dissatisfied patients at a large Michigan health maintenance organization found that more than 90 percent of the problems involved communication. "The most common complaints had to do with a lack of compassion on the physician's part," says Richard M. Frankel, Ph.D., associate professor of medicine at the University of Rochester School of Medicine and Dentistry. "Patients would complain their physician never looked at them during the entire encounter, made them feel humiliated or used medical jargon that left them confused." ...

"Women are patronized and treated like little girls," says Ann R. Turkel, M.D., assistant clinical professor of psychiatry, Columbia University College of Physicians and Surgeons. "They're even referred to as girls. Male physicians will call female patients by their first names, but they are always called 'Doctor.' They don't do that with men. Women are patted on the head, called 'dear' or 'honey.' And doctors tell them things like, 'Don't you worry your pretty little head about it. That's not for you to worry about; that's for me to worry about.' Then they're surprised when women see these statements and reactions as degrading and insulting." ...

There is also a perception among women that physicians don't take women's time seriously. How else to explain what happened to Roberta, a busy magazine editor who was on a tight deadline schedule the day of her doctor's appointment. "My office was just one city block from the doctor's office, so I called them five minutes before my appointment time to see if the doctor was running on schedule," she recalls. The receptionist assured her he was, so Roberta left her office and arrived at her appointment on time—only to be kept waiting for nearly an hour. "When I finally saw the doctor, I was practically shaking with rage, and my blood pressure was sky high," she says. Even though the doctor apologized and spent a lot of time talking with her after the checkup, Roberta decided to find another doctor.

"I think women are kept waiting longer for an appointment than men are," says Dr. Turkel. "I wouldn't go to a gynecologist who kept me waiting in the waiting room for an hour and a half, but I hear these stories all the time from women patients about their gynecologist's office."

Advice columnist Ann Landers even gave a rare interview to *JAMA* to let physicians know how dissatisfied women are with their doctors. "I can't say too often how angry women are about having to wait in the doctor's office," she said. "And, who do they complain to? The office manager, who is also a woman. Then, when the male doctor finally sees them—an hour later—the woman is so glad to see him that she soft-pedals the inconvenience. She wants to see the doctor as a 'knight in shining armor.' This should change. The doctor's time is no more important than the patient's and, while I can understand special circumstances, I can't understand why a doctor is *always* running late."

Doctors may treat women as if they are inferior patients, but studies show that they are anything but. Women tend to ask more questions—and receive more information because of their inquisitiveness. Women also show more emotion during office visits and are more likely to confide a personal problem that may have a bearing on their health to their physicians. Men, on the other hand, ask fewer questions of their physicians, give less information to the doctor, and display less emotion. During a typical fifteen-minute office visit, women ask an average of six questions. Men don't ask any....

Although physicians should be thrilled to have patients who are interested in their health, ask questions, and volunteer personal information, women's concerns are often dismissed as symptoms of anxiety, their questions brushed aside. In business, successful executives are often seen as having forceful, take-charge personalities, while women with similar attributes are described as aggressive or bitchy. In medicine, male patients seem to describe symptoms, while women complain. Instead of valuing women as active, informed patients, doctors are more likely to prefer patients who don't ask questions, don't interrupt, don't question their judgment, and—perhaps most important—get in and out of the office as quickly as possible. Researchers have actually found that physicians *like* male patients better than female ones, even when factors such as age, education, income, and occupation are controlled for.

Perhaps because of these attitudes, women often feel frustrated when they try to ask questions and receive explanations. One study reported that women received significantly more explanations than men—but not significantly more explaining *time*. Wrote the authors, "It is possible that many of the explanations they received were brief and perfunctory. Or, put differently, the men may have received fewer but fuller explanations than the women." The study also found that women were less likely than men to receive explanations that matched the level of technicality of the questions they asked. Doctors tended to talk down to women when answering their questions....

Miscommunication or Mistreatment?

Far more serious than patronizing attitudes and lack of consideration for women's time are the myths about women patients' complaints that jeopardize women's health care.

"Physician folklore says that women are more demanding patients," says Karen Carlson, M.D., an internist at Massachusetts General Hospital in Boston. "From my experience women are interested in health and prevention, desire to be listed to and treated with respect, want the opportunity to present and explain their agenda, and want their symptoms and concerns taken seriously."

But all too often women's symptoms are not taken seriously because physicians erroneously believe that these symptoms have no physical basis and that women's complaints are simply a sign of their demanding natures.

A 1979 study compared the medical records of fifty-two married couples to see how they had been treated for five common problems: back pain, headache, dizziness, chest pain, and fatigue. "The physicians' workups were significantly more extensive for the men than they were for women," reported the authors. "These data tend to support the argument that male physicians take medical illness more seriously in men than in women."

Another study found that women were shortchanged even in general checkups. Men's visits are more likely to include vision and hearing tests, chest X rays, ECGs, blood tests, rectal examinations, and urinalyses.

Dr. Carlson, speaking to a roomful of women physicians at an annual meeting of the American Medical Women's Association, cited evidence to show that women may actually complain *less* than men. "The myth is that women complain more, but studies show another truth," she says. Carlson cited studies showing that, compared with men, women with colon cancer are more likely to delay care and experience diagnostic delay. That women with chronic joint symptoms and arthritis are less likely to report pain. That women have more severe and frequent colds, but men are more likely to overrate their symptoms. That women delay seeking help for chest pain or symptoms of a heart attack. These studies point to women as being more stoic, yet when they finally do show up in the doctor's office, they are apt to be met with skepticism.

Betsy Murphy (not her real name) had been seeing the same doctor for years. "We had a perfectly fine relationship as long as I just went for my yearly checkups and didn't ask a lot of questions," she recalls. "But then I got my first yeast infection and had to go see him for a prescription—the medicine wasn't available over-the-counter then." Betsy told her doctor what she thought she had—she had talked to enough friends and read enough magazine articles to recognize the distinctive cottage-cheeselike discharge, yeasty odor, and intense itching. "But he ignored me when I told him what I thought was wrong. After he took a culture and examined it under the microscope, he sneeringly said, 'Well, Ms. Murphy, it seems as if your diagnosis is correct.'" Although he diagnosed the problem and prescribed the medication, Betsy left his office feeling insulted and patronized.

At a recent workshop on the patient-physician partnership, an auditorium full of physicians was asked how they would handle a "problem" patient. One of these "problems" was the patient who comes in and announces his or her own diagnosis. The physicians, almost unanimously, ridiculed the patient for daring to speculate what was wrong. They preferred that someone just present a description of symptoms, as specifically and articulately as possible. "It's no help for someone to come to me and say, "I have a cold and I just need some medicine,'" said a participating doctor to a journalist in the audience. "Instead the patient should describe how they feel as specifically as possible. And obviously some people are more articulate and some less; that's where the doctor's skill comes in." In other words, a patient should show up for an appointment and tell the doctor, "I have a stuffy nose and I keep sneezing," and then wait for the doctor, in his infinite wisdom, to pronounce, "You have a cold." For a patient, male or female, who is reasonably certain what is wrong, the suggestion seems ludicrous.

Women's dissatisfaction with their medical care can lead to serious health consequences. They may switch doctors so frequently that they receive no continuity of care. Or they may simply avoid seeing doctors altogether because they find the experience humiliating. When men without a regular source of health care are asked why they don't have one, they tend to reply that they don't need a doctor. But women are more apt to say that they cannot find the right doctor, or that they have recently moved, or that their previous doctor is no longer available. In the Commonwealth Fund poll, 41 percent of women (compared with 27 percent of men) said they had switched doctors in the past because they were dissatisfied. "If you brought your car in to be fixed and the person who fixed it did an okay but not great job, but was nasty, wouldn't you go to another mechanic? The same is true of physicians," says Frankel.

Physicians seem to realize there's a problem, but many of their efforts to remedy it are laughable. One 1993 article in the medical newspaper *American Medical News* advised doctors that if they wanted to make their practice "women-friendly," they should "create an atmosphere similar to that of a living room. This includes the seating, lighting and wall decorations." Yet it's difficult to imagine any woman listing "ugly wallpaper" as a reason for being dissatisfied with her health care. It's not the decor women are complaining about when they complain about doctors' offices.

Ob-gyn John Smith lists padded stirrups and speculum warmers as among the improvements women have gotten their doctors to make since the 1960s. But even those superficial improvements are not enough. What women really want are doctors who will listen to them, talk to them, and treat their medical questions and problems with respect and empathy....

THE FUTURE OF WOMEN'S HEALTH

... Despite helter-skelter improvements in the care of women, the move toward special centers, nurse-run practices, and medical school curricula in women's health suggests a larger trend: the feminization of medicine. More women than ever are entering medical school. By the year 2010 the AMA estimates that one-third of all doctors will be women.... Not surprisingly these women are bringing a feminine, and sometimes feminist, sensibility to the practice of medicine.

"Feminism is about empowering all our patients—men, women, and children —and treating them with respect," says Laura Helfman, M.D., an emergency room doctor in North Carolina. "We're doctors, we're not gods up on high." To Helfman this means taking the opportunity to do "a gentle and warm pelvic exam so I can reeducate the person receiving it that it doesn't have to be awful." To a gynecologist friend of hers it means making sure the patients never have to wait and that they always get to speak with the doctor. To a surgeon friend it means holding the patient's hand in the recovery room....

These practitioners are putting the rest of the health care system on notice. Women, both as physicians and as patients, are primed to transform the way medicine is practiced in this country. And so we celebrate the new female norm: the 60-kilogram woman. She has breasts and a uterus and a heart and lungs and kidneys. But she's much more than that. No longer a metaphor for disease, she's the model for health.... The time is right for a new woman-centered health care movement. It's the least women should demand.

NO

Andrew G. Kadar

THE SEX-BIAS MYTH IN MEDICINE

"When it comes to health-care research and delivery, women can no longer be treated as second-class citizens." So said the President of the United States on October 18, 1993.

He and the First Lady had just hosted a reception for the National Breast Cancer Coalition, an advocacy group, after receiving a petition containing 2.6 million signatures which demanded increased funding for breast-cancer prevention and treatment. While the Clintons met with leaders of the group in the East Room of the White House, a thousand demonstrators rallied across the street in support. The President echoed their call, decrying the neglect of medical care for women.

Two years earlier Bernadine Healy, then the director of the National Institutes of Health [NIH], charged that "women have all too often been treated less than equally in... health care." More recently Representative Pat Schroeder, a co-chair of the Congressional Caucus for Women's Issues, sponsored legislation to "ensure that biomedical research does not once again overlook women and their health." Newspaper articles expressed similar sentiments.

The list of accusations is long and startling. Women's-health-care advocates indict "sex-biased" doctors for stereotyping women as hysterical hypochondriacs, for taking women's complaints less seriously than men's, and for giving them less thorough diagnostic workups. A study conducted at the University of California at San Diego in 1979 concluded that men's complaints of back pain, chest pain, dizziness, fatigue, and headache more often resulted in extensive workups than did similar complaints from women. Hard scientific evidence therefore seemed to confirm women's anecdotal reports.

Men more often than women undergo angiographies and coronary-artery-bypass-graft operations. Even though heart disease is the No. 1 killer of women as well as men, this sophisticated, state-of-the-art technology, critics contend, is selectively denied to women.

The problem is said to be repeated in medical research: women, critics argue, are routinely ignored in favor of men. When the NIH inventoried all

From Andrew G. Kadar, "The Sex-Bias Myth in Medicine," *The Atlantic Monthly* (August 1994). Copyright © 1994 by Andrew G. Kadar. Reprinted by permission.

the research it had funded in 1987, the money spent on studying diseases unique to women amounted to only 13.5 percent of the total research budget.

Perhaps the most emotionally charged disease for women is breast cancer. If a tumor devastated men on a similar scale, critics say, we would declare a state of national emergency and launch a no-cost-barred Apollo Project–style program to cure it. In the words of Matilda Cuomo, the wife of the governor of New York, "If we can send a woman to the moon, we can surely find a cure for breast cancer." The neglect of breast-cancer research, we have been told, is both sexist and a national disgrace.

Nearly all heart-disease research is said to be conducted on men, with the conclusions blindly generalized to women. In July of 1989 researchers from the Harvard Medical School reported the results of a five-year study on the effects of aspirin in preventing cardiovascular disease in 22,071 male physicians. Thousands of men were studied, but not one woman: women's health, critics charge, was obviously not considered important enough to explore similarly. Here, they say, we have definite, smoking-gun evidence of the neglect of women in medical research —only one example of a widespread, dangerous phenomenon.

Still another difference: pharmaceutical companies make a policy of giving new drugs to men first, while women wait to benefit from the advances. And even then the medicines are often inadequately tested on women.

To remedy all this neglect, we need to devote preferential attention and funds, in the words of the *Journal of the American Medical Women's Association*, to "the greatest resource this country will ever have, namely, the health of its women."

Discrimination on such a large scale cries out for restitution—if the charges are true.

In fact one sex does appear to be favored in the amount of attention devoted to its medical needs. In the United States it is estimated that one sex spends twice as much money on health care as the other does. The NIH also spends twice as much money on research into the diseases specific to one sex as it does on research into those specific to the other, and only one sex has a section of the NIH devoted entirely to the study of disease afflicting it. That sex is not men, however. It is women.

* * *

In the United States women seek out and consequently receive more medical care than men. This is true even if pregnancy-related care is excluded. Department of Health and Human Services surveys show that women visit doctors more often than men, are hospitalized more often, and undergo more operations. Women are more likely than men to visit a doctor for a general physical exam when they are feeling well, and complain of symptoms more often. Thus two out of every three health-care dollars are spent by women.

Quantity, of course, does not guarantee quality. Do women receive second-rate diagnostic workups?

The 1979 San Diego study, which concluded that men's complaints more often led to extensive workups than did women's, used the charts of 104 men and women (fifty-two married couples) as data. This small-scale regional survey prompted a more extensive national review of 46,868 office visits. The results, reported in 1981, were quite different from those of the San Diego study.

In this larger, more representative sample, the care received by men and women was similar about two thirds of the time. When the care was different, women overall received more diagnostic tests and treatment—more lab tests, blood-pressure checks, drug prescriptions, and return appointments.

Several other, small-scale studies have weighed in on both sides of this issue. The San Diego researchers looked at another 200 men and women in 1984, and this time found "no significant differences in the extent and content" of workups. Some women's-health-care advocates have chosen to ignore data from the second San Diego study and the national survey while touting the first study as evidence that doctors, to quote once again from the *Journal of the American Medical Women's Association*, do "not take complaints as seriously" when they come from women: "an example of a double standard influencing diagnostic workups."

When prescribing care for heart disease, doctors consider such factors as age, other medical problems, and the likelihood that the patient will benefit from testing and surgery. Coronary-artery disease afflicts men at a much younger age, killing them three times as often as women until age sixty-five. Younger patients have fewer additional medical problems that preclude aggressive, high-risk procedures. And smaller patients have smaller coronary arteries, which become obstructed more often after surgery. Whereas this is true for both sexes, obviously more women fit into the smaller-patient category. When these differences are factored in, sex divergence in cardiac care begins to fade away.

To the extent that divergence remains, women may be getting better treatment.

At least that was the conclusion of a University of North Carolina/Duke University study that looked at the records of 5,795 patients treated from 1969 to 1984. The most symptomatic and severely diseased men and women were equally likely to be referred for bypass surgery. Among the patients with less-severe disease—the ones to whom surgery offers little or no survival benefit over medical therapy—women were less likely to be scheduled for bypass surgery. This seems proper in light of the greater risk of surgical complications, owing to women's smaller coronary arteries. In fact, the researchers questioned the wisdom of surgery in the less symptomatic men and suggested that "the effect of gender on treatment selection may have led to more appropriate treatment of women."

As for sophisticated, pioneering technology selectively designed for the benefit of one sex, laparoscopic surgery was largely confined to gynecology for more than twenty years. Using viewing and manipulating instruments that can be inserted into the abdomen through keyhole-sized incisions, doctors are able to diagnose and repair, sparing the patient a larger incision and a longer, more painful recuperation. Laparoscopic tubal sterilization, first performed in 1936, became common practice in the late 1960s. Over time the development of more-versatile instruments and of fiber-optic video capability made possible the performance of more-complex operations. The laparoscopic removal of ectopic pregnancy was reported in 1973. Finally, in 1987, the same technology was applied in gallbladder surgery, and men began to enjoy its benefits too.

Years after ultrasound instruments were designed to look inside the uterus, the same technology was adapted to search for tumors in the prostate. Other pioneering developments conceived to improve the health care of women include mammography, bone-density testing for osteoporosis, surgery to alleviate bladder incontinence, hormone therapy to relieve the symptoms of menopause, and a host of procedures, including in vitro fertilization, developed to facilitate impregnation. Perhaps so many new developments occur in women's health care because one branch of medicine and a group of doctors, gynecologists, are explicitly concerned with the health of women. No corresponding group of doctors is dedicated to the care of men.

So women receive more care than men, sometimes receive better care than men, and benefit more than men do from some developing technologies. This hardly looks like proof that women's health is viewed as secondary in importance to men's health.

*　*　*

The 1987 NIH inventory did indeed find that only 13.5 percent of the NIH research budget was devoted to studying diseases unique to women. But 80 percent of the budget went into research for the benefit of both sexes, including basic research in fields such as genetics and immunology and also research into diseases such as lymphoma, arthritis, and sickle-cell anemia. Both men and women suffer from these ailments, and both sexes served as study subjects. The remaining 6.5 percent of NIH research funds were devoted to afflictions unique to men. Oddly, the women's 13.5 percent has been cited as evidence of neglect. The much smaller men's share of the budget is rarely mentioned in these references.

As for breast cancer, the second most lethal malignancy in females, investiga-

tion in that field has long received more funding from the National Cancer Institute [NCI] than any other tumor research, though lung cancer heads the list of fatal tumors for both sexes. The second most lethal malignancy in males is also a sex-specific tumor: prostate cancer. Last year approximately 46,000 women succumbed to breast cancer and 35,000 men to prostate cancer; the NCI spent $213.7 million on breast-cancer research and $51.1 million on study of the prostate. Thus although about a third more women died of breast cancer than men of prostate cancer, breast-cancer research received more than four times the funding. More than three times as much money per fatality was spent on the women's disease. Breast cancer accounted for 8.8 percent of cancer fatalities in the United States and for 13 percent of the NCI research budget; the corresponding figures for prostate cancer were 6.7 percent of fatalities and three percent of the funding. The spending for breast-cancer research is projected to increase by 23 percent this year, to $262.9 million; prostate-research spending will increase by 7.6 percent, to $55 million.

The female cancers of the cervix and the uterus accounted for 10,100 deaths and $48.5 million in research last year, and ovarian cancer accounted for 13,300 deaths and $32.5 million in research. Thus the research funding for all female-specific cancers is substantially larger per fatality than the funding for prostate cancer.

Is this level of spending on women's health just a recent development, needed to make up for years of prior neglect? The NCI is divided into sections dealing with issues such as cancer biology and diagnosis, prevention and control, etiology, and treatment. Until funding allocations for sex-specific concerns became a political issue, in the mid-1980s, the NCI did not track organ-specific spending data. The earliest information now available was reconstructed retroactively to 1981. Nevertheless, these early data provide a window on spending patterns in the era before political pressure began to intensify for more research on women. Each year from 1981 to 1985 funding for breast-cancer research exceeded funding for prostate cancer by a ratio of roughly five to one. A rational, nonpolitical explanation for this is that breast cancer attacks a larger number of patients, at a younger age. In any event, the data failed to support claims that women were neglected in that era.

Again, most medical research is conducted on diseases that afflict both sexes. Women's-health advocates charge that we collect data from studies of men and then extrapolate to women. A look at the actual data reveals a different reality.

The best-known and most ambitious study of cardiovascular health over time began in the town of Framingham, Massachusetts, in 1948. Researchers started with 2,336 men and 2,873 women aged thirty to sixty-two, and have followed the survivors of this group with biennial physical exams and lab tests for more than forty-five years. In this and many other observational studies women have been well represented.

With respect to the aspirin study, the researchers at Harvard Medical School did not focus exclusively on men. Both sexes were studied nearly concurrently. The men's study was more rigorous, because it was placebo-controlled (that is, some subjects were randomly assigned to receive placebos instead of aspirin); the women's study was based on responses to questionnaires sent to nurses and a review of medical records. The women's study, however, followed nearly four times as many subjects as the men's study (87,678 versus 22,071), and it followed its subjects for a year longer (six versus five) than the men's study did. The results of the men's study were reported in the *New England Journal of Medicine* in July of 1989 and prompted charges of sexism in medical research. The women's-study results were printed in the *Journal of the American Medical Association* in July of 1991, and were generally ignored by the nonmedical press.

Most studies on the prevention of "premature" (occurring in people under age sixty-five) coronary-artery disease have, in fact, been conducted on men. Since middle-aged women have a much lower incidence of this illness than their male counterparts (they provide less than a third as many cases), documenting the preventive effect of a given treatment in these women is much more difficult. More experiments were conducted on men not because women were considered less important but because women suffer less from this disease. Older women do develop coronary disease (albeit at a lower rate than older men), but the experiments were not performed on older men either. At most the data suggest an emphasis on the prevention of disease in younger people.

Incidentally, all clinical breast-cancer research currently funded by the NCI is being conducted on women, even though 300 men a year die of this tumor. Do studies on the prevention of breast cancer with specifically exclude males signify a neglect of men's health? Or should a disease be studied in the group most at risk? Obviously, the coronary-disease research situation and the breast-cancer research situation are not equivalent, but together they do serve to illustrate a point: diseases are most often studied in the highest-risk group, regardless of sex.

What about all the new drug tests that exclude women? Don't they prove the pharmaceutical industry's insensitivity to and disregard for females?

The Food and Drug Administration [FDA] divides human testing of new medicines into three stages. Phase 1 studies are done on a small number of volunteers over a brief period of time, primarily to test safety. Phase 2 studies typically involve a few hundred patients and are designed to look more closely at safety and effectiveness. Phase 3 tests precede approval for commercial release and generally include several thousand patients.

In 1977 the FDA issued guidelines that specifically excluded women with "childbearing potential" from phase 1 and early phase 2 studies; they were to be included in late phase 2 and phase 3 trials in proportion to their expected use of the medication. FDA surveys conducted in 1983 and 1988 showed that the two sexes had been proportionally represented in clinical trials by the time drugs were approved for release.

The 1977 guidelines codified a policy already informally in effect since the thalidomide tragedy shocked the world in 1962. The births of armless or otherwise deformed babies in that era dramatically highlighted the special risks incurred when fertile women ingest drugs. So the policy of excluding such women from the early phases of drug testing arose out of concern, not out of disregard, for them. The policy was changed last year, as a consequence of political protest and recognition that early studies in both sexes might better direct testing.

* * *

Throughout human history from antiquity until the beginning of this century men, on the average, lived slightly longer than women. By 1920 women's life expectancy in the United States was one year greater than men's (54.6 years versus 53.6). After that the gap increased steadily, to 3.5 years in 1930, 4.4 years in 1940, 5.5 in 1950, 6.5 in 1960, and 7.7 in 1970. For the past quarter of a century the gap has remained relatively steady: around seven years. In 1990 the figure was seven years (78.8 versus 71.8).

Thus in the latter part of the twentieth century women live about 10 percent longer than men. A significant part of the reason for this is medical care.

In past centuries complications during childbirth were a major cause of traumatic death in women. Medical advances have dramatically eliminated most of this risk. Infections such as smallpox, cholera, and tuberculosis killed large numbers of men and women at similar ages. The elimination of infection as the dominant cause of death has boosted the prominence of diseases that selectively afflict men earlier in life.

Age-adjusted mortality rates for men are higher for all twelve leading causes of death, including heart disease, stroke, cancer, lung disease (emphysema and pneumonia), liver disease (cirrhosis), suicide, and homicide. We have come to accept women's longer life span as natural, the consequence of their greater biological fitness. Yet this greater fitness never manifested itself in all the millennia of human history that preceded the present era and its medical-care system—the same system that women's-health advocates accuse of neglecting the female sex.

To remedy the alleged neglect, an Office of Research on Women's Health was established by the NIH in 1990. In 1991 the NIH launched its largest epidemiological project ever, the Women's Health Initiative. Costing more than $600 million, this fifteen-year program will study the effects of estrogen therapy, diet, dietary supplements, and exercise on heart disease, breast cancer, colon cancer, osteoporosis, and other diseases in 160,000 postmenopausal women. The study is ambitious in scope and may well result in many advances in the care of older women.

What it will not do is close the "medical gender gap," the difference in the quality of care given the two sexes. The reason is that the gap does not favor men. As we have seen, women receive more medical care and benefit more from medical research. The net result is the most important gap of all: seven years, 10 percent of life.

POSTSCRIPT

Does Health Care Delivery and Research Benefit Men at the Expense of Women?

"Nobody was paying attention to women's health," says Phyllis Greenberger, executive director of the Society for the Advancement of Women's Health Research in Washington, D.C. "For years, women's health issues were ignored because the men who were making the decisions didn't think they were important." This situation may be turning around. In 1987 only 14 percent of the $5.7 billion National Institutes of Health (NIH) budget was spent on women's health research. In 1994 the NIH spent over $1.4 billion dollars on health research related to women's diseases in hopes of finding treatments and cures for osteoporosis (bone thinning), heart disease, and breast cancer. In addition to increased funding, pressure from the Congressional Caucus for Women's Issues forced the NIH, the nation's largest research funder, to include women in all applicable clinical trials of medical treatments. The Food and Drug Administration (FDA) also issued guidelines in 1993 to include women in tests of new drugs.

These reforms, however, are not welcomed by all physicians and researchers. Professor Curtis Meinert of Johns Hopkins University doubts that the new approach will uncover significant differences between the genders either in treatment or in their responses to diseases. Meinert also feels that including women in all studies will require so many additional participants that research will become prohibitively expensive. Benjamin Wittes and Janet Wittes, employees of Statistics Collaborative, a company that designs clinical trials, echo Meinert's view in "Group Therapy," *The New Republic* (April 5, 1993). This viewpoint is also held by Marcia Angell, editor of the *New England Journal of Medicine*. Angell feels that claiming important biological differences between men and women as a rule is not plausible.

The effort to quadruple federal expenditures on breast cancer research has also been criticized. Some scientists have complained that designating so much money for one disease will be at the expense of research into cures and treatment for other illnesses. An article entitled "Equality Law Could Backfire on Researchers," *New Scientist* (August 7, 1993) argues that redressing past inequities by including women and minorities more often in research could backfire.

The claim that women with chest pains or other symptoms of heart disease are treated less aggressively than men has also been disputed. A study reported in "Absence of Sex Bias in the Referral of Patients for Cardiac Catheterization," *The New England Journal of Medicine* (April 21, 1994) found that women were treated as appropriately as men for their specific conditions and that gender was not a significant factor in doctors' deciding on a course of treatment. In "Why Do Women Last Longer Than Men?" *New Scientist* (October 23, 1993), the reasons behind males' shorter life spans are discussed. Life span and longevity are also addressed in "Survey Shows Women May Live Longer, But Not Healthier Than Men," *Nation's Health* (August 1993).

Many articles, in both the popular press and the scientific literature, maintain that there is a gender bias in medicine. These include the following: "Did You Know That Women Continue to Get Shockingly Substandard Medical Care?" *Health Confidential* (January 1995); "Women's Health Falls Through the Cracks," *Shape* (April 1994); "The Neglected Sex," *American Health* (December 1993);"The High Cost of Being a Woman," *Working Woman* (November 1993); "The Identity Politics of Biomedical Research," *Siecus Report* (October/November 1993); "Gender Bias in Biomedical Research," *Journal of the American Medical Women's Association* (September 1993); "Gender Bias in Health Care," *Women Lawyers' Journal* (September 1993); "Survey Shows Poor State of Health Care Offered to Black Women in U.S.," *Jet* (August 9, 1993); "The Gender Agenda," *Economist* (March 20, 1993); "American Women's Health Care," *Journal of the American Medical Association* (October 14, 1992); "Women and Health Care: Unneeded Risks," *USA Today Magazine* (September 1992); "Examples of Gaps in Medical Knowledge Because of Groups Excluded from Scientific Study," *Journal of the American Medical Association* (vol. 263, 1990); "Where Were All the Women?" *New Scientist* (October 27, 1990); and "Medical Studies on Women Are Urgently Needed," *Glamour* (March 1990).

For an overview on women's health, see "Women's Health Issues," *CQ Researcher* (May 13, 1994), which addresses such topics as hormone therapy debates, whether or not women's health should be a separate medical specialty, breast cancer, hysterectomies, and leading causes of death for men and women. Two books on gender bias in women's health are *Women and Health Research: Ethical and Legal Issue of Including Women in Clinical Studies* by Anna Mastroianni et al. (National Academy Press, 1994) and *Unequal Treatment: What You Don't Know About How Women Are Mistreated by the Medical Community* by Eileen Nechas and Denise Foley (Simon & Schuster, 1994).

ISSUE 13

Is AIDS a Major Threat to the Heterosexual, Non-Drug-Abusing Population?

YES: William B. Johnston and Kevin R. Hopkins, from *The Catastrophe Ahead* (Praeger, 1990)

NO: Michael Fumento, from "Heterosexual AIDS: Part VII," *The American Spectator* (July 1994)

ISSUE SUMMARY

YES: William B. Johnston, a senior research fellow and the vice president of the Hudson Institute, and Kevin R. Hopkins, an adjunct senior fellow of the Hudson Institute, describe the rise of AIDS cases among heterosexuals and warn that unless people make a serious attempt to alter behaviors that put them at risk for the disease, this population will be facing an AIDS epidemic.

NO: Michael Fumento, a former AIDS analyst and attorney for the U.S. Commission on Civil Rights, claims that, despite dire predictions in the media, AIDS will not devastate white, middle-class heterosexuals and is in fact on the decline.

AIDS has been called the world's most serious health concern since the bubonic plague killed off one-third of the population of Europe in the fourteenth century. Unless there is a major breakthrough, every person with AIDS will ultimately die (unlike the plague, which some survived). Currently, there is no vaccine or cure for the disease.

It is not clear if AIDS is a "new" disease or one that has been around and has only recently begun to spread. As early as 1977 medical journals carried articles reporting on a pneumonia-like disease that affected mostly young, homosexual males. The disease, first called the "gay plague," was ultimately called "acquired immunodeficiency syndrome," or AIDS. In 1983 scientists isolated the virus responsible for the disease, which eventually became known as the human immunodeficiency virus (HIV). This virus attacks and destroys white blood cells (T-lymphocytes), which are integral to the body's immune system, and damages the body's ability to fight other diseases. Without a functioning immune system to ward off other germs, the HIV-infected person becomes vulnerable to harmful organisms that may cause life-threatening diseases, such as pneumonia.

Although HIV initially appeared to affect mostly male homosexuals, it soon began to spread to intravenous (IV) drug users, persons receiving infected blood products, and the sexual partners of HIV-infected individuals. The virus can also be transmitted to children born to infected mothers. Persons who are infected may not have symptoms of AIDS, but they are still capable of passing the virus on to others.

In the early 1980s about 150 cases of AIDS were reported in the United States. By mid-1995 over 400,000 cases and approximately 250,000 deaths from AIDS were identified by the Centers for Disease Control. AIDS has also spread throughout the world. In Africa over 1 million persons are thought to be infected, and whole villages have fallen victim to the disease. Thousands of Europeans, South Americans, and Asians also are infected with AIDS.

In Africa the disease appears to be transmitted mostly through heterosexual intercourse. In the United States, the reported number of AIDS cases spread in this manner is low. Currently, approximately 83 percent of AIDS cases are linked to either IV drug use or male homosexual behavior. The majority of cases identified as "heterosexual" are attributed to persons having sex with IV drug users.

Not everyone agrees with this analysis. In the following selections, William B. Johnston and Kevin R. Hopkins claim that heterosexually transmitted AIDS is emerging as the second stage of the epidemic. They argue that heterosexual transmission of HIV is now greater than that for homosexual and bisexual men and that, unless they are made aware of the dangers, many heterosexuals will remain at risk because they will not take appropriate precautions. Michael Fumento, in opposition, claims that the number of AIDS cases among non-drug-abusing, middle-class heterosexuals has not grown according to predictions. He argues that reports of rampant heterosexual HIV transmission are based on distorted data and exaggerations by the media.

YES

William B. Johnston and Kevin R. Hopkins

AIDS IS A SERIOUS PROBLEM FOR HETEROSEXUALS

It is distressing to note that the number of new AIDS [acquired immunod-eficiency syndrome] cases in the heterosexual transmission category is now growing more rapidly than the number of AIDS cases among gay and bisexual men. The fact that AIDS cases represent infections that took place five or ten years earlier implies that, even as early as 1980, the number of new infections transmitted among heterosexuals was growing faster than new infections transmitted among gays. It is not certain that the virus will continue to spread as fully through the heterosexual community as it has among gays. What is clear is that the spread of new infections has been proceeding at a faster pace among heterosexuals than it has among gay and bisexual men for at least the last several years.

In addition, it has become apparent recently that the incubation period of HIV [human immunodeficiency virus] may be much longer than originally thought—and thus that the AIDS case data reveal even less about the current state of the epidemic than previously acknowledged. Early reports indicated that most people infected with the virus who were going to contract AIDS would do so within four or five years, with the remainder escaping the debilitating end-state of the disease. Such a long latency period would have caused enough serious complications in using AIDS case data for planning public policy. But more recent findings are even more troublesome. Long-term studies of both homosexual men and heterosexuals infected during transfusion now place the average incubation period at nine years or more, with some people remaining free of symptoms for as long as fifteen years. Hence, people infected today might not show up on the CDC [Centers for Disease Control] AIDS register until the turn of the century, giving them well over a decade to transmit the disease to others....

SOBERING RESULTS

In addition to knowing how many people are now infected with the AIDS virus, it is important to know the distribution of infection among the various population subgroups and the rate at which the disease is spreading within these groups. The government's official position, as stated by the CDC, is that HIV infection "remains largely confined to the populations at recognized risk," including gay men, IV [intravenous] drug users, and heterosexual partners of people known to be infected with the virus.

In the absence of repeated, nationally representative sero-prevalence studies, it is impossible to say definitely whether this optimism is warranted. But there are ways to test the thesis that AIDS and HIV infection are not much of a heterosexual problem—and the results are both surprising and sobering....

The CDC breaks down AIDS case data by sex, race, age, sexual orientation, and presumed means of contracting the virus. Extreme care must be taken in using this disaggregated data, however, particularly with regard to the means by which the AIDS victim is supposed to have contracted the disease. The CDC employs a hierarchical assignment scale that places homosexual contact and drug use at the highest levels. That is, any male AIDS victim who has ever had sex with another man, even once, is generally regarded as having contracted the disease homosexually, and any person who has recently used IV drugs, even once, is generally regarded as having been infected through the IV drug route —regardless of the extent and riskiness of that person's heterosexual activities.

As a result, at least some of those people assigned by the CDC to the gay and IV drug use transmission categories actually may have received the virus through heterosexual contact. While the potential number of such misidentified cases is not large, neither is it trivial. As of mid-1988,

as many as 3.5 percent of AIDS cases attributed to other factors (i.e., gay sex or IV drug abuse) theoretically could have resulted from heterosexual intercourse—a figure, if all cases were misclassified, that would be as high as the entire category of officially recognized heterosexual transmission cases. And even this is a minimum estimate, since the CDC's risk category for "heterosexual contact" is not identical to engagement in heterosexual activity. Rather, the CDC's category includes sex only with AIDS patients or those "at risk" for AIDS (e.g., IV drug users or persons from countries with a high incidence of AIDS)—a very small share of possible heterosexual partners. The category makes no allowance for an AIDS victim's heterosexual contact with people who did not fall into these tightly defined "risk groups," even though these other people also may have been infected and may have been transmitting the virus. Thus, the CDC heterosexual contact category is a rock-bottom estimate of heterosexual transmissions that lead to AIDS. It may understate true heterosexual transmissions by a considerable degree, perhaps by as much as half or more.

A second and more frequently noted source of error in accounting for heterosexual transmissions lies in the "undetermined" group of AIDS cases. This category "includes patients on whom risk information is incomplete (due to death, refusal to be interviewed, or inability to follow up), patients still under investigation, men reported only to have had heterosexual contact with a prostitute, and interviewed patients for whom no specific risk was identified." Most of these people may have been infected by routes other than heterosexual contact, although outside experts estimate that as many as one-sixth to one-third actually were the result of heterosexual intercourse. In any case, it is fair to say that, in assessing the heterosexual dimensions of the epidemic, the CDC has taken the most cautious course possible, excluding virtually everyone from the overtly labeled heterosexual category who possibly could have been infected otherwise—and even excluding those for whom no other obvious infection route could be identified.

HETEROSEXUALS WITH AIDS

But there is a much larger issue, one that is less often recognized. Even if correctly calculated, the number of heterosexually *transmitted* AIDS cases (i.e., people who contracted the disease through heterosexual contact) is not the same thing as the number of heterosexuals *with* AIDS (those people whose primary sexual outlet is heterosexual regardless of how they received the virus). In fact, excluding gay men, who constituted some 63 percent of AIDS cases reported as of mid-1989, the vast majority of the remaining AIDS patients (IV drug abusers, hemophiliacs, transfusion cases as well as heterosexual contact cases) were heterosexuals. And at least some of those men classed as having received the disease through homosexual contacts were predominantly heterosexual in practice. Taking these factors into account, and adjusting the AIDS data for delays in reporting, reveals a sizable heterosexual HIV problem: among the adjusted total of AIDS cases diagnosed through the end of 1988, nearly one-third were heterosexuals. While only about 17 percent of total AIDS cases among whites were heterosexuals, more than half of all minority AIDS cases—some 57 percent of blacks and 52 percent of Hispanics—came from among heterosexuals.

The point is that these people, no matter how they contracted the disease, can pass it on to other heterosexuals. One cannot draw comfort from the small size of the CDC's "heterosexual contact" transmission category for AIDS, not only because it undercounts the number of AIDS cases actually resulting from heterosexual contact, but because it greatly understates—almost by an order of magnitude—the number of heterosexuals who *have* AIDS. William A. Haseltine of Boston's Dana-Farber Cancer Institute has observed, "The infections may not have been acquired by heterosexual sex. However, the patients themselves are heterosexual. To this must be added the statement that most of the people who currently have AIDS and who are heterosexuals have been infected for about ten years and have been transmitting the virus to their partners throughout this period." . . .

A conservative estimate shows that slightly less than half of all infections by the end of 1988 were among gay men, who accounted for some 70 percent of whites with HIV but only 24 percent of blacks and 28 percent of Hispanics. The converse of course, is also true: *about half of all HIV infections have occurred among heterosexuals, with the overwhelming share of infections among minorities taking place among heterosexuals.* Moreover, the number of new infections per year among gay men has fallen by nearly 50 percent since 1984, making theirs a rapidly declining share of the overall epidemic.

By contrast, heterosexual intravenous drug abusers are one of the fastest growing segments of the infected population. Already, as of the end of 1988, they comprised more than one-third of all infected persons. The great majority of these infected drug users were blacks and His-

Figure 1

Heterosexual Contact With Persons With, or at High Risk for, HIV Infection

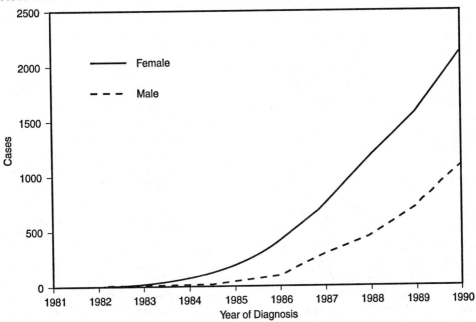

Source: Centers for Disease Control, *Morbidity and Mortality Weekly Report*, June 7, 1991.

panics, with only about a quarter being white. Still, the rate of increase in *new* infections among this group already appears to be slowing down. The number of new infections among drug users may well peak within the next few years, so this group will represent a declining share of the overall epidemic of HIV infection as well.

As serious as this pattern of infection is among gay and bisexual men and IV drug users, it is becoming even more severe among non-drug-using heterosexuals. In total, a best estimate is that there were at least 630,000 heterosexuals infected with HIV as of the end of 1988— a number several times the top-range CDC estimate, and vastly above the most frequently quoted CDC estimate of 30,000 non-hemophiliac, non-drug-

using infected heterosexuals (which is, of course, a much more restrictive measure). To be sure, most of these 630,000 or so heterosexual infections (some two-thirds) have occurred among IV drug users, although that does not change the fact that these people can transmit the disease by heterosexual contact. But the number of infections among heterosexuals who do not use IV drugs is far from minor— a best estimate of nearly 200,000 people. Some 52 percent of these heterosexuals are poor, some 67 percent minorities, and some 67 percent men.

MAINSTREAM POPULATION

These characteristics aside, a substantial number of these people—a best estimate of more than 86,000—are members of the so-called "mainstream" heterosexual population. They are not poor, and they are not IV drug users. Moreover, the number of new infections per year among all non-drug-using heterosexuals has risen by more than three times since 1983, making this group as well one of the fastest growing segments of the HIV-infected population. As Haseltine points out, "AIDS is already a heterosexual problem" in the United States.

How did the spread of HIV infection become so pervasive throughout the heterosexual community? In statistical terms, the answer is simple: as noted, a substantial share, some one-third, of already diagnosed AIDS cases are among heterosexuals, and these represent only a small number of the far larger group of heterosexuals who have been infected but who have not yet come down with AIDS. Moreover, unlike the gay and IV drug-using communities, whose numbers are relatively small, the sexually active heterosexual population is extremely large. And because of the high incidence of divorce and dissolution of other monogamous relationships, heterosexuals move frequently into and out of the pool of sexually active persons, even if they are at times insulated from the virus through celibacy or monogamy.

There also are numerous avenues by which heterosexuals can become infected. Many gay or bisexual men have sex regularly with heterosexual women as well as with men and can infect women in this way. Many otherwise sexually conventional men engage in intercourse with female prostitutes, who generally exhibit high levels of HIV infection. Infected IV drug-using heterosexuals have as sex partners other heterosexuals, many of whom are not IV drug users. Indeed, a study confirms not only that this transfer of HIV infection from drug users to non-users is occurring, but that it is taking place among the middle class as well as the poor, where the majority of drug users apparently are concentrated.

AN UNAVOIDABLE EPIDEMIC

Finally, heterosexuals have sex with other heterosexuals. As with the spread of the disease in the gay community, all that is needed for a self-perpetuating epidemic is for a sufficient number of the most sexually active members of a population to be infected and to pass the virus on to others before they become ill and die. If studies such as that by William Masters, Virginia Johnson, and Robert Kolodny are anywhere near accurate—that is, if as many as 5 to 14 percent of the most sexually active heterosexuals are carriers of the virus—then a breakout of the disease into the nonmonogamous heterosexual population is more than a theoretical possibility. It is almost unavoidable unless dramatic behavioral change or medical progress takes place soon.

NO

Michael Fumento

HETEROSEXUAL AIDS: PART VII

The AIDS [acquired immunodeficiency syndrome] epidemic has peaked—and not everyone wants you to know about it. Especially not the media, which have taken recent CDC [Centers for Disease Control] reports to proclaim yet again that AIDS is exploding, especially among heterosexuals. To quote CNN:

> The number of new AIDS cases in the United States grew even faster than anticipated last year. The Centers for Disease Control and Prevention had expected a 75 percent increase partially because of a new expanded definition of the disease. New AIDS cases actually jumped 111 percent last year because of a sharp increase in infections among heterosexuals.... AIDS resulting from heterosexual contact in 1993 rose 130 percent.

Meanwhile, "NBC Nightly News" reported that "a broader definition of AIDS, [and] a sharp increase in infections among heterosexuals, more than doubled the number of new cases." *Time* said. "The number of new AIDS cases surged unexpectedly last year, more than doubling, owing to a jump in infections among heterosexuals." *Newsweek* jumped in to proclaim that "heterosexual AIDS is no myth," and talk-show host Vicki Lawrence told her audience that 170,000 teenagers had been diagnosed with AIDS in 1991 and 1992. (The actual number was 318.)

Far from a "jump" caused by heterosexual infections, the entire increase in the CDC's findings was due to the expanded definition. By the old definition of AIDS, there was a 2 percent *decrease* in new AIDS cases last year. This is long-awaited news and a monumental relief, but most of the press virtually ignored it: Lawrence Altman in the *New York Times* allowed it part of a sentence on the 107th line of his story.

* * *

The CDC findings appeared in two articles in the agency's official *Morbidity and Mortality Weekly Report*. The first, by John Ward, chief of the surveillance branch, division of HIV/AIDS at the CDC, described the effects of the new case definition. The second, by Pat Flemming, chief of reporting and analysis in the CDC's AIDS division, begins with this sentence, "From 1991 through 1992, persons with [AIDS] who were infected with human immunodeficiency virus (HIV) through heterosexual transmission accounted for the largest proportionate increase in reported AIDS cases in the United States." Note the dates: "1991 through 1992." The new case definition only applied to 1993 cases. Like the horror movie mad scientist who combined man and beast to create a monster, the media spliced the two sets of data together to come up with the latest heterosexual AIDS scare.

Taking each set of data separately, we see that this latest alarm is just as groundless as the ones sounded every year since 1987. While it's true that heterosexual cases did jump 130 percent in 1993, a table in Ward's article shows clearly that the intravenous drug abuser category increased by 136 percent. The largest percentage increase was in the hemophiliac category, which shot up 189 percent.

But headlines like "AIDS Spreading Fastest Among Hemophiliacs" not only don't sell newspapers, they knock down the notion that the heterosexual increase, large as it appears to be, can be attributed to a "sharp increase in infections." That's because hemophiliac infections ceased altogether after 1985, when their clotting factor began to be heat-treated for blood transfusions. If the hemophiliac cases could jump 189 percent with no infections in the past seven years, then clearly the heterosexual jump also has no connection to new infections.

So what's the explanation? Despite the *New York Times's* flat-out assertion that "the new definition does not affect the rate of increase by heterosexual transmission," the CDC data showed that it changed everything. For one thing, the expanded definition added a test whereby persons whose T-cells fall below a certain number are considered to have AIDS. (T-cells are white blood cells that protect the body from infection; generally speaking, the fewer one has the more susceptible one is to deadly infections.) The result is that cases that wouldn't have been diagnosed until 1994 or 1995 were diagnosed in 1993.

Moreover, the definition added three new indicator diseases that, when accompanied by HIV, will prompt an AIDS diagnosis. The new diseases—pulmonary tuberculosis, recurrent pneumonia, and invasive cervical cancer—are found much more often in non-homosexuals than in homosexuals, just as Kaposi's sarcoma is found almost exclusively in homosexuals. Cervical cancer, of course, is strictly a disease of women. The T-cell test has also disproportionately expanded non-homosexual cases because the original indicator diseases tended to be matched to the course of disease in homosexuals, whereas the T-cell depletion affects all AIDS victims.

* * *

Pat Flemming's assertion that heterosexuals accounted for the largest proportionate increase in new infections during 1991–1992 is another failed effort to portray the old and well-explained as something new and mysterious. The heterosexual transmission category has *always* been the fastest-growing, for two simple reasons. First, it's mathematically easier to grow the fastest, in percentage terms, from a low baseline. In other words, if the Eskimo and Mexican populations of Houston in 1992 were two and 50,000 respectively, and in 1993 two more Eskimos moved to town along with 10,000 more Mexicans, the Eskimo increase would be 100 percent while the Mexican increase would be only 20 percent. No one would point to these data as indicating that Houston would shortly be swamped with Eskimos.

The other reason heterosexual cases comprise a larger proportion of the epidemic is that all epidemics, from bubonic plague to smallpox to polio, follow a bell-shaped curve whereby the epidemic's rate of increase is fastest early on, then it progresses at a slower and slower rate until it peaks and cases actually start to decline. Since heterosexual cases lag by a couple of years behind homosexual and intravenous drug abuser cases, they are further down on the upside of that slope. Indeed, by 1992, homosexual cases were already sliding down the right side of the bell curve. Thus, even if heterosexual transmission cases had been exactly the same number as the year before—or even slightly less—as a percentage of the epidemic their share would still have grown.

Prior to the new definition, the trend toward a peaking of heterosexual cases was quite clear. In the early 1980s, heterosexual cases increased by over 100 percent per year. But by 1990, heterosexual cases had increased only 39 percent over the previous year, by 1991 21 percent, and by 1992 only 17 percent. Suddenly there's a 130 percent jump in heterosexual cases.

Not incidentally, this same reasoning also applies to female AIDS cases. Because their numbers are small and because female cases lag behind male ones, female cases have always been increasing more rapidly than male ones. This doesn't stop the media from announcing each and every year, however, that *this* year women's cases are increasing faster than men's. Indeed, it is common to see this presented, as the *Washington Post*'s Boyce Rensberger did last year in a front-page story, in such a way as to make it seem that women now have a greater chance of getting the disease than men. Rensberger wrote: "Last week the [CDC] reported that American women of all ages were coming down with AIDS four times as fast as men." What the CDC actually said was that the *rate of increase* among women was four times greater, the reason being that the rate of increase among men had dropped to almost nothing. But male cases continued to come in at a rate eight times that of female cases.

*　*　*

Did reporters deliberately confuse the two sets of data released by the CDC? Pat Flemming told me that she had fielded over a hundred media phone calls since her article was released. Since she freely acknowledged that the two sets of data were incompatible, there's no reason to believe she would have misled reporters. (Lawrence Altman at the *New York Times* would not return my calls.)

Interestingly, a Nexis search conducted two weeks after the Flemming report's release turned up not a single dissenting reference to the latest heterosexual AIDS myth. By contrast, after a National Research Council (NRC) report last year said AIDS would remain a disease of "marginalized" minorities, the media were filled with critical responses. In its determination to democratize this disease, the press gives little play to its increasing racial and ethnic ghettoization —even within the heterosexual cohort. Charges of racism and homophobia flew. But the NRC was right: Of the 1993 heterosexual contact diagnoses, 78 percent were in black and Hispanic males and 74 percent in black and Hispanic females, even though these groups together comprise only about 20 percent of the population.

If the CDC's new definition has the fingerprints of AIDS activists all over it, that shouldn't surprise: they'd be the first to take credit. As one ACT-UP [AIDS Coalition to Unleash Power] pamphlet notes, "ACT-UP and many public health professionals realized that [the-then] definition was too narrow and pressured the CDC to change it." It continues: "Under activist pressure, CDC announced a proposed expansion of the AIDS definition in the summer of 1991." The Associated Press recognized the activists' influence in this headline two years ago: "CDC Bows to Activists; Adds New Diseases to Proposed AIDS Definition." As the A.P. story noted, "Activists welcomed the proposal, saying it would mean diagnoses for thousands of HIV-infected women and drug users." It was just a matter of time before the new definition pressed for in 1991 became reality in 1993.

* * *

It is also no coincidence that the new definition and its expansion of the heterosexual categories took effect the year that AIDS diagnoses would have otherwise leveled off. Indeed, the latest statistics reveal that the government's projections of an AIDS epidemic increasing on into the late 1990s—along with all the projections of the other AIDS doomsayers —have proved hopelessly wrong. More than that, there was never any reason to think they would be right, as I observed fully five years ago in the May 1989 TAS [The American Spectator].

That article challenged the then-current estimate of HIV infection of one to 1.5 million, citing a large body of infection data and the failure of full-blown AIDS cases to manifest as quickly as would be needed to justify such a number. I proffered instead a lower figure of 500,000–800,000 calculated by Dr. Joel Hay, now of the University of Southern California. For his efforts, Hay was derided by AIDS projectionists at the CDC and elsewhere.

But lo! the next year the CDC did lower its estimate to one million. Yet even that number was too high: last December, authors of the first nationwide survey of AIDS infections estimated that 550,000 Americans were infected. While saying that they thought the figure might be a bit low, the CDC did grant that its one million estimate was too high. As CDC official Dr. Scott Holmberg explained, "Because more than 200,000 people have died of AIDS, we would expect that the current prevalence is below one million." Indeed, the word is out, reported by Lawrence Altman himself, that the CDC is about to lower its official estimate to 800,000. At a glance, Holmberg's explanation makes sense. The problem is, it ignores the impact of the purported new infections that the CDC says are coming in at a rate of 40,000 a year, slightly higher than the highest number of AIDS deaths in any year. By Holmberg's reckoning, the one million figure should actually have been *increasing*, not plummeting.

In 1988 the CDC extended its projected caseload figure to the end of 1993, predicting 450,000 cases by then. The press went wild over the figure, upping it sometimes to half a million. The editor of the Washington Post's Health magazine declared, "No one is questioning the projection that about 450,000 Americans will be diagnosed with AIDS by 1993." But Hay and I and others did question it. Indeed, I cited the CDC's own data indicating that since it appeared that HIV infections peaked around 1991 and 1992 in major cities, the epidemic would peak about ten years later, since lag time from infection to full-blown disease averages about ten years. Now we find that at the end of 1993, even including the new case definition, the CDC projection was too high by about 90,000 cases. Without the new case definition, it would have been too high by fully 50 percent.

My 1989 article also anticipated that the CDC would start talking less and less about its projections "unless CDC keeps expanding the definition of AIDS to catch earlier and earlier stages of HIV infection." And so it did, casting the best news of the epidemic as an utter disaster. Americans have been effectively prevented from learning that in the same year in which the Clinton administration increased AIDS spending by 28 percent —cutting the budget of most every other disease except breast cancer—AIDS cases fell by 2 percent. (The president's proposed budget for next year again favors just these two diseases.)

AIDS remains a horrible disease with no hope of cure on the horizon. A declining epidemic by no means indicates that it is about to end any time soon. Nonetheless, an AIDS campaign that emphasizes heterosexual contact can no more succeed than can a breast cancer detection campaign that singles out men or a prostate cancer program that focuses on men under 30. AIDS prevention efforts can succeed only if the public is told who is at greatest risk, who is at least risk, and what those at greatest risk can do to reduce their peril.

POSTSCRIPT

Is AIDS a Major Threat to the Heterosexual, Non-Drug-Abusing Population?

AIDS was not officially diagnosed until the early 1980s. By that time, doctors had begun noticing rare cancers in young, male homosexuals. Other diseases, such as pneumonia and meningitis, had also begun to disproportionately affect male homosexuals and intravenous (IV) drug users. It wasn't until 1985, however, that President Ronald Reagan ever mentioned the word *AIDS*, even though the number of cases and AIDS-related deaths had risen to epidemic proportions. Finally, in 1986, Surgeon General C. Everett Koop issued a report on the AIDS virus and sent educational materials about AIDS to every household in the United States. Critics claimed, however, that had the government begun AIDS education and research sooner, many lives would have been saved. The late columnist Randy Shilts, in his book *And the Band Played On* (St. Martin's Press, 1987), agreed that the government knew about the AIDS epidemic years before anything was done about it.

Is there an epidemic-to-be among middle-class, non-drug-abusing heterosexuals that is currently being ignored? In 1991 Earvin "Magic" Johnson, the celebrated basketball superstar for the Los Angeles Lakers, disclosed that he was HIV positive. Johnson said that he contracted the disease through heterosexual contact. Is Johnson an early victim of an impending heterosexual AIDS epidemic? Suzanne Fields, a columnist for the *Washington Times*, would say no. In "Misrepresenting AIDS," *Washington Times* (August 17, 1986), Fields claims that AIDS is still primarily related to high-risk behavior practiced by specific population groups. Michael Fumento concurs. For more of Fumento's views on AIDS, see *The Myth of Heterosexual AIDS* (Basic Books, 1990); "Teenaids": The Latest HIV Fib," *The New Republic* (August 10, 1992); and "Media, AIDS, and Truth," *National Review* (June 21, 1993).

AIDS has generated thousands of articles and books since the disease was first diagnosed. Two articles that discuss AIDS among minorities are "The Homecoming: Paranoia and Plague in Black America," *The New Republic* (June 5, 1995) and "The White Cloud: Latino America's Stealth Virus," *The New Republic* (June 5, 1995). The following articles offer several different viewpoints on the seriousness of the epidemic and the government's response to AIDS: "Has AIDS Won?" *New York Magazine* (February 20, 1995); "AIDS: Trends, Predictions, Controversy," *Nature* (June 3, 1993); "Women and AIDS,"*CQ Researcher* (December 25, 1992); "AIDS So Far," *Commentary* (December 1991); "AIDS Poses a Classic Dilemma," *The New York Times* (February 10, 1987);

"AIDS: A Crisis Ignored," *U.S. News & World Report* (January 12, 1987); "AIDS and a Duty to Protect," *Hastings Center Report* (February 1987); "The AIDS Epidemic Has Hit Home," *Psychology Today* (April 1987); and "The Judgement Mentality," *Christianity Today* (March 20, 1987).

PART 5

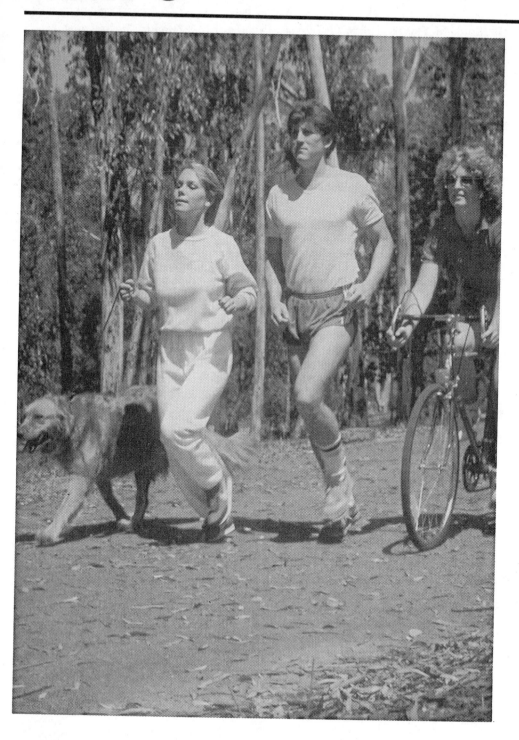

Nutrition and Health

Recently, millions of health-conscious individuals have begun exercising, dieting, and swallowing vitamin pills in an effort to lose weight, prevent disease, and maintain health and well-being. While most physicians support dietary changes and moderate exercise, critics claim that many people who follow diet and nutrition fads may actually develop nutritional deficiencies or a dieting mind-set and increase their risk of physical complications from dieting itself. This section debates some of the controversies that surround diet and nutrition claims.

- Is Yo-Yo Dieting Dangerous?

- Can Large Doses of Vitamin C Improve Health?

ISSUE 14

Is Yo-Yo Dieting Dangerous?

YES: Frances M. Berg, from *Health Risks of Weight Loss*, 3rd ed. (*Healthy Weight Journal*, 1995)

NO: National Task Force on the Prevention and Treatment of Obesity, from "Weight Cycling," *Journal of the American Medical Association* (October 19, 1994)

ISSUE SUMMARY

YES: Nutritionist Frances M. Berg contends that yo-yo dieting, or weight cycling, is associated with an elevated risk of physical and mental health problems and that it increases the risk of regaining lost weight.

NO: The National Task Force on the Prevention and Treatment of Obesity maintains that there is no convincing evidence that weight cycling has any major effects on heart disease risk, the effectiveness of future diets, increased percentage of body fat, or metabolism.

Dieting has become a way of life for many people; close to 50 million Americans are currently dieting. But most will not lose as much weight as they want, and most will not keep off the weight they have lost. So why are so many Americans dieting?

Obesity has become widespread in the United States: 30 percent of the population is considered obese, up from 25 percent 10 years ago. Obesity has been linked with increased risks for certain diseases, including diabetes, heart disease, and some cancers. In addition, there are social and economic implications related to obesity. Many contend that overweight people are less likely to marry, earn less money, and are less likely to be accepted to elite colleges. As a result, more and more people are dieting.

It has been shown that most diets fail. Often, after lost weight is regained, dieters start over again and end up caught in a repeated lose/gain cycle known as "yo-yo dieting" or "weight cycling." Yo-yo dieting is considered by experts to be more dangerous than actually being overweight, and many urge overweight individuals to stop dieting and accept themselves as they are. Some theories as to why yo-yo dieting may be unsafe are that yo-yo dieting lowers metabolic rate, or the rate at which calories are burned; that yo-yo dieting increases the percentage of stored fat and reduces lean muscle tissue; that a lowered metabolic rate and an increase in fat stores can make subsequent dieting more difficult; and that yo-yo dieting may increase one's desire for fatty foods.

Frequent dieting has also been linked with psychological concerns. Some studies have reported a lower level of life satisfaction among weight cyclers. There is also some evidence that frequent dieting may predispose an individual to disordered eating, including binge eating, or compulsive overeating. Research also indicates that among all dieters, both obese and of normal weight, anxiety, depression, and stress are associated with the up-and-down weight cycling that accompanies frequent dieting. These studies conclude that those who maintain a stable weight are better off psychologically, regardless of what they weigh.

Researchers have discerned a relationship between yo-yo dieting and an increased risk of heart disease based on findings from the Framingham Heart Study, a 30-year analysis of weight fluctuations in over 3,000 adults. The study indicated that weight gain or loss in a short period of time increases the risk of a person's dying from heart disease.

Since evidence suggests that most diets fail and that many actually increase the risk of subsequent failure in dieting, is it safer to remain overweight than to try to lose weight? Recent research shows that it *is* more dangerous to remain overweight than to try to lose extra pounds. On the other hand, there is no evidence that *all* diets fail. Some people do lose and maintain weight, although the numbers and dieting methods are unclear. There are also important medical benefits associated with even modest weight loss, including improvements in blood pressure, blood fats (cholesterol), and blood sugar control.

In the following selections, Frances M. Berg asserts that dieting, especially yo-yo dieting, is more dangerous than being overweight. She maintains that people with a history of weight cycling have shown increased stress levels—even those who gained and lost as little as five pounds. The National Task Force on the Prevention and Treatment of Obesity argues that among obese individuals, the benefits of even moderate weight loss are significantly greater than any risks associated with dieting.

YES   Frances M. Berg

WEIGHT CYCLING

The possible risks of repeated bouts of losing and regaining weight, called weight cycling or yo-yo dieting, have gained wide attention in the public press. And for good reason: if weight cycling is harmful and is the almost inevitable result of weight loss, then perhaps weight loss itself is harmful and weight loss an inappropriate goal even for large patients, placing more importance on prevention.

This possibility has major implications for the $30 to $50 billion weight loss industry and for the focus of health care in the United States.

Weight cycling has been under intense investigation at several institutions in the U.S. and other countries since 1986, following studies that suggested losing weight on a very low calorie diet and regaining that weight made subsequent weight loss more difficult.

However, research has shown inconsistent results on several issues. This has led some researchers to conclude weight cycling is not important. Others believe the variables have not yet been found which affect weight cycling changes—perhaps certain subgroups are more likely to be affected, or individuals are more vulnerable at times in their lives, such as during pregnancy.

The Diet and Health report of the National Academy of Sciences notes the possible detrimental effects of weight cycling. Similarly, the Surgeon General's Report on Nutrition and Health recommends that "the health consequences of repeated cycles of weight loss and gain" be given "special priority," and a poll of obesity experts lists weight cycling as one of the key causes of obesity.

There is little doubt that weight cycling is extremely prevalent in the U.S. Sixty to 80 million people are trying to lose weight, and most of those who lose weight apparently regain it fairly quickly.

In a review of weight cycling research, Kelly Brownell and Judith Rodin cite a six-year study which tracked the weight of 153 middle-aged adults and found the women lost an average of 27 pounds and gained 31 pounds during the six years. The men lost and gained an average of more than 22 pounds. For the women, this was a gain of 21 percent of their initial body weight, and a loss of 19 percent. For the men it was about 12 percent lost and gained.

Another study tracked 332 overweight persons and found the vast majority either lost or gained significant amounts of weight.

Weight cycling research focuses on two major issues:

1. Is weight cycling associated with increased risk to physical or mental health?
2. Does weight cycling make weight management more difficult by invoking survival mechanisms?

Major concerns have been raised that cycles of weight variability increase risk factors and the risk of mortality, especially cardiovascular deaths. Other concerns are that weight cycling may lower metabolic rate, decrease the ability to lose weight, increase the body's fat-to-lean ratio and waist-hip ratio, and increase the appetite for dietary fat.

CYCLING MAY THREATEN HEART

Research consistently shows an increase in mortality from all causes and from coronary heart disease with weight cycling.

Weight cycling is associated with greater risks for coronary heart disease and other severe health problems in a major study published recently in the *New England Journal of Medicine* by L. Lissner and colleagues.

The findings are based on a 32-year analysis of weight fluctuations in 3,130 men and women in the Framingham Heart Study.

Individuals with a high weight variability—many weight changes or large changes—were 25 to 100 percent more likely to be victims of heart disease and premature death than those whose weight remained stable. They had increased total mortality, and increased mortality and morbidity due to coronary heart disease.

The relative risk for a high degree of weight variability compared with 1.0 for a low degree of variability is as follows:

Men

Total mortality 1.30

Mortality due to CHD 1.48

Morbidity due to CHD 1.48

Morbidity due to cancer..... 1.04

Women

Total mortality 1.27

Mortality due to CHD 1.47

Morbidity due to CHD 1.42

Morbidity due to cancer..... 1.16

These results seemed to hold true regardless of the individual's initial weight, long-term weight trend and/or cardiovascular risk factors such as blood pressure, cholesterol level, glucose tolerance, smoking and physical activity.

Even though nearly 50 percent of women who diet are not overweight, the researchers note, the weight cycling risks are seen at all weight categories, whether thin or obese.

The degree of weight variability was evaluated in relation to total mortality, mortality from coronary heart disease, morbidity due to coronary heart disease and morbidity due to cancer. Risks were considerably increased for all except cancer, which did not differ significantly.

When age groups were considered separately, weight fluctuation was most strongly associated with adverse health outcomes in the youngest group (age 30 to 40). This is also the group seen as most likely to diet.

The researchers found that a person's weight at age 25 makes an important contribution to whether there will be great variability.

Both men and women gained weight at an average rate of .11 kg per square meter per year.

Researchers from Goteborg, Sweden, and Boston University are involved in the current study. They cite their research in Sweden which found large fluctuations in body weight, measured at three intervals, was associated with heart disease in men and total mortality in both men and women.

In an effort to control for weight changes that may have been caused by illness, diseases and deaths for the first four years were excluded. This study does not distinguish between several weight changes and a single large weight change.

The researchers say weight cycling may account for the observed increase in deaths in these ways:

1. Factors that influence coronary risk (such as cholesterol levels) may change with fluctuating weight and end up worse than before.
2. The amount and distribution of body fat as weight is lost and regained may change. During weight loss, a person loses both fat and lean body mass, but may regain mostly fat. This fat tends to settle in the abdomen, a location linked to increased heart disease risk.
3. People may increasingly prefer high-fat diets when they lose and regain weight. Studies have shown that weight-cycling laboratory animals tend to eat more fat.

In view of their findings, they suggest it may be important to look at public health implications of current weight loss practices. They note that about half of American women and one-fourth of men are dieting at any one time, with many of these efforts unsuccessful. Weight is commonly regained and the cycle repeated.

Kelly Brownell, PhD, a psychologist and weight specialist at Yale University involved in the study, says the harmful effects of weight cycling may be equal to the risks of remaining obese.

"The pressure in this society to be thin at all costs may be exacting a serious toll," Brownell says. The study's findings indicate that weight cycling is "potentially a very serious public health issue" because it affects such large numbers of people.

"It may be equally bad to lose the same five pounds 10 times as to lose 50 pounds and regain it once," he said.

The relative risk of increased risk with weight fluctuation is in the range of 1.25 to 2.00, which is similar to the risk attributed to obesity and to several of the cardiovascular risk factors, say Brownell and Rodin. Thus, determining weight cycling effects is an important question.

HARVARD ALUMS RISK DISEASE BY "ALWAYS" DIETING

Men risk heart disease, hypertension and diabetes by 'always' dieting, regardless of their weight, according to the Harvard Alumni studies reported by Steven N. Blair, an epidemiologist at the Cooper Institute for Aerobics Research in Dallas.

"One of the fundamental tenets of the weight loss industry is if you get people to eat less, they'll lose weight. And if they lose weight, they'll be better off. And there is no evidence to support either one," Blair said at the American Heart Association's annual epidemiology meeting in March 1994.

Earlier, Blair reported higher mortality with weight loss among the Harvard alumni. His latest report investigates non-fatal disease in 12,025 men, average age 67. The men who said they were always dieting had a heart disease rate of 23.2 percent, compared to 10.6 for those who "never" dieted. Their rates for hypertension were 38.3 percent, compared with 23.4 percent for the group who never dieted, and for diabetes 14.6 percent, compared with 3 percent.

Among men who dieted part of the time—"often," "sometimes," or "rarely" —the more they dieted, the higher their rates of disease. These findings held true even among the leanest group of men, and were basically unchanged by weight gain, physical activity, smoking or alcohol intake.

In addition to reporting dieting frequency, the men identified their shape variation at six points through life, total pounds lost, and the number of times they had lost 5, 10, 20 and 30 or more pounds.

In view of his findings, Blair advises people to keep a stable weight and avoid either weight gain or weight loss.

BONE LOSS WITH WEIGHT LOSS

Several studies of large population bases show higher mortality rates with weight loss, causing researchers to puzzle over the possible mechanisms whereby weight loss could cause long-term harm, even though it seems beneficial in reducing obesity-related risk factors in short-term studies.

One possible mechanism may be the bone mineral loss which accompanies weight loss. Weight cycling may increase this loss.

Mineral content in women's bones diminishes with weight loss, even when adequate nutrition and aerobic exercise are present. These findings from the USDA Human Research Center in Grand Forks, N.D., support clues which may explain recent findings in federal studies of potentially higher mortality with weight loss. The Grand Forks Center tested 14 women, age 21–38, in a five-month residential program using dual energy x-ray absorptiometry (DXA) to assess bone mineral status and soft tissue composition. The women lost 8.1 kg on a moderate nutrient-adequate diet with an aerobic exercise program. Both bone mineral content and bone mineral density decreased (36 g and .01 g/cm2 respectively).

Similar results were found at the Osteoporosis Research Centre in Copenhagen, Denmark. Using the DXA method, the study reports 51 obese patients averaged a 5.9 percent loss of total body bone mineral/TBBM during 15 weeks. One patient, who lost 45 kg, lost 754 g bone mineral in nine months. Greater mineral loss was reported in legs than arms. Post-menopausal women who did not get estrogen replacement tended to lose more bone mineral. Bone mineral loss correlated with body fat loss, not with fat-free mass loss, so that as more fat was lost, more mineral was lost as well.

When patients maintained their weight loss, they lost no more bone. If they regained, bone was regained as well. The Danish researchers concluded this level of bone loss was normal for weight loss in obese persons. They suggest an initiating factor in bone loss may be having less weight bearing on the bones.

WEIGHT CYCLING DROPS METABOLISM FOR WRESTLERS

Weight cycling is practiced with single-minded dedication by many high school and college athletes in the sport of wrestling.

Not only must the elite wrestler be talented, fit and superbly trained, but usually he is also actively engaged in weight reduction, even in the lower weight classes of 103 and 112 pounds.

The weight-cycling wrestler commonly loses 10 or more pounds in a few days to make weigh-ins for a match or tournament. He regains this weight quickly, and repeats the cycle many times throughout the wrestling season. Severe water deprivation and dehydration are often a part of his fasting episodes.

Long term effects of such strenuous weight loss efforts on the young wrestler are unknown.

Cold intolerance, weakness, and inability to concentrate are frequently reported. Other reported effects include changes in electrolyte balance, testosterone levels, nutritional status, renal function, thermal regulation, body composition and strength.

Growth and development may be delayed during one of the most active growth periods of a young man's life. The possibility of developing long-lasting eating disorders has been suggested.

FOOD EFFICIENCY

Metabolic effects of this severe weight cycling may cause an increase in food efficiency, and make losing more difficult.

Recent research with high school wrestlers on loss-and-gain cycles gives evidence of a lowered metabolism, as reported in the *Journal of the American Medical Association.*

The wrestlers were attending summer camp at the University of Iowa. It was several months after their last competitive match, and their weight had returned to normal.

The group of 27 wrestlers who cycled their weight were found to have significantly lower resting metabolic rate per unit of lean body mass than those defined as noncyclers.

Weight cyclers were defined as those who:

1. Cut weight 10 or more times during wrestling season.
2. Lost 4.5 kg or more weekly.
3. Reported they cut weight often or always.

Noncyclers

1. Cut weight less than 5 times during the season.
2. Lost no more than 1.4 kg weekly.
3. Reported they cut weight sometimes, rarely or never.

Noncyclers were matched for age, weight, height, surface area, lean body mass, and percent body fat.

The cyclers competed farther below their natural off-season weight than did the noncyclers.

Results showed a significant difference in resting metabolic rate between the cyclers and noncyclers. The difference in resting energy expenditure was 14 percent. Oxygen consumption differed significantly. No differences were shown in respiratory quotient, oral temperature, pulse or blood pressure.

STUDIES NEEDED

The researchers suggest weight cycling was a likely cause of lower metabolic rates, although they grant it is possible that low metabolism came first and even made the severe cycling necessary, as wrestlers with low energy requirements could have had more difficulty controlling weight. They recommended longitudinal studies be conducted to assess any health changes resulting from weight restriction and fluctuation.

Although the body fat for both groups of wrestlers in this study is similar, an increase of fat over lean has been noted during fast weight regain, and a redistribution of fat is suggested as possible. Research is cited that shows increased preference for fat in the diet among weight cycling female rats.

The researchers speculate there may be psychological implications of repeated weight cycling, including frustration over the increasing difficulty in losing weight, which could lead to unhealthy methods of weight loss.

The high school or college wrestler differs from the typical weight cycler in the general population in that he is young, male, physically active, well-muscled, with low body fat. His diet and binge cycle is relatively short, usually lasting about three months a year for perhaps three to six years.

Psychologically, as a successful athlete, he is likely to have high self-esteem and strong social support.

Strong statements against excessive weight loss and the fluid and food deprivation practices often used by wrestlers have been issued by the American College of Sports Medicine and the American Medical Association.

Hank Lukaski, director of the Grand Forks Center, says people have the potential to regain some bone loss when they regain weight. But it is unknown whether bone mineral content and bone density are fully or only partially restored, or whether bone quality is as good as before, or how essential trace elements are affected. Further, the effect on bone quality of repeated bouts of weight loss and regain are unknown, Lukaski says.

WEIGHT CYCLING
INCREASES STRESS

People with a history of weight cycling showed greater pathologic characteristics than those with stable weights, independent of weight, in recent research by John Foreyt, PhD, of Baylor College of Medicine, Houston, TX, and colleagues at Yale and the University of Nevada. The researchers suggest that weight cycling may be causal to the mental distress and pathology they found.

Men and women whose weight fluctuated up or down, as little as five pounds in a year, reported lower feelings of well-being, more out-of-control eating, and higher stress levels than people whose weight was stable in this study. And this was true regardless of their body weight.

The researchers say they did not expect such a large number of significant findings with the tight five-pound categories: "Psychologically, such small shifts in weight in both normal weight and obese individuals may be very important."

In obese women, weight maintenance was associated with fewer significant negative life stressors.

Weight fluctuation was strongly associated with negative psychological effects in both normal weight and obese individuals. Weight change and obesity were also associated with a poorer psychological score.

The researchers studied 497 adults, stratified into five age groups, 25 normal weight and 25 obese in each age and sex category.

The subjects were assessed twice with the Brownell Weight Cycling Questionnaire, which measures current dieting, weight satisfaction, abnormal eating patterns and body image. They reported on health, weight fluctuation, feelings of well-being and depression, stressful life events, and eating self-efficacy (ability to control urges to overeat in high-risk situations). Their weight was assessed over one year to classify them, through a weight change of 5 pounds or more, as maintainers, gainers or losers.

The researchers suggest that attempts at weight loss may be stressful for various reasons, including the self-denial required, the disruption of routine, and a concern about failure. Repeated failures to control weight may reduce one's feeling of self-efficacy, and add to feelings of depression.

"Once inappropriate dieting is initiated, regardless of body weight, fluctuations and increasing obesity may follow," says their report. They cite research that shows that among obese individuals, more than half fluctuate up or down 12 pounds over intervals of 1 to 5 years.

While the researchers suggest that weight change likely causes these adverse effects, they grant the reverse is possible—psychological distress may cause weight change. They recommend further research on assessing and treating weight fluctuation for individuals of all weights.

Weight cycling appears consistently linked to increased psychopathology, lower life satisfaction, more disturbed eating in general, and perhaps increased risk for binge eating in the research, Brownell and Rodin report.

They cite research by Everson and Matthews that found lower levels of life satisfaction related to increased weight cycling in women, but not men. A study of a large sample of runners found weight cycling associated with higher levels of disturbed eating practices. Other studies show repeated or chronic dieting may predispose an individual to disordered eating, including binge eating. One study showed restrained eating (dieting) to be a stronger predictor of weight fluctuation than body weight itself.

FINDINGS STIR CONTROVERSY

The recent findings are likely to be controversial and to further fuel the weight cycling debate among scientists, says Claude Bouchard, PhD, of Laval University, Quebec, in an editorial in the same issue of the *New England Journal of Medicine* as the Lissner study.

Bouchard notes that a recent review of 18 studies of weight cycling in rodents, by Hill and Reed, found no clear evidence that weight cycling makes future weight loss harder and weight gain easier.

They found no evidence that weight cycling increases total body fat or central adiposity, increases subsequent caloric intake, increases food efficiency, decreases energy expenditure, or increases blood pressure, insulin resistance, or cholesterol levels. However, Bouchard suggests there may be a preference for dietary fat in refeeding and that the observed risks could result from higher fat intake.

Rat studies may not provide the weight cycling information needed for humans and, given that human studies are difficult to design, this may be why weight cycling studies give such confusing and conflicting results, says Carolyn Berdanier, PhD, a researcher at the University of Georgia.

Berdanier says rats and mice differ from humans in several important ways. Most critically to weight cycling research, they continue to grow in length throughout their lives. This growth is expensive in calories, and affects the degree of body fat storage, keeping them leaner.

NO

National Task Force on the Prevention and Treatment of Obesity

WEIGHT CYCLING

Weight cycling refers to the repeated loss and regain of weight. When weight cycling is caused by repeated attempts at weight loss, it is popularly known as "yo-yo dieting." Regrettably, with currently available dietary treatments for obesity, many people who lose weight will later regain it. Repeated bouts of weight loss and regain are distressing both to patients and their caregivers, making the search for ways to prevent the development of obesity and for more effective means of long-term maintenance of utmost importance. Much attention has been focused by both the lay press and professional literature on possible physiological and psychological hazards of weight cycling. Standard texts of nutrition and dietetics now present the detrimental effects of weight cycling as established fact. Some have suggested that remaining obese may be preferable to undergoing repeated failed attempts at permanently reducing body weight. The purpose of this article is to address concerns about the effects of weight cycling and to provide guidance on the risk-to-benefit ratio of attempts at weight loss, given current scientific knowledge.

METHODS

Original reports were obtained through MEDLINE and psychological abstracts searches for 1966 through 1994 on weight cycling, yo-yo dieting, and weight fluctuation, supplemented by a manual search of bibliographies. Forty-three English-language articles that evaluated the effects of weight change or weight cycling on humans or animals were reviewed in depth. Studies of human subjects were emphasized. Cited studies were reviewed by experts in the fields of nutrition, obesity, and epidemiology to evaluate study design and the validity of the authors' conclusions based on the published data....

From National Task Force on the Prevention and Treatment of Obesity, "Weight Cycling," *Journal of the American Medical Association*, vol. 272 (October 19, 1994), pp. 1196, 1198–1201. Copyright © 1994 by The American Medical Association. Reprinted by permission. References omitted.

DEFINING WEIGHT CYCLING

Much of the confusion about the effects of weight cycling and the inconsistencies in the outcomes of studies attempting to clarify its effects can be traced to the lack of a standardized definition for weight cycling. At its simplest, the definition of a single weight cycle may seem intuitively obvious: a loss followed by a gain (or vice versa). However, the multiple factors involved in both the definition and measurement of weight cycling are formidable, particularly when the clinically important variables are not yet known. Such confusion is reflected in the multiple definitions of weight cycling found in both cross-sectional and prospective studies seeking to determine metabolic and psychological effects of weight cycling and in observational population-based studies with a primary goal of determining mortality. Although the term "cycling" suggests a more regular pattern of weight change than the more general term "fluctuation," the two are often used interchangeably.

Providing a clinically relevant measure for weight cycling encompasses many components. How many cycles are involved? Is a loss followed by a gain similar in effect to a gain followed by a loss? What is the magnitude of weight change in each cycle? Are several small cycles more or less detrimental than one or two large cycles? What about the duration of each weight cycle? Is a loss that is maintained for 1 year and then regained of greater or less benefit than one that is only maintained for 6 months? Do any detrimental effects of weight cycling on health come about only years after the cycling occurs, or are adverse effects more likely soon after the weight change occurs? Is the effect of a cycle caused by intentional weight change the same or different from a cycle that occurs unintentionally? In which populations (if any) does cycling exert its deleterious effects—in women, in men, in normal-weight vs obese individuals, in ethnic minorities? Despite the numerous studies of weight cycling available, these fundamental questions remain unanswered.

Even such basic information as the normal degree of weight fluctuation during short periods in nonclinical populations is currently unknown. For example, among nine normal-weight women who were recruited as "noncyclers" for an observational study on the basis of self-reports of "rarely or never" dieting and stable weight within 2.3 kg during 5 years, four women experienced weight fluctuations of more than 2.3 kg once or twice during the course of three measurements during 1 year. In a retrospective chart review of 332 overweight adults in a general medical population, Williamson and Levy found significant weight fluctuation. Of all subjects, 34% lost weight (mean, 5.3 kg; SD, 4.8 kg) and 66% gained weight (mean, 5.7 kg; SD, 4.8 kg) between two visits 1 to 5 years apart. Studies to determine the prevalence, magnitude, and frequency of weight fluctuation in the general population are therefore needed. Cutter et al have recently critically analyzed the multiple issues involved in the definition of weight cycling and have proposed that the number of weight cycles be used as the primary measure, using an arbitrary minimal threshold (eg, 2.3 kg [5 lb]) as a cycle (G. R. Cutter et al, unpublished data, 1994). Currently, however, no single definition of weight cycling can be endorsed, and studies should attempt to measure multiple components of weight change with the aim of further clarifying clinically important components.

CONCERNS ABOUT WEIGHT CYCLING

Most concerns about the adverse effects of weight cycling fall into three major areas: the effects on metabolism and weight loss, on morbidity and mortality, and on psychological well-being.

Influence of Weight Cycling on Metabolism

There have been numerous studies that have examined the effects of repeated loss and regain of weight on metabolism and body composition. In 1986, Brownell et al reported that weight-cycled rats showed an increased food efficiency and that weight cycling made weight loss harder and weight regain easier. The authors hypothesized that animals may regain more body fat in relation to lean body mass during each weight cycle, leading to progressive increases in body fat content relative to total weight. Reed and Hill critically reviewed the published literature on weight cycling in rodents and concluded that the existing data did not support the hypothesis that weight cycling promoted obesity, increased body fat, or had permanent effects on metabolism. In fact, the majority of available data suggest that weight cycling in animals does not independently affect any parameter of energy balance (food intake, body composition, or energy expenditure). For example, although it is commonly contended that weight cycling in animals reduces fat-free mass and increases body fat over time, most investigators have reported that weight cycling does not increase body fat or relative adiposity compared with controls. Although the few reports of adverse metabolic effects of weight cycling have been widely quoted both in the lay press and scientific literature, Reed and Hill have described limitations in many of these studies, including choice of control groups, paradigms for producing weight cycling, and effects of gender and aging. They concluded that most, if not all, claims of adverse effects due to weight cycling were not based on strong experimental evidence.

The implication of reports of possible detrimental effects of weight cycling in animals prompted research on the problem in humans. These studies included small prospective trials that evaluated metabolic effects of weight loss in obese women, as well as studies in persons repeating a weight loss program. In one widely cited study, 57 individuals repeating a very low-calorie diet program had a significantly lower rate of weight loss during their second attempt. However, there was a great deal of intersubject variability in time (68 to 2860 days) and in percentage of weight regained (5% to 440%) between diets. Intervening factors, such as changes in body composition with age, make interpretation of the results difficult. In addition, although the authors made attempts to study only adherent patients, differences in compliance to the dietary regimen, particularly among outpatients, may have been a factor in their findings. Smith and Wing found that subjects had significantly worse dietary adherence when repeating a very low-calorie diet program.

Furthermore, other studies have found no relationship between the number of previously reported weight loss cycles and the efficacy of weight loss. Although one study showed that weight-cycling wrestlers had a lower resting metabolic rate than noncycling wrestlers, the cross-sectional nature of this study makes it unclear whether cycling reduced the metabolic rate or whether those whose baseline energy expenditure was low gained weight easily and therefore needed to engage more frequently in efforts to reduce their body weight. Other cross-sectional and prospective studies have not found differences in energy efficiency between cyclers and noncyclers among athletes, nonobese women, or obese women when adjusted for differences in weight and/or lean body mass. Although Manore et al found that cyclical dieters had a lower energy expenditure (per kilogram of body weight) during exercise than weight-stable controls, their weight-cycling subjects were both significantly heavier and fatter than controls, making appropriate comparisons difficult. Lissner et al studied the relationship between weight cycling and metabolic rate in 846 men participating in the Baltimore Study of Aging. They found no evidence that body weight fluctuation was associated with depression in basal metabolic rate; in fact, individuals with the highest variability in body weight had the smallest decreases in metabolic rate over time, whether adjusted for body surface area or for lean body mass.

In addition, neither body composition (percentage of fat vs nonfat tissue) nor body fat distribution appears to be adversely affected by history of weight cycling in humans, independent of body mass index (BMI) (calculated by dividing the weight in kilograms by the square of height in meters). Prentice et al found no detrimental effects on lean body mass as a result of "natural" annual weight cycling in a population of Gambian men. Prospective and cross-sectional studies have generally failed to find differences in body composition between weight cyclers and noncyclers among the obese, those of normal weight, or wrestlers who frequently cycle to "make weight."

Paradoxically, McCargar et al found that the percentage of body fat during three test periods 6 months apart was more stable in cycling than in noncycling normal-weight women.

Because visceral adipose tissue deposition is associated with a variety of adverse health outcomes, the effect of weight cycling on visceral fat deposition is clinically relevant. In a cross-sectional study, Rodin et al found a higher waist-to-hip ratio, often used as a surrogate marker for increased visceral fat deposition, among "high" as compared with "low" weight-cycling women. However, BMI, which is known to be correlated with waist-to-hip ratio, was not adequately controlled for in this study. Lissner et al found an association between body weight variability and increased ratio of subscapular-to-triceps skinfold thickness, suggesting that fluctuators might have greater increases in truncal adiposity. However, the absence of an increased waist-to-hip ratio suggested that the truncal fat deposition they observed did not appear to favor upper vs lower body obesity. In a study of weight-cycling wrestlers, the fat lost during peak season was found to be preferentially lost from the trunk compared with noncycling controls, although no differences existed between groups by off-season. Other studies have found no difference in body fat distribution between weight cyclers vs noncyclers. Anthropometric measures, such as skinfold measurements and body circumferences, do not differentiate between visceral and subcutaneous abdominal fat depots, in contrast with computed tomography and magnetic resonance imaging. When visceral fat measured via magnetic resonance imaging in 14 cycling vs 14 noncycling nonobese and mildly obese women, no difference in visceral adipose tissue deposition existed between groups, although subcutaneous adipose tissue deposition was slightly greater in cyclers. Similar results were observed in a prospective study of obese men and women who underwent one cycle of weight loss and regain during the course of a year.

In summary, the majority of studies did not find a higher prevalence of unfavorable body fat distribution among weight cyclers, and there was no evidence that weight cycling led to increased visceral adipose tissue deposition. In a review of the literature on weight cycling in humans, Wing concluded that most studies showed no adverse effects of weight cycling on body composition, resting metabolic rate, body fat distribution, or future successful weight loss, and subsequently published studies tend to support this conclusion.

Influence of Weight Cycling on Morbidity and Mortality

The potential effects of weight cycling on long-term morbidity and mortality are of greater concern. A number of large population-based observational studies have shown increased risks of variations in body weight for all-cause and cardiovascular mortality, whereas two smaller studies showed no such effect. In some of these studies, variation in weight appeared to be associated with increased mortality, even after control for coronary heart disease risk factors and preexisting disease that might influence weight. In addition to weight cycling, weight loss over time has been found to be associated with increased mortality, even when care has been taken to exclude for smoking and preexisting illness.

These observational studies, however, have several limitations. Only one of these studies attempted to distinguish intentional from unintentional weight loss. In that study, a history of voluntary dieting, although associated with a higher coefficient of variation of body weight, did not predict mortality. None of these studies controlled for variability in body composition and fat distribution, which are known to influence both morbidity and mortality. In addition, the myriad ways in which weight cycling was defined in these studies makes between-study comparisons difficult. For example, use of the coefficient of variation of weight may not be the best means to determine cycling, because this measure is more sensitive to single large changes in weight, rather than frequent small changes. As previously discussed, it is unknown if differences in frequency of weight cycling or amount of weight change per cycle influences outcome. Other potential causes of weight change, such as depression, which significantly affects weight change during long-term follow-up, have rarely been assessed. In fact, general psychological well-being appears to be associated with weight stability rather than weight gain or loss, although assumptions cannot be made about causality.

Finally, mechanisms by which weight cycling might affect mortality in humans remain unexplained. Although studies of changes in cardiovascular risk factors in animals with weight cycling have yielded inconsistent results, human studies have not demonstrated any mechanism by which weight cycling increases risk of cardiovascular disease. In a study of 202 obese men and women, Jeffery et al found no evidence that a history of weight cycling worsened cardiovascular risk factors. Similarly, the majority of cross-sectional and prospective studies have not demonstrated associations between weight cycling and increases in blood pressure, fasting blood levels of glucose or insulin, impaired glucose tolerance measured by oral glucose tolerance test or glycohemoglobin, dyslipidemias or alterations in fat metabolism including fat cell size, basal or stimulated lipolysis, and lipoprotein lipase activity. Schotte et al found no association between weight cycling and glycemic control in 327 men with non–insulin-dependent diabetes mellitus, although differences in the need for hypoglycemic medications may have obscured differences in metabolic control. Holbrook and colleagues, in a study of older adults, found that both self-reported weight gain and weight fluctuation between ages 40 and 60 years were associated with an elevated relative risk (RR) for diabetes mellitus, as evaluated by oral glucose tolerance test. However, a history of dieting to control weight during this time was not associated with increased risk for diabetes. One study did find an association between body weight variability and decreased glucose tolerance after an oral glucose tolerance test, but the magnitude of the increase in plasma glucose (1 mg/dL [0.05 mmol/L] for every 1-kg deviation about the slope) was only about half the size of the effect of 1-kg weight gain per year on glucose tolerance. Although concerns have been raised about the possibility of weight cycling leading to increased fat consumption, the majority of studies in humans have not shown an association between weight cycling and fat preference or fat consumption.

The majority of subjects in population-based observational studies were either nonobese or only mildly obese (BMI<30). If weight cycling has deleterious effects on health, such effects may be limited to those who are not obese. Blair and associates, in an analysis of data from the Multiple Risk Factor Intervention Trial, found that the increased mortality associated with body weight variability was limited primarily to men in the lowest tertile for BMI (<26.08). Similarly, in a study that examined the effects of weight loss on morbidity and mortality, Pamuk and colleagues found that the increase in RR for mortality with weight loss was primarily limited to those in the bottom two tertiles for weight (BMI <29). Among women in the top tertile for weight, all-cause mortality was elevated only among those losing more than 15% of their total body weight. Among men, RR for death was not increased with any degree of weight loss. Moderate weight loss (5% to 14% of initial body weight) was actually associated with reduced cardiovascular mortality among men in the highest tertile for weight. In addition, the proportion of individuals reporting intentional weight loss is greater in obese than in lean individuals. Therefore, weight cycling and weight loss may have both differing causes and effects in obese and nonobese individuals, and caution should be taken in applying the findings of population-based studies to obese patients. The National Institutes of Health Technology Assessment Conference statement on methods for voluntary weight loss and control advised that the data on long-term adverse health consequences of weight cycling, while provocative, were not sufficiently conclusive to dictate clinical practice. This recommendation appears to be appropriate until better data become available.

Psychological Effects of Weight Cycling
Repeated failed attempts at permanent weight loss are obviously distressing. Anecdotes abound regarding the negative effects of such failures on mood and self-esteem. Unfortunately, few well-controlled studies have assessed the impact of weight cycling on psychological functioning. Those that have are generally cross-sectional and cannot distinguish between negative effects of weight cycling and preexisting psychological factors that may predispose individuals to repeatedly lose and regain weight. Currently, scientifically valid data on the psychological effects of weight cycling are not available. Determination of the psychological impact of weight cycling requires further study.

HEALTH RISKS OF OBESITY

In contrast to weight cycling, obesity is associated with increased risks of morbidity and mortality. Furthermore, the biological bases of the increased risk have been well described. Both cross-sectional and cohort studies have shown strong associations between obesity and hyperlipidemia, hypertension, and hyperinsulinemia, leading to an increased prevalence of coronary artery disease and non–insulin-dependent diabetes mellitus. Studies have also clearly documented the amelioration of these conditions with modest weight loss. Certain types of cancer, degenerative joint disease, sleep apnea, gout, and gallbladder disease are also more prevalent with increasing obesity. The economic cost attributable to obesity-related illness has been estimated to exceed $39 billion yearly. The elevations in RR for these conditions are particularly striking in younger adults. One study found that the presence of obesity in adolescent males was associated with increased mortality as long as 50 years later, independent of adult weight. Not all individuals with a given weight or degree of obesity have the same risk for medical complications. Prognostic factors, including gender, amount and location of excess body fat, family history, and the presence of risk factors such as hyperlipidemia, play a role in determining an individual's risk of obesity-related conditions. Evaluation of such risk should determine whether weight loss treatment is medically necessary, as well as the type and intensity of any intervention.

RECOMMENDATIONS FOR FUTURE STUDIES ON WEIGHT CYCLING

Unfortunately, designing studies to correct for the deficiencies identified in this article is exceedingly difficult. For example, even if the issue of voluntary weight loss were to be addressed, not all confounding variables could be adequately controlled. With 40% of all women and 25% of all men in the United States reporting attempts to lose weight at a single point in time, who are the individuals who actually change their weight? Those who consider themselves "chronic" dieters or always on a diet are not necessarily those who lose weight. Unsuspected illness, psychological dysfunction, or deterioration in a known medical condition may contribute to weight change, even in those already attempting weight loss. A randomized, controlled long-term trial weight loss or weight cycling vs weight stability or gain would be extraordinarily complex in design, as well as prohibitively expensive. Thus, innovative approaches to the use of available databases and small-scale clinical studies are needed to determine answers to this important but difficult question.

Descriptive, population-based studies to determine the natural history of weight fluctuation and patterns of weight change in the general population may help to better define the normative level of weight fluctuation and aid the development of a clinically useful definition of weight cycling. Studies examining health risks of weight cycling in obese populations are also needed, particularly because there is some evidence that any adverse effects of weight cycling may be blunted in those at the greatest medical risk for obesity. Animal and human studies that might elucidate putative mechanisms for adverse effects of weight cycling (such as change in fatty acid profile of various tissues would be useful. The roles of physical activity, smoking, stress, and alcohol intake in creating weight cycles also deserve further study.

CONCLUSIONS

Based on the currently available data, we conclude the following:

- There is no convincing evidence that weight cycling in humans has adverse effects on body composition, energy expenditure, risk factors for cardiovascular disease, or the effectiveness of future efforts at weight loss.

- The currently available evidence regarding increased morbidity and mortality with variation in body weight is not sufficiently compelling to override the potential benefits of moderate weight loss in significantly obese patients. Therefore, obese individuals should not allow concerns about hazards of weight cycling to deter them from efforts to control their body weight.

- Determination of the psychological impact of weight cycling requires further investigation.

- Individuals who are not obese and who have no risk factors for obesity-related illness should not undertake weight loss efforts, but should focus on the prevention of weight gain by increasing physical activity and consuming a healthful diet as recommended by the *Dietary Guidelines for Americans*.

- Although conclusive data regarding long-term health effects of weight cycling are lacking, obese individuals who undertake weight loss efforts should be ready to commit to lifelong changes in their behavioral patterns, diet, and physical activity.

POSTSCRIPT

Is Yo-Yo Dieting Dangerous?

The issue of dieting involves the public, health providers, the media, and the diet and food industry. On one hand is the cultural pressure to maintain or achieve a lean body, which is supported by a diet industry valued at more than $30 billion per year that supplies diet foods, books, programs, and videos. On the other hand are health professionals and an increasing number of people among the general public who recognize the growing numbers of obese individuals and their potential health problems but who are concerned that dieting, especially repeated dieting, may have harmful consequences on health and well-being.

The questions remain: Is it better for an overweight person to remain overweight than to yo-yo diet? Does yo-yo dieting increase the probability of regaining lost weight? Is repeated dieting a risk factor for eating disorders and other psychological problems? And is yo-yo dieting linked to heart disease and premature death? Many articles discuss the potential harm related to yo-yo dieting. In "Change in Body Weight and Longevity," *Journal of the American Medical Association* (October 21, 1992), researchers I-Min Lee and Ralph S. Paffenbarger, Jr., report that individuals who cycle between being overweight and normal weight during their lifetime may die sooner than they would if they maintained a steady weight. Other articles concluding that it is more dangerous to diet than to remain overweight include "Yo-Yo Dieting Revisited," *Harvard Heart Letter* (February 1995); "The Great Diet Deception," *USA Today Magazine* (January 1995); "Theories on Yo-Yo Dieting," *Tufts University Diet and Nutrition Letter* (December 1994); "Weight Management," *Better Nutrition for Today's Living* (July 1994); "Quit Watching the Scales," *Consumer Reports on Health* (May 1993); "End Yo-Yo Dieting," *Muscle & Fitness* (February 1993); "Ups and Downs of Dieting May Court Heart Disease," *Environmental Nutrition* (January 1993); "The Dangers of Yo-Yo Dieting," *Total Health* (September/October 1992); and "Rethinking Diets: Breaking the Cycle of the Yo-Yo," *Vogue* (March 1992).

While many studies have found relationships between health problems and yo-yo dieting, there is also a body of research indicating that yo-yo dieting is *not* related to heart disease, decreased metabolism, or an increase in body fat. Some researchers have also found little or no evidence that repeated dieting makes subsequent efforts at weight loss more difficult. Articles arguing that yo-yo dieting is not as harmful as previously thought and that it is better to keep trying to lose weight include "Coasting Downhill," *Prevention* (March 1995); "Yo-Yo Diets Aren't Risky After All," *Health* (January/February 1995); "Don't Let Fears of Yo-Yoing Stop Before You Start," *Environmental Nutrition*

(December 1994); "Yo-Yo Diets May Beat No Diets at All," *U.S. News & World Report* (October 31, 1994); and "Weight Cycling Reviewed," *Obesity & Health* (January/February 1993).

For an overview of weight cycling see "Medical, Metabolic, and Psychological Effects of Weight Cycling," *Archives of Internal Medicine* (June 27, 1994); "Weight Cycling: The Public Concern and the Scientific Data," *Obesity Research* (September 1993); and "Weight Cycling in Humans: A Review of the Literature," *Annals of Behavioral Medicine* (vol. 14, 1992).

While the experts are not in agreement over which is more harmful, yo-yo dieting or remaining overweight, there is further conflict regarding whether or not it is even possible—or advisable—to lose weight. There are also questions over whether or not dieting is the best treatment for obesity. For further information on dieting in general, see "Dieting and Health: Is Dieting the Best Way to Lose Weight?" *CQ Researcher* (April 14, 1995); "The Dieting Maelstrom: Is It Possible and Advisable to Lose Weight?" *American Psychologist* (September 1994); "Consequences of Dieting to Lose Weight: Effects on Physical and Mental Health," *Health Psychology* (vol. 13, 1994); and "Losing Weight: What Works, What Doesn't," *Consumer Reports* (June 1993).

ISSUE 15

Can Large Doses of Vitamin C Improve Health?

YES: Patricia Long, from "The Power of Vitamin C," *Health* (October 1992)

NO: Victor Herbert, from "Does Mega-C Do More Good Than Harm, or More Harm Than Good?" *Nutrition Today* (January/February 1993)

ISSUE SUMMARY

YES: Patricia Long, a journalist who specializes in health issues, presents evidence showing that vitamin C may combat heart disease, aging, birth defects, and cancer. She also suggests that people would benefit from higher levels of vitamin C than those currently recommended by the government.

NO: Physician and attorney Victor Herbert acknowledges that humans have a need for small amounts of vitamin C, but he maintains that megadoses of the vitamin may harm more people than they help.

In 1970 Nobel Prize winner and chemist Linus Pauling (1901–1994) published a book entitled *Vitamin C and the Common Cold,* in which he maintained that huge doses, or "megadoses," of vitamin C can prevent colds by protecting body cells from attack by cold viruses. Pauling believed in taking one or two grams (1,000–2,000 milligrams) of vitamin C per day, which is about 20–40 times the recommended amount. In 1976 Pauling published the second edition of his book, *Vitamin C, the Common Cold and the Flu,* in which he suggested taking even higher doses than he did in the first edition.

Many controlled studies on vitamin C and colds have been performed since Pauling's controversial book first came out. Taken together, they show that the effects of vitamin C, if any, are statistically very small. This does not exclude the possibility that the effects on *some* individuals might be considerable, especially if their vitamin C intakes have previously been low. Research on such effects is not easy to conduct, because people tend to be influenced by what they believe will be the effects of their medicine. In one now-classic study on the effects of vitamin C, for example, a questionnaire given at the end revealed that participants who received placebos (inert substances) and who thought they were being given vitamin C had fewer colds than the subjects who actually received vitamin C.

In addition to the common cold, Pauling also suggested that vitamin C megadoses might be an effective treatment against cancer. However, careful research involving the administration of 10 grams of the vitamin per day to persons with advanced cancer has shown no difference in these patients' symptoms or survival time as compared to patients who were given a placebo.

Although the medical establishment has ridiculed Pauling, recent research has shown that vitamin C and vitamin E together appear to be able to inactivate toxic chemicals in the body known as "free radicals." Free radicals, a byproduct of normal metabolism in cells, create problems by damaging the body's genetic material (DNA), altering biochemical compounds, damaging cell membranes, and killing cells. This chemical destruction is believed to play a major role in diseases such as cancer, heart disease, and even premature aging. Vitamins C and E may help reduce the damage from free radicals by inactivating these dangerous chemicals.

Most experts believe that a balanced diet can provide enough vitamins to meet our needs. A balanced diet, however, consists of at least three to five servings of vegetables and two to four servings of fruit daily, which is currently consumed by less than 9 percent of Americans. For the remaining 91 percent who do not eat enough vitamin-rich fruits and vegetables, vitamin pills may be an answer. Although most experts agree that a daily multiple vitamin will not hurt anyone, opinion is divided over whether or not people should take megadoses of vitamins to prevent disease or to delay aging.

In the following selections, Patricia Long contends that research shows taking large doses of vitamins and following a few other health practices can extend an individual's life by preventing cancer, heart disease, and premature aging. Victor Herbert argues that medical research has not proven that megadoses of vitamin C can help prevent colds and that many people are genetically at risk of causing themselves great harm when they take large doses of the vitamin.

YES
Patricia Long

THE POWER OF VITAMIN C

It's said that God never shuts one door without opening another, and, true enough, when the Linus Pauling Institute sputtered and swerved this past year for lack of funds, researchers at labs elsewhere around the country were just revving up for brand-new studies on the health benefits of vitamin C.

Vitamin C? The nation's most popular placebo? After decades of exaggerated promises and wacky pronouncements—from the vitamin's ability to stave off colds to its power in preventing cancer and heart disease—there's now credible evidence that these claims weren't so farfetched after all.

Pauling, the Nobel Prize–winning chemist, deserves much of the credit, if not the blame, for making vitamin C a household word. In 1976 he unfurled a laundry list of disorders that he said the vitamin could thwart: strokes, mental illness, heart disease, cancer, and infections. With "optimal intake," he said later, we could all probably live an extra 12 to 18 years—his idea of optimal falling somewhere between 3,200 to 12,000 milligrams a day, or what you'd get from 45 to 170 oranges.

Pauling's claims set off the largest uncontrolled (some say "out of control") field study ever. By the late 1980s one of every three Americans was popping vitamin C pills.

It was not a new idea that the vitamin could do more than prevent scurvy. In the mid-1960s an industrial chemist named Irwin Stone had noted that humans, unlike most mammals, lack an enzyme needed to make vitamin C. In his view, the missing enzyme amounted to a genetic disease, one that placed humans at risk for a wide range of illnesses. Still, hardly anyone took the notion seriously until Pauling piped up.

"Pauling had a legendary reputation for being right about all sorts of things, crystal structure, quantum chemistry... the molecular basis of sickle-cell disease," wrote Robert Wittes, a researcher at the National Cancer Institute, in 1985. "One might perhaps do worse than rely at least partly on Pauling's awesome intuition."

That attitude was not universally shared. "Pauling was a physical chemist who plunged into the medical field with no data of his own, making very dogmatic claims," says Kenneth Carpenter, a retired nutrition professor with the University of California at Berkeley and author of *The History of*

Scurvy and Vitamin C. "Many researchers thought, 'Well, Pauling's an old man, he's retired, he's just going bonkers.'"

Those two perceptions of Pauling—genius and crackpot—have kept the fires burning around vitamin C but have also made a lot of researchers nervous about stepping into the light.

"Nutrition doesn't have the greatest reputation in science to start with," says Mark Levine, a physician and biochemist at the National Institute of Diabetes and Digestive and Kidney Diseases. "But vitamin C is considered the flakiest of the flakes."

Qualms aside, Levine is among a growing number of scientists unable to ignore compelling new evidence—mostly from studies on cell cultures and lab animals —that vitamin C may have far-reaching effects in the body. They've noted its abundance in particular organs and cells, including that master shield against illness, the immune system. "You've got to ask yourself," he says, "why is there twenty to a hundred times the amount of vitamin C in the immune cells as in the blood? I mean, why is it there?"

It's the big dose of vitamin C not just in immune cells but in sperm, eyes, and other tissues that's raising eyebrows. Here's the latest on what researchers are now finding:

HEART DISEASE

Vitamin C may help prevent heart disease by inhibiting early damage to the heart's coronary arteries.

This insight springs from new research focusing on oxygen in the bloodstream and on the protective power of "antioxidants" like vitamin C. (Vitamin E and beta-carotene are also antioxidants, as are some enzymes.) When the body uses oxygen it gives rise to substances called "free radicals." These feisty molecules react readily with fats, proteins, and DNA, harming cell membranes and mutating genes.

Enter the antioxidants, which scavenge for the free radicals and render them harmless. But when the body's antioxidants run low, free radicals are at liberty to play a harmful role in the buildup of plaque in the heart's blood vessels. This is how scientists think things go wrong:

Heart arteries clog when low-density lipoprotein (LDL) cholesterol moves from the blood into the artery wall, where it can stay harmlessly for years. Over time, white blood cells may swallow this "bad" lipoprotein and bloat. If these "foam cells" burst, more white cells rush in, creating artery-choking plaque.

None of this would happen if the cells didn't swallow LDL in the first place. And in fact, in laboratory dishes, white cells gulp only LDL damaged by free radicals. So in theory, if antioxidants can snare the radicals before they attack, they should stop the onset of heart disease, or at least delay its early signs.

Sure enough, in 1988, when Daniel Steinberg, an endocrinologist with the University of California at San Diego, gave rabbits the powerful antioxidant drug probucol, the rabbits' arteries showed half the damage of the controls'.

Vitamin C might work as well. Balz Frei, a nutritionist with the Harvard School of Public Health, compared the potency of several antioxidants by exposing LDL cholesterol to cigarette smoke, known to harbor free radicals. Vitamin C halted oxygen damage better than vitamin E and beta-carotene. "No damage occurred until *after* all the vitamin C was used up," Frei says. In another test, the vitamin fought off free radicals as efficiently as the drug probucol.

All these observations could help explain a puzzling fact: Some people with too much LDL cholesterol are never stricken with heart disease. Many researchers now think evidence is strong enough to justify a clinical trial on humans. One group will get antioxidant vitamins, another a placebo—and the researchers will compare their rates of heart attacks, strokes, and cardiac deaths.

CANCER

Vitamin C may prevent or delay the onset of some cancers.

This idea was originally proposed more than a decade ago by Linus Pauling and Scottish surgeon Ewan Cameron. These men envisioned the vitamin's both preventing cancers and halting their spread, but today's researchers focus solely on its potential to keep tumors from forming in the first place.

Biochemist Bruce Ames of the University of California at Berkeley believes cancer begins when the body's cells and DNA are damaged by oxidants—from everyday metabolism, from cigarette smoke, and even from chemicals the body produces to fight infection.

"To protect you from bacteria and viruses, your white blood cells pour out oxides and hydrogen peroxide, which is bleach," says Ames. Unfortunately, the chemicals can't tell a bacterium from a healthy cell. "The price you pay for that defense system is some DNA damage that shows up later as cancer."

Population studies seem to confirm this idea: In areas where diets are low in the antioxidant vitamin C, cancer rates are high—though the evidence is shaky.

Investigators can't actually measure how much vitamin C their subjects eat but estimate it from answers to questions such as "How often to you eat broccoli?"

"It's possible that vitamin C is just a marker for something else in fruits and vegetables, some other vitamin or mineral, or something else entirely," says Gladys Block, an epidemiologist with the University of California at Berkeley.

Despite this weakness, in 46 studies comparing healthy people to those with cancer, 33 found that cancer risk decreases when people get 60 milligrams of vitamin C a day—an orange's worth.

When it comes to fresh foods high in vitamins, Block says, "There's little doubt that there's a protective effect for cancers of the esophagus, oral cavity, and stomach." A diet rich in vitamin C may also protect against cancers of the larynx, pancreas, rectum, breast, cervix, and lung.

As for the vitamin's role in curing existing cancers, the early signs were hopeful. In 1976 Pauling and Cameron gave 100 cancer patients 10,000 milligrams of vitamin C a day throughout their treatment. The researchers then compared the patients' outcomes with those of 1,000 past patients, or "historical controls." (Cameron was so sure of vitamin C's benefits that he refused to withhold it from anyone in treatment.) On average, the controls survived for 50 days, the vitamin C group for 210 days.

The study wasn't conclusive, since it didn't compare identical groups of patients. Yet the large gain in survival time couldn't be ignored. The National Cancer Institute decided to fund a well-controlled study at the Mayo Clinic. In this, 150 cancer patients were given either 10,000 milligrams of vitamin C a day or a placebo. Vitamin C neither shrank tumors nor lengthened survival time any better than the placebo did.

A second study was run, and again vitamin C failed to help. Pauling objected that the researchers hadn't used proper procedures and appealed for a third trial, but the cancer institute declined.

Now, early data from animal studies suggest that vitamin C may lessen the side effects of conventional cancer treatments, perhaps someday allowing higher and more effective doses of radiation or drugs.

COLDS

Vitamin C apparently does have some power against the common cold.

Here's Linus Pauling's legendary advice to cold sufferers: At the first scratchy feeling in your throat, mucus in your nose, or muscle pain and general malaise, take two or more 1,000-milligram tablets of vitamin C. For the next several hours take an additional two tablets or more every hour. If your symptoms persist, push the daily dose up to 10,000 or 20,000 milligrams. Follow this regimen and your cold will be milder and shorter, he says.

At least 20 studies have tried to confirm or refute this claim. The results generally have been conflicting and not wholly trustworthy. One study, which found that vitamin C users suffered fewer colds, relied on vitamin supplements so tart that subjects could easily tell them from placebo pills.

In 1972, however, a well-designed study at the University of Toronto found that volunteers who took a daily 1,000 to 2,000 milligrams of vitamin C caught about the same number of colds as those on a placebo. The vitamin-takers then upped their dose to 4,000 milligrams a day, in a variant of the Pauling pattern, for three days. Their colds lasted a third as long and their symptoms were milder—not exactly something to sniff at. What's more, later studies found it worked just as well to take daily doses of 100 to 200 milligrams, boosting them to 1,000 when a cold hits.

The critics' response? Why, they asked, should people take vitamin C year-round just *possibly* to have milder cold symptoms for the eight days a year the average cold lasts?

Great minds turned elsewhere. But recently, the vitamin maker Hoffmann-LaRoche asked Elliot Dick, a respiratory virologist at the University of Wisconsin in Madison, to reopen the case. Dick agreed to conduct a "miniature" field trial. He took 16 healthy men, gave half 2,000 milligrams of vitamin C daily for three weeks and gave the others a placebo. For the next seven days, the 16 men played poker and slept in the same rooms with eight men infected with a cold virus. Soon everyone was sniffling. Staff noted every sneeze, cough, and drip, day and night.

"Much to our surprise, the vitamin C group got a lot less sick," says Dick. "They caught colds but their symptoms were very mild." Dick repeated the experiment twice with new volunteers and got similar results. Dick concluded that popping vitamin C *can't* keep you from catching a cold, but it *can* reduce the severity of your symptoms.

BIRTH DEFECTS

Vitamin C may prevent birth defects by protecting the father's sperm.

Consider this: Human semen has eight times the vitamin C present in the blood.

"Maybe it's there to protect sperm from DNA damage by oxidants," says Bruce Ames. It's known that children of men who smoke cigarettes are at greater risk for leukemia and immune system cancers.

Ames and toxicologist Cesar Fraga, now with the University of Buenos Aires in Argentina, obtained semen samples from 24 men at a fertility clinic. Semen low in vitamin C showed much more DNA damage. (Vitamin C also improves fertility in men who smoke cigarettes.)

To test the idea that vitamin C might prevent sperm damage, Robert Jacob, a nutritional biochemist at the U.S. Department of Agriculture's research lab in San Francisco, put ten men on a diet yielding a scant 5 milligrams of the vitamin a day. To set a baseline "healthy intake" for comparison, Jacob gave the men 250-milligram supplements—then withheld them so the men got only the basic 5 milligrams. Over the next four and a half weeks, sperm damage doubled and continued to increase, even as Jacob added supplements upping the vitamin to 10, then 20 milligrams. The damage stopped only when the dose reached 60 milligrams a day (the recommended daily allowance).

These findings are provocative evidence that vitamin C may prevent birth defects, but without more studies, with more subjects, no one can yet say so conclusively.

AGING

Vitamin C may actually help people stay healthy longer.

A study published this year in the journal *Epidemiology* reached a conclusion that's hard to ignore: People who get moderately high amounts of vitamin C every day (from food and supplements) have a good chance of living several years longer than people falling short of the daily minimum. Men in the study benefited more than women; still, death rates, mostly from heart disease, fell in both sexes as their daily intake rose toward what the researchers speculated was the 300-milligram range.

What the study didn't tease apart was whether some people lived longer because of vitamin C itself or because of other things in their diet.

Still, vitamin C may deserve some credit, in light of certain novel ideas about aging. According to biochemist Bruce Ames, everyday metabolism—breathing, digesting, thinking—releases oxidants that damage the body's cells and DNA. The body repairs itself, in large part, but over time the damage accumulates. Ames believes antioxidants slow the damage.

"Look at the Seventh-Day Adventists," he says. "They do everything right. They don't smoke, they eat well. But they still get cancer. They just get it later than the rest of us."

Cataracts are another major problem of old age. They form when the eyes' lenses grow opaque, possibly from damage by sunlight and oxygen. Commonly, levels of vitamin C in eye tissues and fluids are up to 20 times as high as in the blood, prompting speculation that vitamin C (and vitamin E) may help prevent cataracts. Cataract sufferers tend to have low blood levels of antioxidant vitamins as well.

HOW MUCH IS ENOUGH?

One thing is clear: If you don't want to suffer scurvy like the old-time sailors, you need around 10 milligrams of vitamin C a day—about what's in a tablespoon of lemon juice. The government, allowing a modest safety margin, stands by its recommended daily allowance (RDA) of 60 milligrams, except for smokers, who are advised to get at least 100 milligrams (to combat the oxidants in smoke).

Beyond that, it's a wide-open field. Several researchers admit to taking anywhere from 500 to 2,000 milligrams a day. Yet when it comes to advice, they stay mum. "Advocating vitamin C can ruin your career, your professional reputation," says one who wishes to remain anonymous.

"Is the current RDA reasonable? asks Mark Levine. "In my opinion as a scientist and a physician, the RDA clearly prevents deficiency. Does that represent optimal? I don't think so. How much higher should it be? I don't know.

"We don't really know how much vitamin C gets in the blood at each dose," Levine says. Besides, he says, blood levels don't always say much about what's going on elsewhere in the body.

Pauling figured his optimum from how much of the vitamin animals make. A goat as big as a 154-pound man, for example, makes 13,000 milligrams of vitamin C each day. But that's a dicey formula. Not all animals produce the same amount. Extrapolating to humans from mice gives 9,000 milligrams; from rabbits, 350 milligrams.

"Forty or fifty years ago, the old-time nutrition researchers realized that we should base requirements on what a vitamin actually does biologically," says Levine. "But they didn't have the foggiest idea of how to measure it." Levine's idea is to start small—with cells, for instance—and focus on something measurable, like how much vitamin C is used by enzymes that need it to work. Until he and others pin all this down, here are some sensible guidelines:

Hit the Minimum

All you have to do to get the daily minimum of 60 milligrams of vitamin C is eat one orange. Yet four out of ten Americans don't do even that much. This national shortfall has many clinicians worried. Some now recommend that anyone who shies away from fruits and vegetables should take a multiple vitamin and mineral supplement.

Get More in Your Meals

If all of us were to eat the recommended two fruits and three vegetables a day, we'd all be getting a daily 100 to 200 milligrams. Even Paleolithic humans got about 440 milligrams daily, simply foraging for wild greens and fruit.

In fact, eating as much as 500 milligrams a day isn't that hard if you make sure each of your meals includes some foods rich in vitamin C. Orange juice in the morning, some fresh salsa on a taco at lunch, cranberry juice for a snack, then a salad with some red cabbage and green pepper at dinner—and you're already well over 300 milligrams.

Don't Go Overboard

For those who want more vitamin C but can't seem to squeeze any more fruits and vegetables into their meals, the experts' best advice on supplements is to hold your daily dose under 1,000 milligrams.

To absorb as much vitamin as possible, divide the pills or powder into small doses and take them with your meals over the course of the day. Stay away from chewable tablets, which can erode your tooth enamel. And don't refrigerate your vitamins; condensed moisture can destroy their potency.

Also, make a point of telling your doctor that you're taking supplements. Vitamin C at the 1,000-milligram-a-day level can skew several medical tests, including diabetics' blood-sugar checks and a common colon-cancer test.

But avoid megadoses totaling thousands of milligrams a day. People who take that much vitamin C are said to have "the most expensive pee in the world," which is to say that at high levels the vitamin is mainly excreted in their urine. American consumers now shell out at least $355 million a year on vitamin C pills and powders.

The cost aside, no one really knows how safe megadoses are. Researchers can't be sure until they've evaluated the risks, and those studies haven't yet been done. A lot of Americans don't care. "Look at Linus Pauling," they say. "He's ninety-one years old and takes eighteen thousand milligrams a day."

That doesn't mean everyone will fare so well. Daily doses of 10,000 milligrams or more aren't ordinarily toxic but can cause heartburn, diarrhea, and gas. Besides, if you begin taking large doses and suddenly stop, you could suffer a dramatic drop in the vitamin C in your blood-possibly to below your initial level.

And for people with inherited disorders (such as hemocromatosis) that lead to large body stores of iron, doses of even 1,000 milligrams can cause serious problems. Normally iron is stored safely inside cells, but vitamin C releases it into the blood, where it can wreak havoc on the liver and heart. Most people who've inherited hemochromatosis don't know it until they suffer irreversible organ damage or until a relative does and the whole family gets checked.

So if health and longevity are your concerns—and why else would anyone care about vitamins?—try to eat more fruits and vegetables. That'll bring your daily C up to several hundred milligrams. If you're looking to supplements for some extra C, don't take more than 1,000 milligrams a day. The skeptics will remind you that promising research isn't proof, but even they're drinking their orange juice these days.

NO
Victor Herbert

DOES MEGA-C DO MORE GOOD THAN HARM, OR MORE HARM THAN GOOD?

The recently reported study by Enstrom, Kanim and Klein[1] demonstrated that a group of individuals *with a healthy life-style,* manifested by **four key healthy life-style markers ("confounding variables" in the jargon of science) that they weigh less (2.2 kg less body fat in the men, 4.4 in the women), smoke less, exercise more, eat more fruits and vegetables** (including oranges, grapefruits, tomatoes and their juices), and *incidentally* also take vitamin supplements (averaging a "best guess" megadose of 800 mg of vitamin C/day), live longer than a group who **weigh more, smoke more, exercise less, eat less fruits and vegetables** and *incidentally* take no regular supplements.

However, Enstrom et al. ignored two of these four (weight loss and eating fruits and vegetables) and lumped the other two confounding variables, smoking and exercise, with eight other variables including total fat and calories consumed. All of these eight variables were identical in the men who took supplements and those who did not and do not appear to be confounding in their study. The differences in the two were obscured by the non-differences in the other eight. Therefore, Enstrom et al. concluded that the supplements were responsible for the much greater longevity in the men in the supplemented compared to the nonsupplemented groups. Because the women taking supplements ate more fat than the women who did not take supplements, their increase in longevity was less.

Before one accepts their conclusion that the supplements were responsible for greater longevity, one would like to see the results if, instead of using the supplements as the index marker, they reevaluated their data, using the four key healthy life-style markers as principal markers in the same supplement and no supplement groups. One would anticipate that such a reevaluation would show an even greater increment in longevity due to those four markers than shown by using the incidental-to-a-healthy-life-style marker of consumption of vitamin C supplements. Vitamin supplement users are more likely to be from a higher socioeconomic status than nonusers. People "into" a healthy life-style often also take vitamin C supplements, because of the relentless hype that vitamin pills are part of a healthy life-style, making vitamin C supplements a surrogate **pseudomarker** for a number of unmeasured variables having to do with a healthy life-style and/or better access to medical care and appropriate nutrition.

One suspects that, if Enstrom et al. reevaluate their data using the above four healthy life-style markers to separate those into two groups (>500 mg/day and 50 to 500 mg/day). The group using mega-C (>500 mg/day) supplements will fare less well than the group using less, because of the harms from megadoses of vitamin C.

Promoters of vitamin C supplements claim that megadoses of vitamin C are harmless. Their incessant repetition of this fiction has so fixed it in concrete in the minds of Americans as "rock logic"[2] that even first-rate epidemiologists like Enstrom believe it. Circulated nationwide was his statement to the media, the day his article in *Epidemiology*[1] was published, that megadoses of vitamin C were harmless.

Nothing could be further from the truth. Vitamin C is a double-edged sword, necessary for health in small amounts and harmful in large amounts. High-*dose* vitamin C supplements, deceptively represented as "high *potency*" to convey an aura of increased value, have produced great harm, ranging from serious illness to death.

The representation of vitamin C and β (beta)-carotene as antioxidants is both truth and misperception, because both are in fact redox agents and pro-oxidant rather than antioxidant in appropriate circumstances. To quote Repka and Hebbel,[3] and as others[4,5] have also pointed out, "lipid peroxidation studies show that at physiologic levels ascorbate acts primarily as an antioxidant; however, as pharmacologic levels are reached, its pro-oxidant effects predominate."

In the presence of iron, vitamin C is one of the most potent pro-oxidants known.[3-13] It converts iron stores to catalytic iron, one of the most oxidant of substances.[6] About 10% of Caucasians and about 8% of African-Americans are born with a gene for increased iron absorption (heterozygous hemochromatosis), and about 1 in 250 have two genes for enhanced iron absorption (homozygous hemochromatosis).[14,15] Vitamin C supplements, which enhance both iron absorption and the release of iron from body deposits, can act as a second gene for iron overload in those born with 1 gene for enhanced iron absorption.[6] By producing iron overload in these people and releasing catalytic iron from their body stores, vitamin C supplements can maim and kill. In her formal statement[16] supporting the position[17,18] that the FDA-proposed lower U.S. RDIs protect consumers, Margit Krikker of the Hemochromatosis Research Foundation wrote: "Vitamin C, which accelerates iron absorption, has also been responsible for cardiac deaths in at least three athletes, unaware of their predisposition to iron-loading or of the hazards of daily megadoses for years."[16]

Some pertinent statistics:

1. Twice as many American adult men (1 in 250) have iron overload disease as have iron deficiency (1 in 500), so vitamin C supplements, which enhance iron absorption, are twice as likely to harm them as help them.[14,19]

2. Almost twice as many Americans (about 10%) have a gene for positive iron balance as are in negative iron balance (about 6%, mainly infants, early adolescents, women in the reproductive years, and pregnant

women), so vitamin C supplements, by enhancing iron absorption, if taken nonselectively by all Americans, are likely to do more harm than good.[6]

3. In a 5-year study of more than 1900 Finnish men, published in *Circulation* in September 1992, Dr. Jukka T. Salonen and his colleagues[20] found that **for each 1% increase in serum ferritin there was a more than 4% increase in risk of heart attack.** Finnish men with serum ferritin above 200 had 2.3 times as many heart attacks as Finnish men with serum ferritin of 100. High low-density lipoprotein (LDL) cholesterol level *per se* was not a risk factor. It only became one when there was concurrent high ferritin, which, particularly in the presence of vitamin C,[6,21] releases catalytic iron which, in turn, converts the harmless LDL cholesterol to oxidized LDL cholesterol, which damages the walls of coronary arteries.

Olson and Hodges noted[22] (and provided pertinent literature references for) all of the following harms from excess vitamin C:

Occasional large intakes of vitamin C may cause stomach cramps, nausea and diarrhea in some fasting persons but have no long-term adverse effects.

When daily large doses are ingested routinely for months or years, however, a number of adverse effects may occur, including uricosuria, reduced bactericidal activity of leukocytes, secondary hyperoxalemia (producing metastatic oxalosis) in hemodialysis patients, enhanced mobilization of bone calcium, impaired blood coagulation time, lowered plasma B_{12} levels, interruption of pregnancy, reduced insulin production and interference with anticoagulant therapy....

These and other possible effects of high doses have been thoughtfully reviewed by Barnes and by Hornig and Moser.[22]

The extent to which the routine ingestion of very high doses of vitamin C impairs health in a serious and lasting way is unknown. The frequency of reported toxic manifestations is unquestionably low relative to the number of persons routinely ingesting large doses. The mortality rate among health-conscious elderly Californians who routinely ingested large doses of nutritional supplements, including vitamin C, is significantly lower than that of one non-smoking reference population but now lower than that of another health-conscious group. The mortality rate was independent of the reported amount of vitamin C ingested daily.[22]

The above section of their discussion[22] on toxicity of vitamin C is quoted *in extenso* because, when the Subcommittee on the RDA edited it, in their enthusiasm for the *ignis fatuus* of vitamin C against cancer,[23] they edited out much of the toxicity section as well as literature references to that toxicity.

Intravenous megadoses of vitamin C can kill within hours that one-eighth of men of Black, Oriental, and Sephardic Jewish and Mediterranean basin-origin born with genetically determined glucose-6-phosphate dehydrogenase deficiency, by instantly oxidatively hemolyzing their red blood cells.[24,25] They can also precipitate acute severe sickle cell crisis in all those with sickle cell disease by causing all their red cells to take the sickle form.[3,24,25]

Luckily, oral megadoses of vitamin C produce less than total hemolysis, less severe sickle cell crises and much less oxalosis than does intravenous mega-C. This is because, while 100% of any size intravenous mega-C dose is absorbed, a genetically calibrated progressively smaller amount of oral mega-C is absorbed the greater the oral dose. The higher the daily dosage, the smaller the percentage absorbed and the higher the amount excreted unchanged in the feces.[26] It is this unabsorbability that produces as a toxic effect the hyperosmotic diarrhea Dr. Linus Pauling proudly states that he gets from the 18 g of vitamin C he takes each day.

It is this same toxic effect that has caused AIDS patients who take mega-C to go into hypovolemic shock, by superimposing the hyperosmotic diarrhea from mega-C on the secretory diarrhea present in about 60% of AIDS patients.[27]

The false claim that mega C is harmless is so pervasive that the Mount Sinai School of Medicine Complete Book of Nutrition[27] carries in its "Vitamins and Minerals" table a heading entitled "Signs of Overdose." The listing for vitamin C includes, "Oxalate kidney stones, oxalate deposits in heart, other body tissues. Urinary tract irritation. Diarrhea. Blood destruction." Other nutrition books seem to follow the practice of not dealing with harms from vitamin C by simply not citing the literature on harms.

A formal request has been sent to the FDA[17] that they require all sellers of vitamin C supplements (and iron supplements), and products with large amounts of additional vitamin C (or iron), to label them as follows:

NOTICE: Before using this product, your serum ferritin should be determined. Millions of Americans, particularly males, but also some females, have a serum ferritin greater than 120 micrograms per liter of blood. If your serum ferritin is greater than 120, this product may be harmful to your health, and you should not take it unless a licensed health professional tells you it is safe to do so.

The cut-off point of 120 is based on the data of Salonen et al.[20] that a serum ferritin level of 200 mg/L or more, more than doubled the relative risk of heart attacks. Additionally, since smokers already have an increased risk of heart attacks, it is likely the Food and Nutrition Board recommendation[28] that they increase their intake of vitamin C to 100 mg daily may further increase their risk of heart attacks, by enhancing iron absorption and increasing release of catalytic iron from ferritin. The latter triggers the oxidation of LDL cholesterol to a form that further narrows coronary arteries already narrowed in response to the nicotine in tobacco smoke.

Much of the commentary[29] on harm from iron supplements was, unfortunately, edited out of the 10th RDAs,[28,30] including the reference to a paper reporting that as little as a 100-mg supplement of iron could produce liver cell wall lipid damage with enzyme leakage.

The Finnish study supports the theory, first advanced in 1981 by J. L. Sullivan,[31] that it is not estrogen which protects women in the childbearing years against heart attacks, but the monthly blood loss, with its concurrent loss of iron.

A good way to bring down a high serum ferritin level in men (when it is due to high iron stores) is to have them donate a pint of blood every few weeks until their serum ferritin level is no longer high to concurrently eat a largely vegetarian diet with a moderate intake of vitamin C and with no supplements of vitamin C or iron. Alternatively, of course, or in addition, iron-chelating agents can be used when appropriate, and when the benefits exceed the harms.[21] Parenthetically, the American Association of Blood Banks says it is up to the individual blood bank director as to whether he/she would use a donation from a person with iron overload.

One suspects the greater fruit and vegetable intake of the supplement group in the Enstrom et al. study is significantly more important to their greater longevity than the supplements of vitamin C.

It is likely that the lesser frequency among vegetarians of heart attacks is in significant part due to the fact that plant iron on average is only about 3% absorbable, whereas animal iron averages 15% absorbable.[29] Thus, vegetarians have substantially lower serum ferritin and iron stores than nonvegetarians.[29]

Each fruit and vegetable is a storehouse of literally hundreds of antioxidants, prooxidants, carcinogens, anticarcinogens, mutagens and antimutagens, all of which tend to balance each other out, but with the balance perhaps in favor of the anticarcinogens, in a sensible diet based on the principles of moderation, variety and balance.[27,32-35]

Talalay's group[34,35] recently isolated and identified the mustard family chemical, sulforaphane, an isothiocyanate not destroyed by microwaving or steaming, from broccoli and other cruciferous vegetables such as Brussels sprouts, cauliflower, and kale, as well as noncruciferous carrots and green onions. It is a highly potent inducer of so-called phase II detoxication enzymes, which are involved in the inactivation of carcinogens; related isothiocyanates also have anticarcinogenic properties.

A variety of chemicals naturally present in foods and preservatives added to food cause cultured cells to generate a variety of enzymes, some of which (phase II detoxication enzymes) bond to and thereby inactivate and flush out carcinogens, others of which (phase I enzymes, such as cytochrome P-450)[36] transform otherwise innocuous chemicals into mutagens and carcinogens. Some chemicals induce both kinds of enzymes to a variable degree, depending on various factors.[27,32-36] An example of creation of a carcinogenesis promoter from a dietary per se nonpromoter is what our liver xanthine oxidase does to the acetaldehyde our livers produce from alcohol, by generating superoxide from it, a process accelerated by iron and vitamin C.[4,5,36] Our genetic blueprint determines our individual potential for maximal generation of each of our enzymes and whether we generate a normal or warped enzyme.[37]

It has been known since the late 1950's that oral vitamin C dramatically releases iron from body stores, sharply raising the serum iron level.[38] For that reason, physicians started adding intravenous vitamin C to the chelating agents used to lower the high iron stores of patients in whom iron built up because of monthly transfusions for chronic anemias. A number of young people died suddenly while the vitamin C needle was still in the vein, because the vitamin C released into their bloodstreams lethal amounts of free iron, above the ability of the chelating agents to bind and thereby inactivate it. This free iron circulated to their hearts, producing fatal cardiac arrhythmias.[39] Due to this potential lethality, intravenous and oral vitamin C can only be used very cautiously to help lower body iron stores in young people with thalassemia and sickle cell disease.

At the 1992 annual meeting of the American Society for Clinical Nutrition,

Elaine Feldman's group[40] reported that in normal individuals supplements of 1 g daily of vitamin C for 1 month decreased systolic and diastolic blood pressure. In the discussion period, they were responsive to our observation that nitrous oxide, the "endothelial relaxing factor" our own cells generate,[41] has the same effect, as well as to our suggestion that large doses of vitamin C acted as an *oxidant* to increase the few seconds of lifespan of nitrous oxide after its manufacture in endothelial cells, allowing more nitrous oxide to attach in the presence of excess vitamin C to its "receptor" iron bound to enzymes,[41] and our suggested methodology for checking this possibility.

At the April 1992 FASEB Symposium on Nutritional Epidemiology of Chronic Disease, a presentation titled "Results of a Metabolic Study of Response to Vitamin C, Population Implications," based on blood levels, showed once again that if you eat more vitamin C, you get higher vitamin C blood levels, and if you eat less, you get lower blood levels. It promoted vitamin C supplements based on a number of epidemiologic studies. In the discussion, it was pointed out to the author that those epidemiologic studies showed the value of fruits and vegetables, not of vitamin C. A subsequent editorial[42] by the same author produced nationwide headlines.

In her editorial,[42] accompanying the Enstrom et al. paper,[1] Gladys Block ignored the life-style factors. Her statement, "Their data indicate that those who take supplements containing vitamin C *and* have a reasonable dietary intake of vitamin C do better than those who simply have a reasonable dietary intake," was misleading because the supplement takers ate substantially **more** fruits and veg-etables (including substantially more dietary vitamins A and C) than those who did not take supplements. Instead of using creative "water logic"[2] to objectively assess epidemiologic data, the editorial misinterpreted the Enstrom paper to fit the "rock logic"[2] preconception that vitamin C supplements prevent disease and extend life.

The Bottom Line: Both oxidants and antioxidants are needed in the biochemical economy of human cells. We need to inhale oxygen because it is the fundamental oxidant we use; without it we would die. Cells walk a balance between essential oxidant and essential antioxidant processes. That is the fundamental reason moderate antioxidation is helpful and excessive antioxidation is harmful. Vitamin C is a redox agent, usually antioxidant in the moderate quantities found in food, but often oxidant in the large quantities found in many supplements.[6,21] As a supplement, it can be antioxidant or oxidant, depending on circumstances and is particularly oxidant when taken with iron or when body iron stores are high.

NOTE ADDED IN PROOF

Because of the potential lethality of vitamin C supplements in persons with iron overload, the "1992 Management Protocol for the Treatment of Thalassemia Patients" distributed by the Thalassemia International Federation, states (page 15):

Role of Vitamin C
Iron-loaded patients usually become vitamin C deficient, probably because iron oxidizes the vitamin. When this is the case, administration of vitamin C increases excretion of iron in response to

Desferal®.* Vitamin C increases the availability of iron, and so may increase its toxicity if large doses are taken without simultaneous Desferal® infusion. Therefore the following precautions are recommended:

a. Start treatment with vitamin C only after an initial month of treatment with Desferal®.

b. Give vitamin C supplements only if the patient is receiving Desferal® regularly.

c. Do not exceed a daily dose of 200 mg. The minimum effective dose of vitamin C is about 2–5 mg/kg (N. Di Palma, A. Piga unpublished data). In general, 50 mg suffice for children under 10 years of age, and 100 mg for older children. Vitamin C should be given only on days when Desferal® is taken, ideally when the pump is set up.

The Protocol is available in the United States from the Cooley's Anemia Foundation, Box CEP, 105 East 22nd Street, New York, NY 10010.

REFERENCES

1. Enstrom JE, Kanin LE, Klein MA. Vitamin C intake and mortality among a sample of the United States population. *Epidemiology* 1992;3:194–200.
2. De Bono E. *I am right—you are wrong.* New York: Viking, 1991.
3. Repka T, Hebbel RP. Hydroxyl radical formation by sickle erythrocyte membranes: role of pathological iron deposits and cytoplasmic reducing agents. *Blood* 1991;78:2753–8.
4. Herbert V. Jayatilleke E, Shaw S. Alcohol and breast cancer. *N Engl J Med* 1987;317:1287–8.
5. Shaw S, Herbert V, Colman N, Jayatilleke E. Effect of ethanol-generated free radicals on gastric intrinsic factor and glutathione. *Alcohol* 1990;7:153–7.
6. Herbert V. Iron disorders can mimic anything, so always test for them. *Blood Rev* 1992;3:125–32.
7. Sadrzadeh SMH, Eaton JW. Hemoglobin-mediated oxidant damage to the central nervous system requires exogenous ascorbate. *J Clin Invest* 1988;82:1510–5.
8. Ottolenghi A. Interaction of ascorbic acid and mitochondrial lipids. *Arch Biochem Biophys* 1959;79:353–63.
9. Barber AA. Lipid peroxidation in rat tissue homogenates: interaction of iron and ascorbic acid as the normal catalytic mechanism. *Lipids* 1966;1:146–51.
10. Sharma SK, Krishna Murti CR. Production of lipid peroxide by brain. *J Neurochem* 1968;151:147–9.
11. Sharma SK, Krishna Murti CR. Ascorbic acid: a naturally occurring mediator of lipid peroxide formation in rat brain. *J Neurochem* 1976;27:299–301.
12. Zaleska MM, Floyd RA. Regional lipid peroxidation in rat brain in vitro: possible role of endogenous iron. *Neurochem Res* 1985;10:397–410.
13. Bucher JR, Tien M, Morehouse LA, Aust SD. Redox cycling and lipid peroxidation: the central role of iron chelates. *Fundam Appl Toxicol* 1983;3:222–6.
14. Herbert V. Prevalence of abnormalities of iron metabolism in the U.S.A. In *Serum ferritin: a technical monograph.* La Jolla, CA: National Health Laboratories, 1989:3–8.
15. Edwards CQ, Griffen LM, Kushner JP. Disorders of excess iron. *Hosp Pract* 1991;26(suppl 3):30–6.
16. Krikker MA. *A joint statement in support of RDIs replacing US RDAs.* Submitted February 24, 1992, to FDA Dockets Management Branch, Docket No. 90N–194.
17. Herbert V. *Statement in support of RDIs replacing US RDAs.* Submitted February 23, 1992, to FDA Dockets Management Branch, Docket No. 90N–194.
18. Anonymous. Herbert says FDA-proposed US RDIs protect consumers. *Food Chem News* 1992;March 9:11–2.
19. Herbert V. Introduction and medicolegal considerations: symposium on diagnosis and treatment of iron disorders. *Hosp Pract* 1991;26(suppl 3):4–6.
20. Salonen JT, Nyyssönen K, Korpela H, Tuomilehto J, Seppänen R, Salonen R. High stored iron levels are associated with excess risk of myocardial infarction in Eastern Finnish men. *Circulation* 1992;86:803–11.
21. Herbert V. Everyone should be tested for iron disorders. *J Am Diet Assoc* 1992;92:1502–9.
22. Olson JA, Hodges RE. Recommended dietary intakes (RDI) of vitamin C in humans. *Am J Clin Nutr* 1987;45:693–703.

*[Desferal® is the iron-chelating agent, desferrioxamine.]

23. Herbert V. The 1989 RDA is mainly the work of the 1980–85 (10th) RDA Committee, but with 9th RDA numbers for vitamins A and C. *FASEB J* 1990;4:A374.

24. Herbert V. Vitamin C and iron overload. *N Engl J Med* 1981;304:1108.

25. Cohen A, Schwartz E. Vitamin C and iron overload. *N Engl J Med* 1981;304:1108.

26. Marshall CW. In: Barrett S, ed. *Vitamins and minerals: help or harm?* Mount Vernon, NY: Consumers Union, 1985.

27. Herbert V, Subak-Sharpe G, Hammock D, eds. *The Mount Sinai School of Medicine complete book of nutrition.* New York, St. Martin's Press, 1990.

28. Subcommittee on the Tenth Edition of the RDAs (Eds). Recommended Dietary Allowances, 10th Edition. Washington, DC, National Academy Press, 1989.

29. Herbert V. Recommended dietary intakes (RDI) of iron in humans. *Am J Clin Nutr* 1987;45:679–86.

30. Stone R. NAS plagiarism fight to go another round. *Science* 1992;258:19.

31. Sullivan JL. Stored iron and ischemic heart disease: empirical support for a new paradigm. *Circulation* 1992;86:1036–7.

32. Ames B, Profet M, Gold LS. Dietary pesticides (99.99% all natural). *Proc Natl Acad Sci USA* 1990;87:7777–81.

33. Ames B, Profet M, Gold LS. Nature's chemicals and synthetic chemicals: comparative toxicology. *Proc Natl Acad Sci USA* 1990;87:7782–86.

34. Prochaska HJ, Santamaria AB, Talalay P. Rapid detection of inducers of enzymes that protect against carcinogens. *Proc Natl Acad Sci USA* 1992;89:2394–8.

35. Zhang Y, Talalay P, Cho C-G, Posner GH. A major inducer of anticarcinogenic protective enzymes from broccoli: isolation and elucidation of structure. *Proc Natl Acad Sci USA* 1992;89:2399–2403.

36. Lieber, CS. Alcohol, liver and nutrition. *J Am Coll Nutr* 1991;10:602.

37. Simopoulos A, Herbert V, Jacobson B. *Genetic nutrition: designing a diet based on your family medical history.* New York: Macmillan, 1993.

38. Zalusky R, Herbert V. Megaloblastic anemia in scurvy with response to fifty micrograms of folic acid daily. *N Engl J Med* 1961;265:1033–8.

39. Herbert V. Vitamin C and iron overload. *N Engl J Med* 1981;304:1108.

40. Feldman EB, Gold S, Greene J, Moran J, Xu G, Shultz GG, Feldman DS, Hames CG. Vitamin C administration and blood pressure regulation. *Clin Res* 1992;40:627A.

41. Hoffman M. A new role for gases: neurotranmission. *Science* 1991;252:1788.

42. Block G. Vitamin C and reduced mortality. *Epidemiology* 1991;3:189–91.

POSTSCRIPT

Can Large Doses of Vitamin C Improve Health?

An article in the *Journal of the National Cancer Institute* (April 17, 1991) provides an overview of a 1990 symposium sponsored by the National Cancer Institute and the National Institute of Diabetes and Digestive and Kidney Diseases on the biological functions of vitamin C and its possible relation to cancer. These organizations report that vitamin C is protective against cancers of the esophagus, larynx, oral cavity, pancreas, stomach, rectum, lung, breast, and uterus. In "The New Scoop on Vitamins," *Time* (April 6, 1992), research is presented that links several different vitamins to the prevention of many diseases, including heart disease, cataracts, cancer, and even aging.

While many respected scientists involved with vitamin research maintain that these nutrients may be the answer to disease prevention and treatment, there are many skeptics who disagree. In "Vitamin Pushers and Food Quacks," *Nutrition Forum* (March/April 1993), Victor Herbert argues that vitamin pills do not do any good. He feels that Americans get all the vitamins they need in their diets and that taking supplements is a waste of money. Other physicians contend that taking large amounts of vitamins is costing people unnecessary millions of dollars and may be costing people their health. The American Medical Association and the National Institutes of Health maintain that Americans, in general, eat a healthy diet that provides all the necessary nutrients for good health and well-being.

While experts disagree, consumers continue to be confused about exactly how much of each specific vitamin is needed and what the best way is to get them (from food or from pills?). Supplements could certainly furnish the nutrients missing from the diet. However, supplements can only supply certain nutrients, such as vitamins, minerals, and amino acids; pills do not contain the fiber, carbohydrates, or calories necessary for maintaining the body and supplying energy. While in theory these nutrients could be put into pill form, it would be an impractical and tasteless substitute! Real food also supplies a variety of other, more obscure nutrients that may have some value.

Additional readings on the subject include "Antioxidant Vitamin Intake and Coronary Mortality in a Longitudinal Population Study," *American Journal of Epidemiology* (June 15, 1994); "The Truth About Vitamins," *Consumers Digest* (May/June 1994); "Can Vitamin C Save Your Life?" *Consumer Reports on Health* (March 1994); and "Vitamin Supplements: Current Controversies," *Journal of the American College of Nutrition* (April 1994).

PART 6

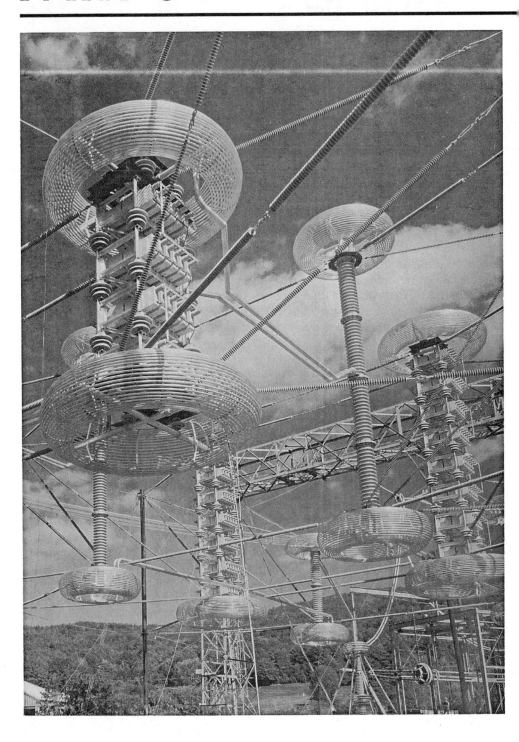

Environmental Issues

Many of today's environmental concerns are related to modern technology. Since World War II, thousands of new chemicals have been developed for the manufacturing and agricultural industries and for the military. But technological growth often has negative effects. Persian Gulf War veterans, for example, returned from the conflict claiming that environmental exposure to chemicals in the Persian Gulf have caused both minor and severe health problems in the soldiers. Also, as the world population continues to grow, how can food production keep pace without increasing environmental degradation and exposure to toxic pesticides? And is exposure to electromagnetic fields from outdoor power lines and indoor home appliances safe? This section discusses controversies related to environmental health issues.

- Is the Gulf War Syndrome Real?

- Are Pesticides in Foods Harmful to Human Health?

- Does Exposure to Electromagnetic Fields Cause Cancer?

ISSUE 16

Is the Gulf War Syndrome Real?

YES: Dennis Bernstein and Thea Kelley, from "The Gulf War Comes Home: Sickness Spreads, But the Pentagon Denies All," *The Progressive* (March 1995)

NO: Michael Fumento, from "What Gulf War Syndrome?" *The American Spectator* (May 1995)

ISSUE SUMMARY

YES: Journalists Dennis Bernstein and Thea Kelley claim that there are some four dozen disabling, sometimes life-threatening medical problems related to environmental and chemical exposure affecting thousands of soldiers who fought in the Persian Gulf War.

NO: Michael Fumento, a science and economics reporter, argues that medical experts have not found any evidence to support the existence of a syndrome related to the war and that the illnesses and symptoms suffered by Gulf War veterans are more likely caused by stress and other natural causes.

Since Operation Desert Storm—the 1991 international effort to drive invading Iraqi forces out of Kuwait—more than 45,000 veterans out of the approximately 650,000 troops who served in the Persian Gulf War have complained of symptoms that have collectively become known as the Gulf War Syndrome. These symptoms include rashes, fatigue, headaches, vision problems, infections, joint and bone pain, birth defects in babies conceived after the war, and cancer.

The syndrome has been compared to the afflictions suffered by veterans of the Vietnam War. During that conflict, the defoliant Agent Orange was released over the jungles. Agent Orange contained dioxin as a contaminant, a substance that is toxic to humans and animals. Numerous studies have linked dioxin exposure to skin rashes, nervous system disorders, muscle aches, digestive problems, and certain cancers. Despite these studies, it took the Department of Veterans Affairs 10 years of debate before it finally connected Agent Orange to the similar health concerns suffered by Vietnam War veterans.

Unlike the health problems of the Vietnam veterans, the causes of the Gulf War veterans' varied symptoms are less clear. A number of entities are currently searching for an explanation. The American Legion claims that toxins from a long list of possible environmental origins—including fumes from burning oil wells and landfills, contact with hydrocarbons, pesticides sprayed over military vehicles, poor sanitary conditions, local parasites, inoculations, and insect bites—may be to blame. The U.S. government is exploring other causes, such as the drug *pyridostigmine bromide*, an experimental pharmaceutical issued to soldiers to protect them against a possible nerve gas attack. The drug (as yet not approved for general use) was administered under a special waiver from the Food and Drug Administration. It was to be distributed with the informed consent of soldiers after the Department of Defense conducted its own research. Troops ordered to take the drug were reportedly never warned about its possible side effects, such as memory loss and respiratory problems. In addition, research on the drug was conducted only on men, so the drug's effects on women were unknown.

Another explanation being proposed is that veterans' health problems are the result of exposure to depleted uranium. Uranium was used to coat some artillery shells and tanks to protect them from enemy fire. However, on impact, depleted uranium releases radioactive particles of a related compound. The government claims that a relatively small number of personnel were exposed to this material and that none of them have shown any adverse symptoms. Nevertheless, the dangers of depleted uranium exposure have become a major issue among U.S. veteran groups as well as among war veterans in Britain.

Despite widespread reports of health problems among Gulf War veterans, the Department of Veterans Affairs and the Pentagon insist that the symptoms are either psychological or due to chance. Major-General Ronald Blanck, commander of the Walter Reed Army Medical Center in Washington, D.C., in addressing Congress said, "Extensive evaluation and thorough epidemiological investigations have failed to show any commonality of exposure or unifying diagnosis to explain these symptoms." Many politicians, however, are fighting back and have vowed not to allow the Gulf War Syndrome to become another Vietnam-style denial by the government.

In the following selections, Dennis Bernstein and Thea Kelley argue that although the Pentagon denies it, exposure to environmental and toxic substances in the Persian Gulf is responsible for illnesses experienced by thousands of veterans and their families. Michael Fumento argues that the many illnesses suffered by Gulf War veterans have been attributed to the so-called syndrome without sufficient evidence. He blames veterans' health complaints on post-traumatic stress disorders rather than on exposure to environmental contaminants, and he faults the media for contributing to the hysteria.

YES

Dennis Bernstein and
Thea Kelley

THE GULF WAR COMES HOME:
SICKNESS SPREADS, BUT THE
PENTAGON DENIES ALL

The Persian Gulf War is not over. It drags on in the lives of tens of thousands of Gulf War veterans. Gulf War Syndrome, or Desert Fever as it is often called in Britain, is a set of some four dozen disabling, sometimes life-threatening medical conditions that afflict thousands of soldiers who fought in the war, as well as their offspring, their spouses, and medical professionals who treated them.

The symptoms suggest exposure to medical, chemical, or biological warfare agents, but the Pentagon denies such exposure occurred and claims it can't identify any common link among those who suffer from Gulf War Syndrome. Don Riegle, the recently retired Senator from Michigan who held hearings on the subject beginning in the fall of 1992, doesn't buy it. He believes the Pentagon may be engaged in a massive cover-up of this serious health problem.

The scale of the problem is enormous. More than 29,000 veterans in the United States with symptoms of Gulf War Syndrome have signed onto the Veterans Administration's Persian Gulf War Registry, 9,000 more have registered separately with the Pentagon, and the Pentagon's list is growing by 1,000 veterans a month.

"These are horrendous statistics that show the true scale of this problem," said Riegle last October when he released his final report on Gulf War Syndrome. Riegle condemned "the heartlessness and irresponsibility of a military bureaucracy that gives every sign of wanting to protect itself more than the health and well-being of our servicemen and women who actually go and fight our wars. To my mind, there is no more serious crime than an official military cover-up of facts that could prevent more effective diagnosis and treatment of sick U.S. veterans."

Birth defects are one of the most alarming problems associated with Gulf War Syndrome. One National Guard unit from Waynesboro, Mississippi, reported that of fifteen children conceived by veterans after the war, thirteen had birth defects. An informal survey of 600 afflicted veterans conducted by Senator Don Riegle's Banking, Housing, and Urban Affairs Committee last fall found that 65 percent of their babies were afflicted with dozens of medical problems, including severe birth defects.

Another disturbing phenomenon is the apparent transmission of the syndrome from soldiers to their family members. Riegle's study found that 77 percent of the wives of these veterans were also ill, as well as 25 percent of the children conceived before the war.

Riegle believes the Pentagon knows that U.S. veterans were exposed to chemical or biological weapons in the Gulf War. "The evidence available continues to mount that exposure to biological and chemical weapons is one cause of these illnesses," Riegle said. "I have evidence that despite repeated automatic denials by the Department of Defense, chemical weapons [were] found in the war." Riegle added that "laboratory findings from gas masks" showed the presence of biological warfare materials "that cause illnesses similar to Gulf War Syndrome."

The cover-up is not limited to the U.S. Government, however. Britain's Ministry of Defense is also being less than forthcoming. It has "a policy of denying Desert Fever for fear of big compensation claims," the British newspaper *Today* reported on October 10. A British Defense spokesperson told the paper, "We have no evidence that this illness exists." More than 1,000 of the 43,000 British troops who served in the Persian Gulf have cited symptoms of Gulf War Syndrome.

*   *   *

At 3 A.M. on January 19, 1991, Petty Officer Sterling Symms of the Naval Reserve Construction Battalion in Saudi Arabia awakened to a "real bad explosion" overhead. Alarms went off and everybody started running toward their bunkers, Symms said. A strong smell of ammonia pervaded the air. Symms said his eyes burned and his skin was stinging before he could don protective gear. Since that time, he has experienced fatigue, sore joints, running nose, a chronic severe rash, open sores, and strep infections. Symms and other soldiers described several such chemical attacks to Riegle's committee in May 1994.

One of the men interviewed by the committee who requested anonymity wrote home to his mother about the attack: "I can deal with getting shot at, because even if I got hit, I can be put back together—a missile, I can even accept that. But gas scares the hell out of me.... I know they detected a cloud of dusty mustard gas because I was there with them, but today everyone denies it. I was there when they radioed the other camps north of us and warned them of the cloud."

Front-line officers assured their troops that it was not a chemical attack, that what they heard was a sonic boom. "Members of Symms's unit were given orders not to discuss the incident," says Senator Riegle's report dated May 25, 1994.

Former U.S. Army Sergeant Randall L. Vallee served in the Persian Gulf as an advance scout. Vallee told Congress back in 1992 that he was convinced Iraqi Scud missiles were armed with chemical or biological warfare agents. "I was in numerous Scud missile attacks when I was in Dhahran," says Vallee. "It seemed like every time I was back there we'd come under fire."

Vallee has been afflicted by at least a half dozen serious medical conditions that started shortly after the Scud attacks. He had been in "perfect health" before his Gulf War service. Vallee supported what scores of veterans have already told Congress: that after every Scud attack, hundreds of alarms signaling chemical and biological attacks would sound, to the point where they were routinely shut off and reset as a matter of course.

Vallee and other members of his detail questioned their superiors about the alarms and about the presence of chemical-warfare agents in the Gulf. "After the whole ordeal was over, we asked about it and they said, 'No, the alarms are just acting that way because they're sensitive.' They gave us stories like, 'Oh, it's because of supersonic aircraft' or 'sand in the alarms.' There was always a story as to why the alarms sounded."

Last August, Vallee received a phone call from the Pentagon's Lieutenant Colonel Vicki Merriman, an aide to the Deputy Assistant Secretary of Defense for Chemical and Biological Matters.

"She asked me about my health and my family," says Vallee. But after some small talk, "the colonel's attitude turned from one of being concerned about my well-being to an interrogator trying to talk me out of my own experiences. She started using tactics of doubt regarding my statements. She said in regard to chemical and biological agents that there was absolutely no way that any soldiers in the Gulf were exposed to anything. Her exact words were, 'The only ones whining about problems are American

troops, why aren't any of our allies?' And that was her exact word, 'whining.'"

* * *

British Gulf war vet Richard Turnball was surprised to hear Lieutenant Colonel Merriman's suggestion that only U.S. vets complained of Gulf War Syndrome. Turnball, who lives just outside Liverpool, served eighteen years in the British Royal Air Force. During the war against Iraq, Turnball built nuclear, biological, and chemical shelters, and instructed British troops in use of chemical monitoring and protective clothing. Turnball was based in Dhahran, Saudi Arabia.

Turnball is convinced there was widespread use of chemical-warfare agents. "People got sick in the chest and eyes, they got infections and skin rashes," he says. "One lad had his whole body covered with spots from head to toe" soon after a Scud attack that Turnball is convinced was chemical in nature.

"Within seconds of the warhead landing on January 20, every chemical-agent monitoring device in the area was blasting the alarm. We were put into the highest alert for twenty minutes," says Turnball, "and then we were told it was a false alarm caused by the fuel from aircraft taking off."

Corporal Turnball carried out two residual-vapor-detection tests for chemical and biological agents on January 20, shortly after the Scud hit "and both were positive," he says. Field supervisors dismissed the test results, claiming that jet fuel set off the indicators. Turnball was skeptical. "We tried on umpteen occasions, when aircraft were taking off in mass numbers," he says. "We stood on the side of the runway closer to the area where the aircraft were taking off, we carried out tests, and we got no readings."

At one point, Turnball says, he was warned to drop the case, and that if he kept it up he might be subject to secrecy laws under which he could be imprisoned. "I've had a very, very senior officer friend of mine ring me up and say, 'Richie, back off, you're kicking over a can of worms.'"

Before he went to war, Turnball said, he was in top condition, worked out every day, and was an avid scuba diver. Since his return, he has had twenty-four separate chest infections, and he has been forced to give up scuba diving because he "can't take the pressure below a few feet." Turnball can no longer run or swim or even take long walks. He said he has been put on steroids and uses two inhalers to help ease serious respiratory complications.

Turnball says the allies "used us as guinea pigs for new drugs" and chemical-weapons testing. He believes "probably both" chemical warfare agents and experimental drugs are responsible for his illness. "I feel we were subject to a chemical attack that affected us," he says. "As a serviceman, I can accept that, it's my job. But I believe more damage was done due to experimentation by our government. Many people got sick after taking some of the drugs. I came down with a high fever, I was sweating excessively. I actually stopped breathing a couple of times."

After three years of illness and fighting with the defense ministry, Turnball is still amazed by the denials that come out of the various bureaucracies. "We were always told that there was a 99.999 percent possibility of a chemical attack. We were expecting it. That was in our intelligence briefings. 'Inevitable' was the word used. And now they deny it."

* * *

Dr. Vivian Lane has never been to the Persian Gulf and is not a wife or mother of a Gulf War vet. The forty-three-year-old former squadron leader and former chief medical officer at the Royal Air Force base in Stafford, England, said she became seriously ill after treating a half dozen "very sick" British soldiers upon their return from the Persian Gulf. Dr. Lane says she was forced to move in with her elderly parents after she could no longer care for herself. Her parents, now in their eighties, are sick and suffering from lesions "very similar" to the ones she is suffering from, she says. "Nobody in this country can tell us why or what they are."

From December 1990 through June 1991 Dr. Lane treated at least six veterans who had the syndrome. Since that time, the aviation medical specialist, a former athlete, has been in great pain. She remembers waking up at four o'clock in the morning "with a terrific, excruciating, crushing type of chest pain and abdominal pain. When I got to the toilet, I didn't know whether to sit on it or stand over it. It just got worse from there. I managed somehow to get myself down to the medical center on base. All I remember was the excruciating chest pains. Next thing I know, I'm in intensive care. My parents had been brought to my bedside because everyone thought I was going to die. They didn't know what was wrong with me."

Dr. Lane offers a different angle on the hundreds of inoculations the soldiers were given before they left for the Persian Gulf. The protective shots were issued by the fistful, says Lane, and it's a wonder more people didn't have serious reactions. "With the amount we were banging into them, I'm surprised we didn't have more people falling over. We were attacking both arms, both buttocks, and their legs to get it all into them all at once. I think anybody with that amount of injections being shoved into them all within a couple of minutes of each other, would not feel terribly well."

Dr. Lane is one of several hundred former British soldiers suing the Ministry of Defense for medical redress. She says she is not holding her breath for results, though. "Frankly, I don't mean to be nasty, but I think they've bitten off more than they can chew."

Corporal Terry Walker was in the Persian Gulf from January to April 1991. Walker was a driver for the British Army's Fourth Armoured Brigade, First Armoured Division in Saudi Arabia. He has been sick ever since. He says his whole family suffers from Gulf War Syndrome.

In a recent interview, Walker described what he, too, believes was the Iraqi chemical Scud attack on January 20. "I was at the docks at Al-Jubayl about 2:30 in the morning," he said. "There was a couple of mighty bangs above our heads and suddenly all the chemical alarms went off and there were soldiers just running around in sheer panic, running around trying to get on their chemical suits." He says an "ammonia-like smell" filled the air after the sirens went off.

Walker, who had trouble getting his gas mask on, became ill soon after the Scuds hit. "I was feeling the burning sensation under the chin, around the back of the head as well. And ever since I've come back from the Gulf I've been ill." Walker suffers from chest infections, rashes, and headaches. Many of the people he served with were also sick after the attack, he says.

"As soon as the bangs happened, all these alarms went off and it was obvious that there was a chemical attack," says Walker, "but our superiors told us it was the jet fighters flying over with the sonic booms, and that it was also the fumes from the jets that set the alarms off."

"The thing is," says Walker, "they never went off before. The planes were flying day in and day out, and the alarms never went off at all, and on January 20, for about a ten-mile, fifteen-mile radius, these alarms went off."

Walker, who has since left the military, is furious with the military establishment in his country for "covering up what happened and the real risks" that would be faced by allied forces. "When they sent us out to fight the war, we expected them to look after us. Instead, when we came back they just tried to cover it up. They said there was nothing wrong at all because the general public would go against them if they found out about the exposures to chemical and biological warfare and how it gets into your whole family."

It is his family's illnesses that he objects to the most. "We knew there was a risk of being killed," he says, "but we didn't know that we would come back from the war so ill, and that our families would be getting sick, too. The wife has been ill since I've come back."

Walker's wife has had chronic abdominal pain and has been hospitalized at least seven times in the last three years. "She's been cut open twice but they couldn't find what was wrong," says Walker. The Walkers are extremely troubled about the health of their six-week-old child who has been plagued with a cold and respiratory problems "from day one."

* * *

Canadian legislator John O'Reilly recently raised the issue of Gulf War Syndrome in the House of Commons. O'Reilly asked the Defense Minister's Parliamentary Secretary, Fred Mifflin, what the government was doing to assist "deserving Canadians" who have been ill after serving in the Persian Gulf. Mifflin responded that the veterans had been cared for by Defense Department doctors and were experiencing "no difficulty whatsoever."

If Mifflin had spoken to Canadian Navy Lieutenant Louise Richard, he might have thought twice before painting such a rosy picture. Lieutenant Richard is an active-duty medical officer stationed at the National Defense Medical Center in Ottawa, the largest military hospital in Canada. Lieutenant Richard volunteered for service in the Persian Gulf as an operating-room nurse. She treated Americans, Britons, and Iraqi prisoners of war.

After eight years of commended service, Richard will be discharged from the Canadian Navy in September because of severe illness. She suffers from many of the same medical conditions afflicting some two dozen veterans interviewed for this article: severe respiratory problems, short-term memory loss, bronchitis, asthma, and pneumonia.

When Richard began to make a ruckus over her war-related illness and threatened to take it to the media, she ran into a stone wall of official denials and intimidation. "They've basically threatened me and said, 'It's all in your head, it's bullshit, don't go forward with it in the media.'" Richard says the threat from her medical superiors, whom she refuses to name for fear of further retribution, ran the gamut of intimidations. "It was the whole thing," says Richard, "your career, your pension—you know, the package."

She's frustrated at the lack of attention to the problem in Canada. "There doesn't seem to be anything happening since we're back," she says. "There's no research, no follow-up, there's nothing going on to help us." She said that she knows of many people in her position who have chosen to remain silent. "People fear to disclose anything because they don't want to ruin their pension or their career or whatever," she says. "I'm angry, because we were valued individuals when we were sent there, and now we're back, and we're not valued individuals at all. We're basically treated like mushrooms in a dark room."

* * *

Dr. Saleh Al-Harbi is an immunologist in Kuwait's Ministry of Public Health, and director of the immunogenetics unit of Kuwait University Medical Center. He says many people in Kuwait and Iran are suffering from what appear to be illnesses involving exposure to chemical and biological warfare agents.

"After the war we were getting diseases, respiratory diseases and unknown blood diseases such as leukemia, but not the typical kind, and for unknown reasons," he says. He is currently investigating with U.S. researchers the underlying causes of the medical conditions that have been plaguing Kuwaitis since the war. "Birth-related problems increased dramatically after liberation," he says, "and those kinds of cases have been reported to me."

He, too, is under pressure to keep a lid on his findings and concerns. "The authorities here are also standing with the Europeans' and Americans' point of view, but we believe that this is something political. I'm independent in mentioning this, and hopefully I will not get any threats from the superiors regarding this matter. They don't want the bad news and rumors to go around."

Dr. Al-Harbi characterizes the syndrome as a form of multiple chemical sensitivity, an explanation that is gaining favor in the United States as well.

Senator Riegle's report says that British and U.S. Army specialists, using sophisticated detection devices, made at least twenty tests that were positive for the presence of chemical-warfare agents. According to his report, "The Kuwaiti, U.S., and British governments all received reports on the discovery and recovery of bulk chemical agents."

Riegle's report also confirms than the alarms used in the war to warn troops of the presence of chemical warfare agents sounded thousands of times. In some cases, the report says, the alarms were sounding so frequently that they were simply turned off.

"The Defense Department told us at a hearing that they were all false alarms," says a former Riegle aide. "There were 14,000 of those chemical-alarm-monitoring units used during the war, and they're telling us that every time they went off, on all 14,000, they were false alarms. That's a little hard to believe."

According to a letter from Riegle to Veterans Affairs Secretary Jesse Brown, eighteen chemical, twelve biological, and four nuclear facilities in Iraq were bombed by the U.S.-led allied forces. Debris from the bombings was dispersed upwards into upper atmospheric currents, as shown by a U.S. satellite videotape obtained by Congress.

The Veterans Administration has only recently admitted that there is a problem with some "mystery illness" afflicting vets and their families. But the Pentagon denies there is any connection to chemical or biological warfare exposures.

In a May 25, 1994, "Memorandum for Persian Gulf Veterans," Defense Secretary William Perry and Joint Chiefs Chairman John Shalikashvili wrote:

"There have been reports in the press of the possibility that some of you were exposed to chemical or biological weapons agents. There is no information, classified or unclassified, that indicated that chemical or biological weapons were used in the Persian Gulf."

On June 23, 1994, the Defense Department's science board reported the results of an investigation into chemical and biological exposures in the Persian Gulf War. According to the report, "there is no evidence that either chemical or biological warfare was deployed at any level, or that there was any exposure of U.S. service members to chemical or biological warfare agents."

* * *

On December 13, 1994, the Pentagon released a report that says there was no single cause for Gulf War Syndrome. Veterans' groups were highly critical of this report. "It is more lies by the Pentagon to confuse and cover up the real causes of Gulf War Syndrome," says Major Richard Haines, president of Gulf Veterans International. In January, the Institute of Medicine of the National Academy of Sciences released a report critical of the Pentagon's research on Gulf War Syndrome.

Pentagon spokesman Dennis Boxx still maintains "we do not have any indication at this point that these things are transmittable to children or spouses."

Such declarations are consistent with the official British Ministry of Defense line. According to a July 14, 1994, letter from the Chemical and Biological Defense Establishment to the Pentagon's Lieutenant Colonel Vicki Merriman, "there was no evidence of any chemical warfare agent being present" in the Persian Gulf.

Ironically, when Senator Riegle first approached officials at the Department of Defense about veterans' possible exposures to chemical and biological warfare agents in the Persian Gulf, he was told by Walter Reed Army Medical Center commander Major General Ronald Blank that the issue was not even explored because "military intelligence maintained that such exposures never occurred."

While the Pentagon has refused to admit that chemical and biological warfare agents were present during the Gulf War, Senator Riegle stated on October 8, 1994, that "these Department of Defense explanations are inconsistent with the facts as related by the soldiers who were present, and with official government documents prepared by those who were present, and with experts who have examined the facts."

According to official Pentagon documents, at least eight members of the U.S. military who served in the Persian Gulf, in fact, received letters of commendation for locating and identifying chemical-warfare agents during the war. Army Captain Michael Johnson was awarded the Meritorious Service medal for overseeing the "positive identification of a suspected chemical agent." The certificate that accompanied Private First Class Allen Fisher's bronze star medal stated that his discoveries were the "first confirmed detection of chemical-agent contamination in the theater of operation."

In a memorandum dated January 4, 1994, to "Director, CATD," Captain Johnson of the Nuclear Biological and Chemical Branch of the Army wrote to his superiors: "Recent headlines have aroused considerable interest in the possible exposure of coalition forces to Iraqi chemical agents. Much of this interest is the result of health problems by Gulf War veterans that indicated exposure to chemical agents. Although no government officials have confirmed use, there is a high likelihood that some coalition forces experienced exposure to chemical agents."

Captain Johnson stated that he believed "coalition soldiers did experience exposure to Iraqi chemical agents." Johnson, who was commander of the 54th Chemical Troop, had cited in his report an example of a British soldier who was exposed. According to Johnson, "the soldier had an immediate reaction to the liquid contact. The soldier was in extreme pain and was going into shock." Captain Johnson first notified his superiors of his concerns in August 1991.

"This official dissembling and effort to obscure the facts are a continuation of Defense Department tactics," said Riegle in a written statement accompanying his October report. "The serious question remains as to why we were not provided with an official report dating from the time of the incident by the Department of Defense."

"If you look at the symptoms associated with biological and chemical contamination," says a former aide to Senator Riegle, "you'll see the same symptoms that are present in these veterans to varying degrees. The common denominator in all their illnesses is the breaking down of their immune system just as AIDS [acquired immunodeficiency syndrome] does, making them sicker and sicker as the days and years go by, and eventually incapacitating and killing some of them. And it's somehow being passed along to other people. We were getting hundreds of calls from people saying, 'He brought home this duffel bag, and we opened it up, and my eyes and hands started burning, and now I'm sick. What's wrong? What's happened?' "

NO

Michael Fumento

WHAT GULF WAR SYNDROME?

It has become a ritual by now. Each morning they inspect their skin, study their gums, feel their neck and armpits for swollen lymph nodes. When they cough, when their joints ache a bit, when they itch or whenever anything doesn't seem quite right with their bodies, they panic—and for good reason. Having stood down the fifth-largest military in the world, the men and women who served our country in the Persian Gulf are being told their fate will be forever linked to that line they guarded in the sand. For they are at risk of suffering one of the most insidious afflictions of the late twentieth century —Gulf War Syndrome.

Or so they've been told by over 500 newspaper and magazine stories, and a slew of television shows ranging from "20/20" to "Nightline" to "60 Minutes." No fewer than three respected men's magazines have featured the story, with such titles as GQ's "Cover-Up: U.S. Victims of the Gulf War." What vets haven't been told is the source of their fear may lie a bit closer to home than the windswept deserts of the Middle East.

That which is called Gulf War Syndrome comprises ailments diagnosed in some of the almost 700,000 men and women assigned to the Gulf region in 1990 and 1991. More than 50,000 vets have now signed on to the Persian Gulf Registry. While some of these vets say they are perfectly healthy and simply want to be monitored, the majority have joined the registry because they believe they may be suffering from the alleged syndrome.

BURNING SEMEN

According to Rep. Lane Evans (D-Ill.), "The commonality of experiences that [Gulf War veterans] have faced seem to be fairly convincing that they are suffering serious problems...." Likewise, CNN titled one of its interview segments "Gulf War Veterans Complain of Common Symptoms."

Yet their symptoms are anything but similar. They include, among others: aching muscles, aching joints, abdominal pain, facial pain, chest pain, blood clots, flushing, night sweats, blurry vision, photosensitivity, jaundice, bruising, shaking, vomiting, fevers, sinus growths, irritability, fatigue, swollen lymph nodes, weight loss, weight gain, loss of appetite, heartburn, nausea, bad breath, hair loss, graying hair, rashes, sore throat, heart disease, diverticulitis and other intestinal disorders, kidney stones, a growth in the eye, tingling and itching sensations, sore gums, cough, cancer, diarrhea with and without bleeding, constipation, testicular pain, epididymitis, unspecified swelling, memory loss, dizziness, inability to concentrate, choking sensation, depression, lightheadedness, hot and cold flashes, labored breathing, sneezing, sensitive teeth and other dental problems, neurological disorders, nasal congestion, bronchitis, leg cramps, twitching, hemorrhoids, thyroid problems, welts, rectal and vaginal bleeding, colon polyps, increased urination, a "bulging disk" in the neck, hypertension, blood in urine, insomnia, headaches, and "a foot fungus that will not go away."

The symptom list reads like the index of a medical self-help book. Veterans have even blamed the syndrome for their having contracted malaria, herpes, and tuberculosis, diseases heretofore thought to have been spread by mosquitoes, sexual intercourse, and coughing. Many symptoms are highly subjective, such as "lumps under the skin" or "thick saliva." Readers or viewers of news reports don't know this, however, because whenever they see or hear a list of symptoms it's rarely more than about five items long, implying the syndrome spectrum is fairly small.

Yet the definition of the syndrome has been widened even beyond Gulf vets to include their wives and children. In addition to suffering most of the illnesses of their husbands, these women also claim to suffer yeast infections, menstrual cramps, and irregular periods, while the children's attributed ills include earaches and rashes, among others. Some wives and girlfriends of vets have even complained that their men's semen burned their skin, rather like the blood of the creatures in the *Alien* films.

* * *

If the definition of this syndrome is murky, the cause is hardly more clear. Theories as to the specific cause or causes of the illnesses have ranged from the use of depleted uranium in American shells to fumes from burning oil fires. A 1994 Centers for Disease Control (CDC) study found that while firefighters did have increased exposure to certain toxics from the burning wells, personnel in nearby Kuwait City had essentially the same exposure as persons living in the United States. Yet few American soldiers were even as close as Kuwait City. Likewise, a National Institutes of Health report issued in April 1994 made short order of the uranium theory, noting among other things that the use of the material was highly localized.

At a hearing on May 6, 1994, Sen. John D. Rockefeller IV (D-W.Va.), then-chairman of the Senate Veterans' Affairs Committee, implicated the drug Pyridostigmine bromide, which had been given Gulf troops as "pretreatment" for nerve agent poisoning. But a National Institutes of Health (NIH) report released on June 22, 1994, noted this drug has been used by some patients for decades—in doses of up to 6,000 milligrams a day—with "no significant long-term effects. By contrast, the troops received a mere thirty milligrams for up to three weeks."

Nonetheless, Rockefeller continues to hammer at Pyridostigmine bromide as being the syndrome's most likely cause, which says something about the even less likely causes. On a December "Nightline" broadcast focusing on the offspring of Gulf War vets, Rockefeller went on to claim that the drug causes birth defects in Gulf vet offspring. But no birth defects have been associated with women who used the drug before or during pregnancy, much less with the more tenuous exposure of the male.

GAS PAINS

The most chilling theory, and the one to which the media has given the most credence, was suggested by the *USA Today* headline, "Trail of Symptoms Suggests Chem-arms." Chemical weapons were the focus of a 160-page report from the Senate Banking Committee. Don Riegle (D-Mich.), then-chairman of the committee, had been among the minority who voted against the resolution authorizing President George Bush to take military action against Iraq—as were four of the most vocal congressmen on the issue of Gulf War Syndrome.

The Riegle report includes testimony from a number of vets who appear convinced that they were exposed to chemical weapons and believe they are now suffering as a result. The media reported statements such as the one by a fellow who told *USA Today*, "I know in my heart I was gassed."

But chemical weapons experts such as Dr. George Koelle, professor emeritus at the University of Pennsylvania and a former chemical warfare specialist for the military during World War II, have pointed out that if the men were really exposed to such weapons, they would darned well know it. Koelle says, "None [of the Gulf War vets] exhibit symptoms characteristic of either blistering agents like mustard or organo-phosphates, those types of agents which would be primarily in use."

Koelle's experience with chemical warfare victims from World War II indicates that, as he put it, "Blistering agents or mustard leave very little in the way of residual effects. Acute effects, yes, even fatal ones, but lasting effects are not characteristic." He recalls that during the Second World War he tried recruiting into a study chemical-weapons victims who were still suffering from the attack but couldn't find any. Further, he notes, this was the case with soldiers who had suffered massive acute exposure, much less soldiers who by their own statements could not have received a high dosage.

He is also aghast that chemical weapons could be blamed, as they are in the Banking Committee report, for illnesses in family members of exposed persons; only a contagion could accomplish this, he notes.

In a "60 Minutes" segment on Gulf War Syndrome broadcast on March 12, reporter Ed Bradley, who six years earlier began the Alar apple scare, suggested that the veterans' symptoms could have been the result of poisoning by sarin. Sarin is a nerve agent the Germans developed before World War II but never deployed. Eight days later, the world was horrified to find out what the real symptoms of sarin poisoning are when terrorists planted the gas aboard several Tokyo subway cars. Passengers fainted, vomited, and went into convulsions. Over 5,000 needed immediate hospitalization, and eight died within hours.

This is what chemical weapons do; they incapacitate an enemy. Conversely, vets who have now become convinced they suffered gas attacks in the Gulf say that at the time they had symptoms no more serious than tingling on the back of the neck or dry mouth or perhaps a burning sensation in the lungs. In contrast with the thousands of Japanese subway riders, no U.S. soldier in the Gulf was ever hospitalized or incapacited by any unseen weapon.

* * *

Admitting as much was Dr. Charles Jackson of the Tuskegee VA Medical Center in Huntsville Alabama. Jackson brought great publicity to the issue of Gulf War Syndrome in 1993 by using the syndrome, and exposure to chemical-biological warfare, as a diagnosis for numerous ailing members of a Naval Reserve Seabee unit. "But suppose they'd developed something that was insidious so they didn't need to incapacitate in the field," he told *USA Today*, "something that would get you when you got home." For a guy as wily as Saddam Hussein has proved to be, inventing a chemical weapon that didn't even begin working until years after the war was lost would be pretty stupid indeed.

Neither the NIH report, nor another produced by the Department of Defense in June—by a task force chaired by Nobel prize winner Dr. Joshua Lederberg of Rockefeller University—was able to pinpoint a specific cause for the mysterious syndrome. A third report, released in December by the Defense Department's Comprehensive Clinical Evaluation Program, declared, "There is no clinical evidence for a single or unique agent causing a 'Gulf War Syndrome.'" Rather, it said, "unexplained illnesses reported by Persian Gulf veterans are not a single disease or apparent syndrome, but rather multiple illnesses with overlapping symptoms and causes."

An Institute of Medicine report released in January criticized the government's efforts to study the problem and reach scientific conclusions. It then made the seemingly bizarre recommendation that Vice President Al Gore be in charge of coordinating the Gulf War Syndrome research effort. Gore has no scientific or medical background. But even the Institute of Medicine panel said it couldn't find evidence to support the argument that chemical weapons and medicine dispensed to vets were the chief causes of the syndrome.

THE EXPERTS AGREE

If these various reports could find no syndrome, how to explain all those sick men, with their sick wives and sick children?

Lost in the rush to find the most quotable or pathetic victim is the notion that everybody occasionally becomes ill. Says Edward Young, former chief of staff at the Houston VA Medical Center, one of the three centers set up to investigate ailments among Gulf War vets, "We're talking about people who have multiple complaints. And if you go out on the street in any city in this country, you'll find people who have exactly the same things, and they've never been to the Gulf."

An early Army study of seventy-nine Indiana reservists who served in the Gulf and complained of a variety of symptoms found "no objective evidence for an outbreak of disease." It said, "Problems and symptoms like those found here would be expected to occur throughout the Reserve forces which deployed."

A wider, on-going VA study has compared over 7,000 Gulf War veterans with 7,000 veterans who had served elsewhere during the same period. While the controls are not scientifically matched and the results have not been prepared in proper form for publication, there seems to be no difference in illnesses. As Lederberg observes, "You can't even take numbers as we have seen them and draw the conclusion that anybody's sicker from serving in the Gulf than comparable people elsewhere," though he adds that doesn't necessarily "mean it isn't true."

* * *

One advocacy group that opposed the Gulf War deployment, the Military Family Support Network of Fort Bragg, North Carolina, has attributed both miscarriages and birth defects to exposures in the Gulf. But a combined study of pregnancies at several bases found the miscarriages of Gulf vets' wives to be at the same level as that population had before deployment to the Gulf. This was about half the civilian rate.

Yet in a December 1994 "Nightline" broadcast focusing on the children of Gulf War vets, the show's reporter made the alarming claim, "In Waynesville, Mississippi, thirteen of fifteen babies born to returning members of a National Guard Unit were reported to have severe and often rare health problems."

Reported, yes—but without substantiation. The Mississippi Department of Health investigated the alleged cluster and found that of fifty-four births to returning Guardsmen in that state, there were three major defects, with two to four expected in a group that size. They also found four minor defects, with three to five expected. There were no more premature or low birth-weight children than would be expected.

A larger study of 620 pregnancies at Robins Air Force Base in Georgia also found defects and miscarriages among Gulf vets' children to be at or below normal levels. In the Persian Gulf Registry of veterans, the reported rates of miscarriage are below that of the general population.

THE REAL CAUSE

The thing unspoken in the Gulf syndrome allegations is that somehow the vets, their wives, and their offspring are supposed to be immune to illness. If they are not, then the illness must be from exposure to something in the Gulf. The fallacy employed is the one universally used to show causation where none is otherwise apparent. It is the bulwark of scare-of-the-weekism, as in "My wife began using a cellular phone and then developed a brain tumor, therefore the phone caused the tumor."

Does all this mean that, for all categories of illness, Gulf vets, their wives, and offspring have no more problems than other people? Not at all. Gulf veterans show extraordinarily high rates of post-traumatic stress, and they also suffer disproportionately from drug and alcohol dependency.

But with a few exceptions, the vast number of symptoms attributed to Gulf War Syndrome can be brought on by stress. While the Allies ultimately won a quick, lopsided victory, the soldiers had no idea that would be the case. What they did know was that, in facing Saddam Hussein's Iraq, they were threatened by horrible weapons which no American had faced since World War I.

A further stressor for many was the quick transformation from civilian to combatant—as was the case with reservists and National Guardsmen. The Indiana reservist study concluded that, to the extent there were abnormalities, they appeared to be related to the stress of being ripped quickly out of civilian life and being sent to a war zone, and then a few months later being thrust back into civilian life. This may explain why reservists and National Guardsmen are far more likely to complain of Gulf War-related ills than are active duty soldiers.

* * *

Massive illness brought on by stress among veterans is nothing new. Stephen E. Straus, of the National Institute of Allergies and Infectious Diseases, told *Science News*, "There is a spectrum of this illness that is seen with all military adventures." Civil War veterans had undiagnosable symptoms, including fatigue, breathlessness, and gastrointestinal symptoms. In World War I, some 60,000 British troops were found to suffer from a mysterious "effort syndrome," a problem that recurred in World War II. Similar phenomena have been called variously "soldier's heart," "neurasthenia," "combat fatigue," "shell shock," or the Vietnam-era "post-traumatic stress disorder." But a major difference between then and now is that now there is a mass media to publicize the claims.

Indeed, the closest Gulf War Syndrome comes to having a prime cause may be the American media. The study of the seventy-nine Indiana reservists found that many of the symptoms appeared to arise in response to reports of other people being sick. "When we have media reports of a particular symptom that hasn't been reported before," said Army spokeswoman Virginia Stephanakis, "suddenly by God we'll get plenty of those."

Hillary Clinton surely understands the power of the media in this regard. Since her health-care reform setback, she has adopted Gulf War Syndrome as a personal cause and pledged to do whatever she could to bring more attention to the plight of the ailing Gulf vets. The *Washington Post* reported that the first lady "has become the Clinton administration point-person on the Gulf War Syndrome issue." In March, her husband announced he was forming a special panel of physicians, scientists, veterans, and unspecified "others" to investigate the mystery ailment. Even the mainstream media found the president's announcement a bit much, with several newspapers referring to Clinton's act, combined with an effort to prevent trimming the Veterans' Affairs budget, as a move to "outflank his GOP rivals on veterans' issues."

There are plenty of veterans' issues at play. Under the enacted legislation, veterans can receive anywhere from $89 to $1,823 a month, depending on the extent of their alleged disabilities. To qualify, they must have been symptomatic at least six months and be found to suffer fatigue, skin problems, headaches, muscle pains, joint pains, nerve disorders, neuropsychological problems, respiratory problems, sleep disturbances, stomach problems, heart problems, and menstrual disorders that began during or within two years after the war and lasted at least six months.

Other vets may simply have succumbed to the lure of litigation. Some 2,000 of them have joined a $1 billion lawsuit against both American and foreign companies, alleging that these companies gave Iraq the chemicals needed to produce the weapons that they claim caused their illnesses.

HYSTERIA, BUT NO LAUGHING MATTER

There's no reason to think, however, that most of those vets who say they are sick from exposure in the Gulf are not sincere. Indeed, most may be truly sick. As Dr. Dimitrios Trichopoulos, the head of the Department of Epidemiology at the Harvard School of Public Health, explains it, when many people hear they should be ill, they become ill—the flip side, as it were, of the placebo effect. "If you keep telling people they should be sick, of course they believe it," Trichopoulos says.

Phantom epidemics in which many people fall ill upon hearing they may have been exposed to something harmful are not uncommon. Two years ago, more than 2,000 children in and around Cairo fell suddenly ill in an epidemic of fainting that some blamed on chemical and biological agents. The "epidemic" proved to be only psychological.

In 1986, reports of hundreds of girls in the Israeli-occupied West Bank hospitalized with symptoms of nausea, dizziness, headaches, abdominal pains, and fatigue sparked an international incident. At least one newspaper blamed the maladies on nerve gas; others pointed to a pesticide. Ultimately, medical investigators found nothing to blame for the epidemic other than mass hysteria. U.S. schools are also occasionally swept by such hysterias.

The illnesses attributed to Gulf War Syndrome also seem to have a peculiar way of targeting Americans. Although there are some ill Canadian, British, and Australian troops, as of last year no more than a few dozen of the 42,000 British troops who served in the war reported any kind of mysterious illness.

The British Surgeon General has denied that any "medical condition exists that is peculiar to those who served in the Gulf conflict."

Brian McMahon, who was Trichopolous's predecessor as head of the Department of Epidemiology at the Harvard School of Public Health and is now professor emeritus at the school, says, "We've been through this before. We saw this broad array of symptoms with PCBs in Michigan. When you get such an array with the only thing in common being exposure," he said, you're seeing psychosomatic illness. "People are looking at clouds and trying to see faces instead of looking at data," he said.

Still, some veterans—and their terrified wives—are truly suffering. Stress-related illness is "a devastating problem with physical consequences," says Dr. Barry Rumack, a toxicology expert and clinical professor at the University of Colorado School of Medicine. "It's just not anything chemical."

WEIRD SCIENCE

Unfortunately, with rare exceptions, scientific evidence, statistical data, and mundane explanations have lost out to exotic theories, lobbyists' demands, politicians' polemics, and numerous unsubstantiated anecdotes. The Banking Committee report found no room for discussions of background rates of illness, yet it devoted seventeen pages to personal testimonies. These are emotional, sad and compelling anecdotes—but they're anecdotes just the same.

Naval Reserve Seabee Nick Roberts is one of the Seabees diagnosed under the auspices of Dr. Charles Jackson. Roberts suffers from lymphoma, a cancer of the lymph glands. In November 1993, he told a congressional panel that of the thirty-three members in his military reserve unit, ten have been diagnosed with the same illness. He also held up a list of what he said were 173 cancer-stricken Gulf veterans. The media promptly reported his testimony. Yet a Persian Gulf Registry update five months later showed only eight lymphomas out of all Gulf vets in America, with thirty-eight cancers of all types. This cancer rate was about fifty percent *below* that of the comparison non-Gulf veterans, although the control group was not scientifically matched.

Lymphomas are thought to usually develop decades after their instigation (although with AIDS patients who have suffered almost a complete collapse of their immune system, this can be shortened to a few years). What may be the most celebrated case of Gulf War Syndrome—and the only one with death widely attributed to it—is that of lymphoma victim Michael Adcock. But Army spokeswoman Stephanakis said Adcock had just arrived in Saudi Arabia when he was diagnosed with his first symptom. "He [Adcock] had rectal bleeding six days after arriving and the family blamed it on the Gulf," she said skeptically.

"Beyond a shadow of a doubt, I believe Michael died of multiple chemical exposure," Adcock's mother told the *Washington Times* in May 1993. She cited exposure to oil well fires, paint used to insulate vehicles from chemical weapons exposure, and lead in the diesel fuel used in lanterns and heaters as probable causes for her son's lymphoma. Six months later, in congressional testimony, she was convinced the cause was a chemical weapon released in a Scud missile explosion—which authorities said was actually a sonic boom—the day before her son's rectal bleeding began.

No reporter or congressman dared suggest it was more probable that Adcock's cancer was merely one of the almost 50,000 lymphomas diagnosed that year. No one dared consider the possibility that Mrs. Adcock's statements were one woman's sad effort to cope with the unexpected loss of a child. Surely much of why the coverage of Gulf War Syndrome has been so lopsidedly unskeptical is that to do otherwise is to be branded a rotten human being, not unlike those who, a decade earlier, questioned what proved to be the outrageous estimates of missing and kidnapped children.

THE REAL COVER-UP

Just ask the Houston VA center's Edward Young. In an interview with the *Birmingham Daily News*, he said he had seen enough alleged victims of the disease to be convinced there wasn't one. "It really rankles me when people stand up and call it 'Persian Gulf Syndrome,'" said a clearly frustrated Young. "To honor this thing with some name is ridiculous." Although he later asked that his comments not be printed, the American Legion, the chief lobbying group for the syndrome, got wind of them and complained to the VA, which unceremoniously yanked Young from his position. The VA cited his lack of compassion.

The CBS program "Eye to Eye with Connie Chung" originally expressed great interest in doing a show debunking the alleged syndrome, or at least telling both sides of the story. Producer Mary Raffalli collected a great deal of information on the subject and said the show would definitely be done. But it wasn't

—according to Susan Zirinski, a CBS producer, the program at the time was understaffed and the piece seemed time-sensitive, although she now concedes it was not.

Some syndrome proponents, however, are willing to concede that science is not on their side. Last year, after Congress passed legislation providing compensation without a clear definition of the ailment, Veterans' Affairs Secretary Jesse Brown admitted, "This legislation is revolutionary. We have never before provided payment for something we're not even certain exists." Jay Rockefeller, asked if there was a definite connection between Gulf War service and defective offspring, said, "If you were to ask as a human being, I would have to say absolutely. If you were to ask me as a scientist, I would have to say we cannot yet prove there is a link." Seen any non-human scientists lately? Rockefeller was saying the problem with scientists is they insist on using science to draw conclusions. And the science here, as he admits in his own way, does not support his position.

* * *

Nor will it ever, which may be what those "others" to be appointed to President Clinton's panel are all about. As Mary R. Stout, then-national president of Vietnam Veterans of America, once testified before a congressional panel:

> I guess, to sum up all of what this means to us and what it means to... veterans, is that if we must now presume that the scientific community cannot be trusted —and in some cases obviously—we are assuming that—a political decision must be made on this issue to provide compensation to veterans.

The year was 1990 and the issue wasn't Gulf War Syndrome but the defoliant Agent Orange, and the vets in question were from Vietnam. Study after study found that, other than stress, there was no difference in levels of illness between soldiers who could have been exposed to the herbicide and those who were not, and that many convinced they'd been exposed clearly hadn't been. The scientific community thus became untrustworthy and was overridden by the political "community." The case of the Gulf War Syndrome is currently following a similar course.

Where does this leave the vets? Dr. Russell Tarver, who led the Mississippi National Guard birth-defect investigation, strayed from his data during an interview just long enough to offer an opinion. "I think it's unconscionable to frighten people out of reproducing unless you have some good data to support that contention," he said. "I think you're committing a crime against those veterans."

POSTSCRIPT

Is the Gulf War Syndrome Real?

The article "Walking Wounded," by Gregory Jaynes, *Esquire* (May 1994) begins with the following heading: "The real casualties of Desert Storm may have been the soldiers who came back alive. A haunting account of a mysterious malady: Gulf War Syndrome." Jaynes and many other journalists, veterans, and doctors believe that exposure to toxic biological and/or environmental agents in the Persian Gulf during Operation Desert Storm are responsible for a variety of symptoms experienced by thousands of veterans of the Gulf War in 1991. The U.S. government, however, has tried to deny ill veterans disability pay because it maintains that there is no proof that these illnesses are connected with service in the gulf. The government is not alone in its view that the Gulf War Syndrome does not exist. Articles that question the legitimacy of the syndrome include "Research Is Incomplete and Inadequate," *Chemistry and Industry* (January 16, 1995); "Pentagon Study Finds No Clinical Evidence for a Single Cause of "Gulf War Syndrome," *Chemical and Engineering News* (December 19, 1994); and "Gulf War Syndrome: Is It a Real Disease?" *The New York Times* (November 23, 1993). In "The Truth About Health Scares," *Health Confidential* (May 1993), Michael Fumento discusses several media-hyped environmental causes of death, and he describes how people can protect themselves from other health scares.

Agent Orange, the herbicide used during the Vietnam War, has been linked to several health problems among veterans of that conflict. Although the U.S. government initially denied any relationship between exposure to Agent Orange and illness, it was eventually accepted that there is a link. The National Academy of Science's Institute of Medicine released a report in 1993 showing a link between herbicides like Agent Orange and three types of cancer, including Hodgkin's disease, and two types of skin disease. See "Agent Orange Risks Reassessed," *Science* (August 6, 1993). Many people feel that the government's denial of any relationship between environmental factors present in the Persian Gulf and subsequent health concerns among Gulf War veterans is similar to the government's original denial of the adverse effects of Agent Orange on Vietnam veterans. See "Congress Cites Agent Orange Coverup," *Science* (August 31, 1990). Additional articles about the health effects of exposure to Agent Orange during the Vietnam War are "Agent Orange Benefits Still Available from the VA," *Jet* (March 6, 1995); "Vietnam Aftermath: An Admiral's Ordeal," *U.S. News & World Report* (September 26, 1994); and "List of Diseases Linked to Agent Orange Expanded," *Jet* (November 1, 1993).

Other articles calling for more and better research into the Gulf War Syndrome and Agent Orange include "The Gulf War Syndrome," *British Medical*

Journal (vol. 310, 1995); "Institute of Medicine Calls for Coordinated Studies of Gulf War Veterans' Health Complaints," *Journal of the American Medical Association* (February 8, 1995); "The Persian Gulf Experience and Health," *Journal of the American Medical Association* (August 3, 1994); "Push for Gulf Syndrome Research," *Nature* (August 19, 1993); and "US Congress Urged to Back Further Agent Orange Studies," *Nature* (July 29, 1993)

Readings that support the existence of the Gulf War Syndrome include "A Lingering Sickness," *The Nation* (January 23, 1995); "Mal de Guerre," *The Nation* (March 7, 1994); "Mystery Illness and the Gulf War," *Maclean's* (August 23, 1993); "House Bill Would Guarantee Care for Victims of Gulf War Ills," *Congressional Quarterly Weekly Report* (July 31, 1993); and "Coming Home to Pain," *Newsweek* (June 28, 1993).

ISSUE 17

Are Pesticides in Foods Harmful to Human Health?

YES: Lawrie Mott and Karen Snyder, from "Pesticide Alert," *Amicus Journal* (Spring 1988)

NO: Bruce Ames, from "Too Much Fuss About Pesticides," *Consumers' Research* (April 1990)

ISSUE SUMMARY

YES: Pesticide researchers Lawrie Mott and Karen Snyder maintain that the very foods consumers are trying to eat more of—fresh fruits and vegetables—are those that are most contaminated with harmful pesticide residues.

NO: Professor of biochemistry and molecular biology Bruce Ames argues that any risks from pesticides in foods are minimal and that fears are greatly exaggerated.

Throughout history, farmers and other food growers have fought with insect and weed pests that invade the food supply and cause disease and discomfort. Early attempts to reduce pest damage included purely physical attacks—burning and stepping on the pests—as well as saying prayers and performing ritual dances. A few more effective measures were discovered before modern times. These included sulfur compounds, plant extracts, wood ashes, and natural pest enemies.

For the past 50 years, the battle against pests has escalated, and some of the most lethal and sophisticated chemicals ever invented have been used against them. When modern pesticides, such as DDT, were first introduced in the late 1940s, scientists proclaimed total victory against crop destruction and diseases carried by insects. Many dispute this victory, but the evidence of these chemical weapons against insects is present in streams, rivers, and soils —and in our bodies. Most of us carry traces of several chemical pesticides in our body tissues. Moreover, although pesticides are used specifically to kill insect pests, many of them are quite toxic to humans as well. Pesticides are responsible for an estimated 25 million human poisonings each year, mostly of children under 10.

To cause harm to humans, a pesticide must be taken internally through the mouth, skin, or respiratory system. Eating unwashed fruits or vegetables that were recently sprayed with pesticides or entering a field too soon after pesticide application are ways in which pesticides may enter the body. Symptoms of acute or one-time exposure include headache, fatigue, abdominal pain, coma, and death. Long-term exposure may cause cancer, mutations, or birth defects.

Pesticide poisoning from sprayed fruits and vegetables became a national issue when reports of the contamination of apple crops made headlines. Since 1968 some red varieties of apples have been sprayed with a chemical growth regulator that prevents the apples from dropping off trees before they ripen, improves color and firmness, and extends shelf life. The chemical, known as daminozide, is marketed under the trade name Alar. Alar penetrates the pulp of the apple and cannot be washed, cooked, or peeled off. In 1986 processors and stores in the United States, bowing to consumer pressure, vowed not to accept apples treated with the chemical. It was reported that a breakdown product of Alar, which is formed when treated apples are heated, is a low-level cancer-causing agent.

A report released in the spring of 1987 by the National Academy of Sciences claimed that pesticides may be responsible for as many as 20,000 cases of cancer a year. In their report, the academy identified 15 foods (tomatoes, beef, potatoes, oranges, lettuce, peaches, pork, wheat, soybeans, beans, carrots, chicken, corn, grapes, and apples) treated with a small group of pesticides that pose the greatest risk of cancer. While these figures are certainly frightening, many scientists believe that too much fuss is being raised about pesticides. They point out that many foods contain natural cancer-causing agents, and they argue that people are still better off with a high intake of fruits and vegetables—ironically because they contain nutrients that may help prevent cancer.

In the following selections, Lawrie Mott and Karen Snyder contend that a lot of the food that is sold in supermarkets is not safe and that the government does not adequately test the fruits and vegetables that are sold to the public. Bruce Ames maintains that while it is good for consumers to be concerned about what they eat, the hysteria about pesticide residues may not be warranted by the actual risk they pose.

YES   Lawrie Mott and Karen Snyder

PESTICIDE ALERT

If you are like most Americans, when you go to the supermarket, you try to choose foods that are healthy. Instinctively, you steer your shopping cart towards the produce section. The typical produce section currently stocks over five times the number of items displayed a decade ago. The increased availability and variety of fresh fruits and vegetables is due, in part, to the extensive use of chemical fertilizers and pesticides. Yet, residues of these agricultural chemicals can remain in our food. The fruits and vegetables in your supermarket may contain invisible hazards to your health in the form of residues of pesticides.

All of us are exposed to pesticides on a regular basis. The food we eat, particularly the fresh fruits and vegetables, contains pesticide residues. In the summer of 1985, nearly 1,000 people in several western states and Canada were poisoned by residues of the pesticide Temik in watermelons. Within two to twelve hours after eating the contaminated watermelons, people experienced nausea, vomiting, blurred vision, muscle weakness, and other symptoms. Fortunately, no one died, though some of the victims were gravely ill. Reports included grand mal seizures, cardiac irregularities, a number of hospitalizations, and at least two stillbirths following maternal illness.

In 1986, the public grew increasingly concerned over the use of the plant-growth regulator, Alar, on apples. Primarily used to make the harvest easier and the apples redder, Alar leaves residues in both apple juice and apple sauce. The outcry led many food manufacturers and supermarket chains to announce they would not accept Alar-treated apples.

Also in 1986, approximately 140 dairy herds in Arkansas, Oklahoma, and Missouri were quarantined due to contamination by the banned pesticide, heptachlor. Dairy products in eight states were subject to recall. Some milk contained heptachlor in amounts as much as seven times the acceptable level. Those responsible for the contamination were sentenced to prison terms.

Last year, the National Academy of Sciences issued a report on pesticides in the food supply which concluded that pesticides in our food may cause more than 1 million additional cases of cancer in the United States over our lifetimes. Although some have argued that this theoretical calculation is excessively high, the number was based on the presence of fewer than thirty carcinogenic pesticides in our food supply (many more pesticides applied to food are carcinogens) and does not consider potential exposure to carcinogenic pesticides in drinking water.

The repetition of the Temik, Alar and other stories suggests that the government programs designed to protect us from pesticide residues may be inherently flawed. These events also demonstrate the need for information on a series of fundamental issues concerning pesticide residues in food. As it now stands, you have no way of knowing if your food contains dangerous residues or whether the amount of residue you are eating is hazardous. Not only is government testing of food for residues spotty and inadequate, not only are some levels of pesticides allowed in food being challenged by leading scientists as too high, but no state or federal government agency really attempts to answer your most basic questions about pesticide residues in food—questions such as what pesticides are found in your food, what level of residue is safe, and who should make these decisions.

Each year, approximately 2.6 billion pounds of pesticides are used in the United States. Pesticides are applied in countless ways throughout the United States, not just on food crops. They are sprayed on forests, lakes, city parks, lawns, and playing fields, and in hospitals, schools, offices, and homes, and are contained in a huge variety of products from shampoos to shelf paper, mattresses to shower curtains. As a consequence, pesticides may be found wherever we live and work, in the air we breathe, in the water we drink, and in the food we eat. A former director of the federal government's program to regulate pesticides called these chemicals the number one environmental risk, because all Americans are exposed to them.

By definition, pesticides are toxic chemicals—toxic to insects, weeds, fungi, and other unwanted pests. Most are potentially harmful to humans and can cause cancer, birth defects, changes in genetic material that may be inherited by the next generation (genetic mutations), and nerve damage, among other debilitating or lethal effects. Many more of these chemicals have not been thoroughly tested to identify their health effects.

Pesticides applied in agriculture—the production of food, animal feed, and fiber, such as cotton—account for 60 percent of all U.S. pesticide uses other than disinfectants and wood preservatives. Pesticides are designed to control or destroy undesirable pests. Insecticides control insects; herbicides control weeds; fungicides control fungi such as mold and mildew; and rodenticides control rodents. Some of these chemicals are applied to control pests that reduce crop yields or to protect the nutritional value of our food; others are used for cosmetic purposes to enhance the appearance of fresh food.

As a result of massive agricultural applications of pesticides, our food, drinking water, and the world around us now contain pesticide residues; they are literally everywhere—in the United States and throughout the world. In fact, though all these chemicals have been banned from agricultural use, nearly all Americans have residues of the pesticides DDT, chlordane, heptachlor, aldrin, and dieldrin in their bodies. Ground water is the source of drinking water for 95 percent of rural Americans and 50 percent of all Americans; yet, according to a 1987 Environmental Protection Agency (EPA) report, at least twenty pesticides, some of which cause cancer and other harmful effects, have been found in ground water in at least twenty-four states. In California alone, fifty-seven different pesticides were detected in the ground water. The banned pesticide DBCP remains in 2,499 drinking water wells in California's San Joaquin Valley—1,473 of these contaminated wells are not considered suitable for drinking water or bathing because the DBCP levels exceed the state health department's action level. As more states conduct ground water sampling programs for pesticides, more pesticides are expected to be found. Surface water supplies have also been found to contain pesticides. For example, the herbicide alachlor, or Lasso, has contaminated both ground and surface water in the midwest, primarily as a result of use on corn and soybeans. The federal government must provide financial assistance to cotton and soybean farmers because enormous surpluses of these crops exist in the United States.

The extent of contamination of our food is unknown. The federal Food and Drug Administration (FDA) monitors our food supply to detect pesticide residues. Between 1982 and 1985, FDA detected pesticide residues in 48 percent of the most frequently consumed fresh fruits and vegetables. This figure probably understates the presence of pesticides in food because about half of the pesticides applied to food cannot be routinely detected by FDA's laboratories, and the agency samples less than one percent of our food.

The cumulative effect of widespread, chronic low-level exposure to pesticides is only partially understood. Some of the only examples now available involve farmers and field workers. A National Cancer Institute study found that farmers exposed to herbicides had a six times greater risk than nonfarmers of contracting one type of cancer. Other studies have shown similar results, with farmers exposed to pesticides having an increased risk of developing cancer. Researchers at the University of Southern California uncovered startling results in a 1987 study sponsored by the National Cancer Institute. Children living in homes where household and garden pesticides were used had as much as a sevenfold greater chance of developing childhood leukemia.

Another frightening consequence of the long-term and increasing use of pesticides is that the pest species farmers try to control are becoming resistant to these chemicals. For example, the number of insects resistant to insecticides nearly doubled between 1970 and 1980. Resistance among weeds and fungi has also risen sharply in the last two decades. In order to combat this problem, greater amounts of pesticides must be applied to control the pest, which in turn can increase the pest's resistance to the chemical. For example, since the 1940s pesticide use has increased tenfold, but crop losses to insects have doubled.

Pesticides can also have detrimental effects on the environment. The widespread use of chlorinated insecticides, particularly DDT, significantly reduced bird populations, including bald eagles, ospreys, peregrine falcons, and brown pelicans. DDT is very persistent and highly mobile in the environment. Animals in the Antarctic and from areas never sprayed were found to contain DDT or its metabolites. Though most of the organochlorines are no longer used in the United States, continuing use in other nations has serious environmental consequences. Other types of pesticides now applied in the United States have adverse effects on the environment.

* * *

A February 1987 EPA report, entitled *Unfinished Business*, ranked pesticides in food as one of the nation's most serious health and environmental problems. Many pesticides widely used on food are known to cause, or suspected of causing, cancer. To date, EPA has identified fifty-five pesticides that could leave residues in food as being carcinogens. Other pesticides can cause birth defects or miscarriages. Some pesticides can produce changes in the genetic material, or genetic mutations, that can be passed to the next generation. Other pesticides can cause sterility or impaired fertility.

Under today's scientific practices, predictions of the potentially adverse health effects of chemicals on humans are based on laboratory testing in animals. Unfortunately, the overwhelming majority of pesticides used today have not been sufficiently tested for their health hazards. The National Academy of Sciences estimated, by looking at a selected number of chemicals, that data to conduct a thorough assessment of health effects were available for only ten percent of the ingredients in pesticide products used today.

A 1982 congressional report estimated that between 82 percent and 85 percent of pesticides registered for use had not been adequately tested for their ability to cause cancer; the figure was 60 percent to 70 percent for birth defects, and 90 percent to 93 percent for genetic mutations. This situation has occurred because the majority of pesticides now available were licensed for use before EPA established requirements for health effects testing.

In 1972, Congress directed EPA to reevaluate all these older chemicals (approximately 600) by the modern testing regimens. Through reregistration, EPA would fill the gaps in required toxicology tests. By 1986, however, EPA still had not completed a final safety reassessment for any of these chemicals. Roughly 400 pesticides are registered for use on food, and 390 of these are older chemicals that are undergoing reregistration review. To make matters worse, scientists are uncovering new types of adverse health effects caused by chemicals. For example, a few pesticides have been found to damage components of the immune system—the body's defense network to protect against infections, cancer, allergies, and autoimmune diseases. Yet testing for toxicity to the immune system is not part of the routine safety evaluation for chemicals. In short, pesticides are being widely used with virtually no knowledge of their potential long-term effects on human health and the human population is unknowingly serving as the test subject.

The lack of health effects data on pesticides means that EPA is regulating pesticides out of ignorance, rather than knowledge. This poses particularly serious consequences for EPA's regulation of pesticides in food. Pesticides may only be applied to a food crop after EPA has established a maximum safe level, or tolerance, for pesticide residues allowed in the food. However, EPA's tolerances may permit unsafe levels of pesticides for five reasons:

1. EPA established tolerances without necessary health and safety data.

2. EPA relied on outdated assumptions about what constitutes an average

diet, such as assuming we eat no more than 7.5 ounces per year of avocados, artichokes, melons, mushrooms, eggplants or nectarines, when setting tolerance levels.

3. Tolerances are rarely revised when new scientific data about the risks of a pesticide are received by EPA.

4. Ingredients in pesticides that may leave hazardous residues in food, such as the so-called "inert" ingredients, are not considered in tolerance setting.

5. EPA's tolerances allow carcinogenic pesticide residues to occur in food, even though no "safe" level of exposure to a carcinogen may exist.

The EPA is not solely responsible for the flaws in the federal government program to protect our food supply. The FDA monitors food to ensure that residue levels do not exceed EPA's tolerances. Food containing pesticide residues in excess of the applicable tolerance violates the food safety law and FDA is required to seize the food in order to prevent human consumption. However, FDA is not always capable of determining which foods have illegal pesticide residues. For instance, FDA's routine laboratory methods can detect fewer than half the pesticides that may leave residues in food. Some of the pesticides used extensively on food that cannot be regularly identified include alachlor, benomyl, daminozide and the EBDCs. Furthermore, FDA's enforcement against food with residues in excess of tolerance is ineffective: according to a 1986 General Accounting Office report, for 60 percent of the illegal pesticide residue cases identified, FDA

did not prevent the sale or the ultimate consumption of the food.

* * *

To get a better picture of the pesticides that occur in the foods most commonly eaten, NRDC [Natural Resources Defense Council] analyzed representative federal and state pesticide monitoring data. From 1982 to 1985, FDA analyzed 19,515 samples of the twenty-six types of fruits and vegetables nationwide. Forty-eight per cent contained detectable residues. In the same period, the California Department of Food and Agriculture (CDFA) analyzed 17,237 produce samples. Pesticide residues were detected in 14 percent of the samples. These numbers most likely understate the amount of pesticides in food because the laboratory tests cannot detect all the chemicals applied to our food. The discrepancy between FDA and CDFA results is probably due to FDA's ability to detect a greater number of chemicals in lower amounts and the greater number of imported samples analyzed by FDA.

Over 110 different pesticides were detected in all these foods between 1982 and 1985. Of the twenty-five pesticides detected most frequently, nine have been identified by EPA to cause cancer (captan, chlorothalonil, permethrin, acephate, DDT, parathion, dieldrin, methomyl, and folpet). And two of these carcinogens, DDT and dieldrin, are now banned from use in the United States (DDT and dieldrin were banned in 1972 and 1974, respectively, due to their carcinogenicity and environmental persistence); residues occurring in food result either from the continued use of these chemicals in foreign nations exporting food to this country, or from contamination by trace levels of the chemicals persisting in the U.S. environment.

Certain fruits and vegetables are more likely to contain pesticides more frequently than others. For some fruits and vegetables, including strawberries and peaches, high standards about the cosmetic appearance of the food result in greater pesticide use. Foods with edible portions grown directly in contact with soil, such as celery, carrots and potatoes, may act as sponges and absorb chemical residues from the soil. Other fruits and vegetables have naturally occurring barriers to some pesticide residues, including thick skins on bananas, husks on corn, and wrapper leaves on cauliflower.

Between 1982 and 1985, approximately 40 percent of all FDA's sampling of these fruits and vegetables was of imported foods. Of the imported foods analyzed, pesticide residues were detected in 64 percent; in comparison, 38 percent of the domestic foods were found to have pesticide residues.

For all but six of the individual food commodities, imported foods contained more pesticide residues than the domestically grown foods. In some cases, the imported foods had pesticide residues over twice as frequently. For example, 23 percent of the domestically grown tomatoes contained pesticides, whereas 70 percent of the imported tomatoes had residues. Thirty percent of the domestic cucumbers had residues, while 80 percent of the imported cucumbers contained residues.

In the short run, here are a few tips on how to limit your exposure to pesticides in fresh foods:

- Wash all produce. This will remove some but not all pesticide residues. A mild solution of dishwashing soap and water will help remove additional residues.
- Peel produce when appropriate. Unfortunately, this may reduce the nutritional value of some produce and will not help if the pesticide has been absorbed.
- Grow your own vegetables.
- Buy organically grown fruits and vegetables.
- Buy domestically grown produce.
- Buy produce in season.
- Beware of perfect-looking produce.

You can accelerate the transition to a less chemically dependent method of agriculture by meeting with your supermarket manager and alerting him to your concerns. Also, write your congressional representatives, the FDA, and EPA.

In the long run, we need to reduce agriculture's reliance on chemicals substantially. Methods to produce food with little or no pesticides have existed for many years. But more research needs to be done to expand these techniques, and the nation's food producers must be encouraged to switch to these methods. You can participate directly in resolving the problems posed by pesticide residues in food. If consumers begin to look for and demand safer food, farmers will be forced to reduce their use of pesticides and make changes that will significantly benefit our health and protect the environment.

Through your choices in the supermarket of foods with less chemicals, you can send a direct message to the food industry that will speed the transition away from hazardous pesticides in agriculture. Even food companies can now take steps to reduce the levels of pesticides in their products. The H.J. Heinz Company, in a March 13, 1986, letter to growers, an-

PEACHES

Over half of all fresh peaches sampled were found to contain residues of one or more pesticides. Altogether, thirty-six different pesticides were detected. (The routine laboratory method used by the federal government can only detect fifty-five of the nearly 100 pesticides that can be applied to peaches.) Dicloran residues were detected in 30 percent of all samples, and captan residues were detected in 20 percent of the FDA samples. Here are the five pesticides detected most frequently in order of decreasing occurrence:

Pesticide	Health Effects	Can residue be removed by washing?	Residue removal
Dicloran DCNA, Botran	No observed reproductive toxicity in one animal study. According to EPA, has not been sufficiently tested for carcinogenicity, birth defects, or mutagenic effects.	YES	Residues remain on surface following foliar treatment but are absorbed and translocated to edible tissue, following soil treatment Incorporation of dicloran into wax formulations reduces the effectiveness of washing. Washing, peeling, cooking, or heat processing may reduce residues.
Captan Merpan, Orthocide	Probable human carcinogen. Some evidence of mutagenic effects in laboratory test systems. EPA initiated Special Review in 1980 due to carcinogenicity, mutagenic effects, and presence of residues in food.	YES	Residues remain primarily on the produce surface. However, the metabolite THPI, a suspected carcinogen, may be systemic. Washing, cooking, or heat processing will reduce residues.
Parathion Phoskil	Possible human carcinogen. Some evidence of mutagenic effects in laboratory studies. No observed reproductive toxicity or birth defects in animal studies.	UNKNOWN	Residues remain primarily on the produce surface. Washing, peeling, cooking, or heat processing may reduce residues slightly.
Carbaryl Sevin	Some evidence of adverse kidney effects in humans, and mutagenic effects in laboratory test systems. No observed carcinogenicity or reproductive toxicity in animal studies.	YES	Residues remain primarily on the produce surface. Washing, peeling, or cooking will reduce residues.
Endosulfan	Some evidence of adverse chronic effects including liver and kidney damage and testicular atrophy in test animals. No observed mutagenic effects in laboratory test systems.	UNKNOWN	Residues remain on the produce surface; however, endosulfan metabolites may be systemic. Peeling, cooking, or heat processing may reduce residues slightly. No information on removal with water.

nounced that food treated with any of thirteen pesticides EPA is reviewing as a potential health hazard will not be used to manufacture baby food. You can also make the government do a better job of protecting your food supply and regulating these chemicals.

The ideal solution to the current problems posed by pesticide residues in our food has five different components:

- Organic food should be made available in regular supermarkets. You should have the right to choose between different types of produce.

- All produce should be labeled to identify where the food was grown and what pesticide residues it contains. This information would allow you to make more informed choices when purchasing produce.

- The Environmental Protection Agency should regulate pesticide use more stringently, and set tougher limits on pesticide levels in food.

- The Food and Drug Administration should improve and expand its monitoring for pesticides in food.

- Agricultural production methods should be modified to reduce reliance on chemical pesticides. Food should be grown without chemicals used to improve the cosmetic appearance of our fruits and vegetables. Sustainable agriculture—farming that renews and regenerates the land—would be better for our health and the environment.

* * *

These changes will not come overnight, but some already are occurring. Several California supermarkets have adopted an independent program to identify pesticides in the produce sold in their stores. Organic produce is available in certain Boston food stores. Some national chain stores have said they would offer organic produce if requested by customers. By our efforts individually and together, we can ensure that these goals become reality.

NO
Bruce Ames

TOO MUCH FUSS ABOUT PESTICIDES

In the wake of the Alar-in-apples scare last year [1989], consumers have become highly concerned about the threat posed to their health by the ingestion of trace amounts of man-made pesticides. While it is good for consumers to be concerned about what they eat, the hysteria about pesticide residues may not be warranted by the actual risk they pose. In helping consumers develop a fuller picture of the true risk of man-made pesticides (or other chemical additives to food), we present below an excerpt of a letter from Dr. Bruce Ames to *Consumer Reports* magazine. The letter was in response to an article run in that magazine (October 1989), which, according to Dr. Ames, "distorts my views and misstates facts." ...

—Ed. [of *Consumers' Research.*]

Consumer Reports' four-page attack on my scientific work both distorts my views and misstates the facts on which they are based. Good scientists are committed to challenging assumptions rigorously, and this is particularly important in the prevention of cancer, a murky, complex, multidisciplinary field to which I have devoted much of my scientific career. Sound public policy should be based on sound science, and new data or theory may require altering some prevailing assumptions.

In our efforts to prevent human cancer, it makes no sense to apply a double standard for human exposures to natural vs. synthetic chemicals. My colleagues and I have therefore attempted to provide an overview of possible carcinogenic hazards.

The following points clarify my views and their factual and theoretical basis:

1) Discovering the Causes of Cancer. Epidemiologists are continually coming up with clues about the causes of different types of human cancer, and these hypotheses are then refined by animal and metabolic studies. This approach will, in my view, lead to the understanding of the causal factors for the major human cancers during the next decade. Current epidemiologic data point to the major risk factors for human cancer as cigarette smoking (which is responsible for 30% of cancer), dietary imbalances, hormones, viruses, and lifestyle factors—not to such factors as water pollution or synthetic pesticide residues.

For example, epidemiologists in many countries have identified excessive salt as a risk factor for stomach cancer, one of the major types of cancer. Extensive experimental work in rodents on salt as a co-carcinogen supports the epidemiology. Yet *Consumer Reports* unfairly criticized Edith Efron for saying that salt is a carcinogen.

Consumer Reports criticized me for calling alcohol a carcinogen, yet alcoholic beverages, of numerous types, are carcinogenic in humans at a level of 5 drinks/day. Alcohol itself was positive in one rat test and also was co-carcinogenic in other tests. Acetaldehyde, the main metabolite of alcohol, is a carcinogen in rodents. Most of the leading scientists in the field believe that the active ingredient in alcoholic beverages is alcohol itself. I think that chronic high doses of alcohol are active by causing cell proliferation and inflammation and that, therefore, low doses are not of much interest.

2) Animal Cancer Tests.

There are three fundamental problems with the use of animal cancer tests in trying to prevent human cancer from low-dose human exposures.

a) There are millions of chemicals in the world that we are exposed to in low or moderate doses, 99.9+% of which are natural. To identify significant risks, we need to identify the right chemicals to test in rodents.

b) About half of the chemicals tested in long-term bioassays in both rats and mice have been found to be carcinogens at the high doses administered, the maximum tolerated dose (MTD). Synthetic industrial chemicals account for almost all (82%) of the chemicals (427) tested in both species. However, despite the fact that humans eat vastly more natural than synthetic chemicals, only a small number (75) of *natural* chemicals have been tested in both rats and mice. For the 75 natural chemicals the proportion of positive results (47%) is similar, also about *half*. While some synthetic or natural chemicals were selected for testing precisely because of suspect structures, most chemicals were tested because they were natural or synthetic food additives, colors, high volume industrial compounds, pesticides, or natural or synthetic drugs. Thus, the high proportion of carcinogens among synthetic test agents in rodent studies is not simply due to selection of suspicious chemical structures, and the natural world of chemicals has never been looked at systematically. Recent research into the mechanism of carcinogenesis (see #4 below) supports the idea that when tested in rodents at the MTD, a high proportion of all chemicals we test in the future, whether natural or synthetic, will prove to be carcinogenic.

c) The problem of knowing whether there is any risk at all from the very low doses of human exposure to chemicals causing tumors in rodents at very high doses has been argued by toxicologists and regulators for years, precisely because one cannot measure effects at low doses. Regulators have opted for worst-case estimates, using assumptions that increasing scientific evidence suggests may be incorrect.

Because conventional risk assessment is focused mainly on man-made chemicals and is based on worst-case assumptions that we believe are proving to exaggerate hazard greatly, many leading scientists have argued that it is misleading to the public to try to present estimates of "worst-case risk" from animal studies in terms of expected numbers of human cancers. Our HERP [Human Exposure/Rodent Potency, Dr. Ames's index for estimating carcinogenic risk] uses essentially the same information as that in conventional risk assessment, but is explicitly intended as a relative scale. We have attempted to achieve some perspective on the plethora of possible hazards to humans from exposure to known rodent carcinogens by establishing a scale of the possible hazards for the amounts of various common carcinogens to which humans might be chronically exposed. We view the value of our calculations not as providing a basis for absolute human risk assessment, but as a guide for priority setting.

Carcinogens clearly do not all work in the same way, and as we learn more about the mechanisms, HERP comparisons can be refined, as can risk assessments.

Thus, if the public is told that the possible hazard of the UDMH residue [the breakdown product of Alar] in a daily glass of apple juice (about 30 parts per billion) is 1/18 that of aflatoxin (a mold carcinogen) in a daily peanut butter sandwich (the Food and Drug Administration [FDA] allows 10 times that residue level), 1/50 that of a daily mushroom, and 1/1,000 that of a daily beer, it puts these items in perspective. The possible relative hazard of a daily apple is at least 10× less than the apple juice. This is quite different from showing a witch's hand holding an apple [as was depicted on the May 1989 *Consumer Reports* cover on Alar—Ed].

3) **Pesticides, 99.99% All Natural.** All plants produce toxins to protect themselves against fungi, insects, and animal predators such as man. Tens of thousands of these natural pesticides have been discovered, and every species of plant contains its own set of different toxins, usually a few dozen. In addition, when plants are stressed or damaged, such as during a pest attack, they increase their natural pesticide levels many fold, occasionally to levels that are acutely toxic to humans. We estimate that Americans eat about 1,500 mg/day of natural pesticides, 10,000 times more than man-made pesticide residues, which FDA estimates at a total of 0.15 mg/day. Their concentration is usually measured in parts per thousand or million, rather than parts per billion (ppb), the usual concentration of synthetic pesticide residues and pollutants in water. We estimate that Americans are ingesting 5,000 to 10,000 different natural pesticides and their breakdown products, a subset of the tremendous number of natural chemicals we ingest. For example, there are 49 different natural pesticides (and breakdown products) ingested in eating cabbage.

Surprisingly few plant pesticides have been tested in animal cancer bioassays, but among those tested, again about *half* (25 out of 47) are carcinogenic. A search for the presence of just these 25 carcinogens in foods indicates that they occur naturally in the following (those at levels over 50,000 ppb are listed in parentheses); anise, apples (50,000+ ppb), bananas, basil (4 million ppb), broccoli, Brussels sprouts (500,000 ppb), cabbage (100,000 ppb), cantaloupe, carrots (50,000+ ppb), cauliflower, celery (50,000+ ppb), cinnamon, cloves, cocoa, coffee (brewed) (90,000 ppb), comfrey tea, fennel (3 million ppb), grapefruit juice, honeydew melon, horseradish (4 million ppb), kale, lettuce (300,000 ppb), mushrooms, mustard (black) (40 million ppb), nutmeg (5 million ppb), orange juice (30,000 ppb), parsley, parsnips (30,000 ppb), peaches, black pepper (100,000 ppb), pineapples, potatoes (50,000+ ppb), radishes, raspberries, strawberries, tarragon (1 million ppb), and turnips.

There is every reason to expect that we will continue to find mutagens and carcinogens among nature's pesticides if we ever test them systematically. In short-term tests for detecting mutagens, the proportion of natural pesticides that turn up positive is just as high as for synthetic industrial chemicals. In a compendium on the ability of 950 chemicals to break chromosomes in animal tests, there were 62 natural pesticides: half of them were positive. Thus, it seems highly probable that almost every plant product in the supermarket will contain natural carcinogens at much higher levels than those of man-made pesticides. We have suggested that many more natural pesticides (and chemicals from cooking of food) be tested in long-term bioassays.

Additionally, there is a fundamental trade-off between nature's pesticides and man-made pesticides. We can easily breed out many of nature's pesticides to protect our crops from being eaten by insects. In contrast, growers are currently breeding some plants for insect resistance and unwittingly raising the levels of natural pesticides. A new variety of insect-resistant celery that is being widely sold is almost 10× higher in carcinogens (6,200 ppb) than standard celery.

4) Mechanisms of Carcinogenesis. In the rapidly advancing field of mechanisms of carcinogenesis, there is now evidence to suggest that cell proliferation is extremely important. A large number of the major human carcinogens such as hormones, chronic viral infection, salt, asbestos, and alcohol are likely to be primarily active through causing cell proliferation. A cell is at considerably greater genetic risk during division, so chronic cell proliferation in itself is a mutagenic and carcinogenic stress. Cancers induced in animal cancer tests done at high doses seem to be primarily caused by cell proliferation, in part due to chronic cell killing, and inflammation that results from high toxic doses. This would be in agreement with the high proportion of all chemicals that are turning out to be carcinogens at high doses and the relation of toxicity to carcinogenic potency. The induction of cell proliferation is restricted to high doses, and this strongly suggests that low doses of carcinogens are of no risk, or are very much less hazardous than has been assumed.

In addition, humans, who live in a world of natural toxins, are well protected by many layers of inducible general defenses against low doses of toxins—defenses that do not distinguish between synthetic and natural toxins. Therefore, even the high levels of natural plant pesticides may not be of much concern in a balanced diet.

5) Trade-offs. Identifying and controlling the major causes of human cancer are not a matter of blame. We have tried in our scientific work to put into perspective the tiny exposures to pesticide residues by comparing them to the enormous background of natural substances. Minimizing pollution is a separate issue, and is clearly desirable, aside from any effect on public health, but it involves economic trade-offs. As a society, efforts to regulate pesticides or other synthetic rodent carcinogens down to the ppb level inevitably involve understanding these trade-offs. Synthetic pesticides (and chemicals such as Alar) have markedly lowered the cost of our food, a major advance in nutrition and, thus, health. Every complex mixture from gasoline to cooked food to orange juice contains rodent carcinogens. When people drive to work, put logs on a fire, or make a barbecue they are putting carcinogens into the air. There are costs and benefits to all of these. Exaggerating the risks from man-made substances, ignoring the natural world, and converting the issue to one of blaming U.S. industry does not advance our public health efforts. If we spend all our efforts on minimal, rather than important, hazards, we hurt public health. The Environmental Protection Agency (EPA) is trying to prevent hypothetical risks of 1 in a million at enormous economic cost. Yet the leading scientists trying to prevent cancer are working on numerous possible carcinogenic risks in the 1 in a 100 to 1 in 10 range: my lab is working on 4 that we think are in this range.

POSTSCRIPT

Are Pesticides in Foods Harmful to Human Health?

Increased consumer fear of pesticide residues on food has encouraged many activists to push for a ban on pesticide use. Although doing so might provide some health benefits, Ronald Knutson, director of the Agricultural and Food Policy Center at Texas A & M University, believes that such a ban would cause a significant rise in food prices. In "Pesticide-Free Equals Higher Food Prices," *Consumers' Research* (November 1990), Knutson and his colleagues argue that if there were a complete ban on the use of pesticides, food bills would rise at least 12 percent, crop yields would fall, and there would need to be a 10 percent increase in cultivated acreage, which would result in a corresponding rise in soil erosion.

An investigation by Constance Matthiessen challenges the opinions of Knutson and others. Matthiessen, writing in *Mother Jones* (March/April 1992), takes the position that despite the widespread use of pesticides, insects and weeds seem to be doing as much damage as ever. The reason: insects and weeds have the ability to adapt and evolve to become pesticide-resistant. As a result, the share of crop yields lost to pests has almost doubled over the last 40 years. Environmentalist Shirley A. Briggs agrees that pesticides have failed to decrease crop losses while causing widespread environmental damage. In "Silent Spring: The View from 1990," *The Ecologist* (March/April 1990), Briggs argues that we must find ways to reduce pesticide dependence.

Robert J. Scheuplein, a scientist with the Office of Toxicological Sciences at the Food and Drug Administration, shares the opinions of Ames. In "The Risk from Food," *Consumers' Research* (April 1990), Scheuplein argues that the public has an unrealistic view of pesticides and that other factors, particularly overall diet, contribute much more to the development of different cancers than pesticide-treated foods.

Most scientists agree that pesticide residues can affect human health to *some* degree. Many experts, however, maintain that current levels of residues are insignificant and that our food supply is safe. Others argue that pesticides pose health risks, are environmentally unsound, and do not work in the long run, because many pests have become resistant to them. Researching alternatives to pesticides, as described in "A New Crop of Pest Controls," *New Scientist* (July 14, 1988) and "Getting Off the Pesticide Treadmill," *Technology Review* (November/December 1985), may be a safer, more ecologically sound, and ultimately more successful approach to limiting pest damage than maintaining a total reliance on chemicals.

ISSUE 18

Does Exposure to Electromagnetic Fields Cause Cancer?

YES: Paul Brodeur, from "Annals of Radiation: The Cancer at Slater School," *The New Yorker* (December 7, 1992)

NO: Gary Taubes, from "Fields of Fear," *The Atlantic Monthly* (November 1994)

ISSUE SUMMARY

YES: Journalist Paul Brodeur argues that exposure to electromagnetic fields (EMFs) emitted from high-voltage power lines can cause cancer and that the utility industry has gone to great lengths to cover it up.

NO: Reporter Gary Taubes contends that because people want to believe that EMFs are dangerous, they do. He further argues that selective reporting of scientific evidence has generated unnecessary public anxiety about electromagnetic fields.

This issue examines the theory that there is a relationship between exposure to electromagnetic fields (EMFs) around power lines and the development of childhood leukemia and other cancers. Research on EMFs began in the late 1970s, when scientists Nancy Wertheimer and Ed Leeper reported that children living in areas of high EMF exposure were twice as likely to develop leukemia as children in low exposure areas. Their research did not generate much interest, however, until 10 years later, when Paul Brodeur published a series of articles in the *New Yorker* entitled "Annals of Radiation" claiming that EMFs cause cancer. Frightened consumers demanded to know if the EMFs generated from power lines and home appliances were a threat to their health. In response, several studies have attempted to assess the risks of EMFs, including a $65 million research program organized by the Department of Energy and a five-year study conducted by the National Cancer Institute.

Currently, about 2,600 new cases of childhood leukemia develop each year in the United States. The chance of any given child developing this disease is about 1 in 20,000, with most cases occurring by the age of five. Do EMFs increase this risk? If so, by how much, and is it worth worrying about?

All electric current produces two types of fields, electric and magnetic. The *electric* field part of an EMF is mostly blocked by building materials and is not a major concern. The primary issue is the *magnetic* field, which easily passes through anything, including human bodies and buildings. Magnetic fields increase in strength in proportion to the electric current, and their intensity falls off quickly with distance from the source.

A number of ordinary household appliances can generate relatively strong magnetic fields in their immediate vicinities. A few of these appliances have come under scrutiny because of the strong EMFs they generate. Cellular phones, in particular, have come under study because they are considered by some to be particularly risky. Portable phones carry their own power supply (an EMF source) and antenna in a single handset that is held very close to the user's head. Some reports have linked the usage of cellular phones with brain cancer.

Electric blankets manufactured before 1991 exposed users to strong magnetic fields all night long. A 1990 study published by David Savitz and his colleagues at the University of North Carolina reported that children whose mothers slept under electric blankets during pregnancy had a 70 percent greater chance of developing leukemia than children whose mothers did not. Such reports forced manufacturers to produce low-EMF electric blankets, labeling them as having "reduced fields" for the consumer's benefit. Other electric appliances identified as having strong EMFs include the microwave oven and the computer monitor, which, as personal home computers become more and more common, increases the urgency of this issue.

Those who believe that EMFs can increase the risk of cancer cite evidence that magnetic and electrical fields in a laboratory can produce measurable changes in cellular activity. Detractors point out that our bodies *naturally* contain electrical energy that causes our muscles to contract and our hearts to beat. Some argue that EMFs probably do not directly cause cancerous cells but promote the development of cancer begun by some other means. Another theory is that magnetic fields cause disease by suppressing the hormone melatonin, which has been shown to prevent tumor growth. Although these theories may sound plausible, they have not been proven, and the final word on the safety of EMFs remains open.

In the following selections, two writers present opposite viewpoints on the dangers of EMFs. Paul Brodeur claims that there is a real danger to exposure to electromagnetic fields from high-voltage power lines. Gary Taubes argues that the reporting of EMF risks has generated considerable anxiety at great expense to the public.

YES

Paul Brodeur

ANNALS OF RADIATION: THE CANCER AT SLATER SCHOOL

On a Friday afternoon in mid-December of 1990, half a dozen women who taught at the Louis N. Slater Elementary School, in Fresno, California, were interviewed in the teachers' lounge there by Amy Alexander, a staff writer for the Fresno *Bee*, who wanted to know if they were concerned about the presence of two high-voltage transmission lines that ran past the school on Emerson Avenue. That morning, the *Bee* had published an Associated Press story about an attempt by the Bush Administration to delay the release of a report compiled by the federal Environmental Protection Agency [E.P.A.] which linked residential and occupational exposure to the alternating-current magnetic fields given off by power lines with the development of cancer in children and adults. Earlier in the week, a mother whose child attended the Tobey B. Lawless Elementary School, about a mile northwest of the Slater school, had asked the principal there to get in touch with the Pacific Gas & Electric Company [P.G.&E.], of San Francisco—the utility that serves Fresno and is the largest in the nation—about the potential hazard of high-voltage transmission lines running along Corona Avenue, within three hundred feet of the school. The mother also mentioned her concern to an acquaintance on the *Bee's* staff, who passed it along to Alexander. After making a few telephone calls, Alexander learned that the Slater school sits only a hundred feet or so from the same high-voltage power lines that run past Lawless. It was then that she arranged to meet with teachers at Slater.

Up to the time of Alexander's visit, none of the forty-three teachers at the Slater school had apparently ever entertained any doubts about working close to power lines. When Alexander told the women she met with in the teachers' lounge about the E.P.A. report, however, they were quick to inform her that at least nine teachers and teachers' aides at Slater had developed cancer in recent years. Two days later, an article by Alexander about the possible hazard at Slater appeared on the front page of the *Bee*, under the headline "POWER LINES WORRY SCHOOL." Alexander said in her article that the transmission lines on Emerson Avenue supplied power for more than forty thousand Fresno homes, and that transmission lines had been there

YES Paul Brodeur / 305

since the nineteen-twenties. She also reported that since 1987 the California Department of Education had required new schools to be situated at least a hundred and fifty feet from such lines.

Earlier in the article, Alexander quoted the E.P.A. official in San Francisco as saying that President George Bush's national science adviser had expressed reservations about releasing the agency's report on the potential carcinogenicity of power-line emissions, because he feared that it could cause "widespread panic." She then quoted the Slater principal, George Marsh, as cautioning that "we need to allay people's fears rather than have them become hysterical." After reporting that P.G.&E. representatives would be taking measurements at the Slater and Lawless schools the next day, Alexander quoted a spokesman for the California Department of Health Services as saying that he was unfamiliar with concerns about health risks from power lines near schools in the Fresno area, and the Fresno Unified School District's director of health services as saying that she was unaware of any unusual incidence of cancer at any of the district's schools. But Loretta Hutton, one of the women Alexander interviewed in the teachers' lounge, declared that the high incidence of cancer at Slater had been noted by some of her colleagues in the school district. "They say, 'Oh, you teach at Slater? Well, that's certainly the kiss of death,'" Hutton told Alexander.

Alexander's article was the topic of considerable discussion among the teachers at Slater during the next week. Nothing much came of it, however, because on the following Friday the faculty and pupils began a two-week Christmas vacation. Moreover, because Slater is a year-round school, teachers

there are required to take two six-week vacations during the year, so nearly a dozen teachers, including several whom Alexander had interviewed, did not return to work until the middle of February. Among them was Patricia Berryman, a first-grade teacher and the mother of two grown children. An attractive woman in her late forties, Berryman had special reason to find Alexander's piece unsettling. She had come to Slater in August of 1975, three years after the school opened, and had since been teaching reading, writing, math, science, and social studies to first graders in Pod A—an octagonal area at the southeast corner of the school. Pod A, which faces Emerson Avenue, contains three first-grade classrooms and two kindergarten rooms. Slater has four such pods: they are situated at the four corners of the school building, and surround a large rectangular area that houses offices for the principal, the vice-principals, the administrative secretaries, and nurses, and also a kitchen, a faculty room, an all-purpose room, a patio, and several workrooms. Pod B, at the southwest corner of the building, also faces Emerson Avenue, and contains five classrooms for fifth and sixth graders. Pods C and D, at the northwest and northeast corners of the school, respectively, are, of course, farther away from Emerson Avenue; they contain ten classrooms for second, third, and fourth graders.

"During the mid-nineteen-eighties, I began to realize that cancer and various other tumors were striking a lot of people who worked around me at Slater," Berryman said recently....

[W]hen I learned about the E.P.A. report and the fact that it specifically cited brain cancer as being associated with exposure to power-line magnetic fields,

I began to wonder for the first time about the huge transmission lines I could see through the window of my room in Pod A, running down Emerson Avenue."

* * *

The E.P.A. report—a three-hundred-and-sixty-seven-page document entitled "Evaluation of the Potential Carcinogenicity of Electromagnetic Fields"—had come to light in March of 1990, when someone in the agency sent a draft version of it to Louis Slesin, the editor and publisher of a pioneering and influential newsletter called *Microwave News*, which since the early nineteen-eighties has been reporting on the hazards of exposure to radiation from power lines and other sources.... Chief among the conclusions was one specifying that power-line electromagnetic fields should be classified as a "probable" human carcinogen. Slesin also learned that... this conclusion [was] to be deleted from the report.

In spite of the deletion, the summary-and-conclusions section of the draft E.P.A. report contained a persuasive indictment of power-line magnetic fields as a cancer-producing agent. Its authors stated that five of six case-control studies published in the peer-reviewed medical literature showed that children who lived near power lines giving off strong magnetic fields were developing cancer more readily than children who did not live near power lines. This association was statistically significant in three of the studies; and in two studies in which magnetic-field measurements had been made children exposed to fields of between two and three milligauss or above were experiencing a significantly increased risk of developing cancer. (A gauss is a unit of measure for magnetic-field strength; a milligauss is a thousandth of a gauss. Ambient levels of between two and three milligauss can be measured routinely in buildings within fifty to a hundred and fifty feet of wires carrying strong electric current.) The E.P.A. researchers declared that a "consistently repeated pattern of leukemia, nervous system cancer and lymphoma in the childhood studies" argues "in favor of a causal link" between the development of these diseases and the exposure of children to power-line magnetic fields. They went on to say that they had reviewed more than thirty reports dealing with cancer or mortality among workers exposed to such fields, and had found that the statistical results of the occupational studies tended to support the statistical results of the childhood studies, with leukemia, brain cancer, and malignant melanoma of the skin predominating among the exposed workers.

After determining that magnetic fields were the most likely cause of the excess cancer found in the epidemiological studies, the authors of the E.P.A. report described a body of experimental research—it included studies showing that weak magnetic fields could change the chemistry of the brain, impair the immune system, and inhibit the synthesis of melatonin, a hormone known to suppress several types of tumors and to be present in reduced amounts in women who develop breast cancer—and declared that it furnished "reason to believe that the findings of carcinogenicity in humans are biologically plausible." The final paragraph of the section contained this sentence: "With our current understanding we can identify 60 Hz magnetic fields from power lines and perhaps other sources in the home as a possible, but not proven, cause of cancer in people."...

During [subsequent] hearings, eighteen oral comments were given, and more than half of them were delivered by people who represented the utility industry or the Air Force, which for years had opposed any suggestion that the electromagnetic radiation emitted by its radars and communications equipment could be hazardous, or by people who had stated publicly that there was no evidence of an association between exposure to electromagnetic fields and cancer. Among the latter was Robert Adair, of Yale: he claimed that universally accepted laws of physics made it virtually impossible that sixty-hertz magnetic fields at levels below a hundred milligauss could cause any observable biological effects. Moreover, there were only half a dozen comments by people who were concerned that power-line fields might pose a health risk, and not one was delivered by anyone with a scientific-research background, let alone by any of the scientists who had conducted any of the dozens of studies that had been cited in the E.P.A. report as showing that electromagnetic fields were a possible cause of cancer....

* * *

On February 25, 1991, Thom DeYoung, a service-planning analyst for Pacific Gas & Electric, sent a thirty-two-page report of the magnetic-field measurements that the utility had taken at the Lawless and Slater schools in December, together with some background material on the electromagnetic-field hazard, to Wayne McMillen, the director of the Fresno Unified School District's Benefit and Risk Management Department....

On March 1st, McMillen forwarded a copy of the P.G.&E. report to... an assistant superintendent of the school district, with a cover letter assuring him that not enough scientific information existed to make a judgment regarding magnetic-field exposure levels. To understand how McMillen may have come to this conclusion, one need only read the background material.... It included a public-policy statement that had been published by P.G.&E. in October of 1990 and a pamphlet that had been written earlier that year by Dr. Raymond Richard Neutra, the chief of the California Department of Health Services' Special Epidemiological Studies Program, and three of his colleagues, who supported the utility's position at almost every turn.

Neutra and his co-authors started out by declaring that, given the scientific information now available, it was not possible to set a standard for exposure to electromagnetic fields or to say that any particular level was either safe or dangerous. In a later section of the pamphlet, they implied that epidemiological studies with findings that supported a link between exposure to power-line magnetic fields and the development of cancer were balanced by a similar number of studies with findings that did not support such a link. The fact is that, as the E.P.A. draft report clearly stated, five out of six studies of childhood residential exposure and most of thirty or so occupational studies that has been conducted since 1979 showed a positive link between exposure to power-frequency magnetic fields and cancer. Neutra and his colleagues said almost nothing about the research demonstrating that weak electromagnetic fields could affect the brain, the immune system, and the synthesis of melatonin—the research that had provided the chief basis for the E.P.A.'s conclusion that the findings of carcinogenicity were "biologically plausible."

Neutra and his colleagues emphasized the fact that the childhood epidemiological studies had relied on rough estimates of magnetic-field exposure based on the proximity of homes to power lines, rather than on spot measurements of actual magnetic-field strength, but they failed to point out that most leading researchers consider such estimates to be historically more accurate and to give a better idea of actual exposure at the time of and before diagnosis than spot measurements. They concluded their pamphlet by stating that public concern about the power-line health hazard was based on "incomplete and inconclusive" data, and that until better data were available any concerned individuals might wish to limit their exposure to electromagnetic fields "when this can be done at reasonable cost and with reasonable effort."

Like Neutra and his colleagues, the authors of the P.G.&E. statement emphasized that estimates of magnetic-field exposure in the childhood studies had been based on proximity to power lines, and not on actual magnetic-field measurements, and thus did not prove a link between exposure to the fields and the development of cancer. In addition, like Farland and Trichopoulos, they suggested that if power-line magnetic fields really caused or promoted cancer "the fivefold increase in electrical usage during the past 30 years would have been expected to have produced an epidemic of childhood leukemia." The utility industry stopped making this argument in June of 1991, after the National Cancer Institute released a report saying that in recent years there had been unexplained increases of nearly eleven per cent in

childhood leukemia, and of more than thirty per cent in childhood brain cancer.

As it happened, evidence of the cancer hazard associated with exposure to power-frequency emissions had been accumulating steadily during the previous two years. On January 30th and 31st of 1991, a panel of epidemiologists attending a workshop on the health effects of electromagnetic radiation that was being held in Cincinnati by the National Institute for Occupational Safety and Health strongly urged that the association of female breast cancer and exposure to electromagnetic fields be given high priority in future research programs. Just a month earlier, a Norwegian study had been published which showed that male breast cancer—a disease so rare that only about one case had been diagnosed in every hundred thousand men each year—was occurring at twice the expected rate in men whose occupations involved exposure to electromagnetic fields, and at four times the expected rate in electric-transport workers, such as railway-engine drivers, tram operators, and trackwalkers.

The Norwegian study was the third investigation in little more than a year to observe an exceptional rate of breast cancer among men exposed to electromagnetic fields. Seven months earlier, epidemiologists at the Fred Hutchinson Cancer Research Center, in Seattle, had reported that telephone linemen, electricians, and electric-power workmen were developing breast cancer at six times the expected rate, and in November of 1989 [epidemiologist Genevieve] Matanoski and her colleagues at Johns Hopkins had announced that there was an increased incidence of male breast cancer among central-office telephone technicians, who were exposed to magnetic fields of between two and three milligauss being given off by switching equipment. (The increase proved to be six times as great as expected.) In spite of the fact that Louis Slesin had reported all these findings in *Microwave News*, almost no word of them had found its way into the nation's newspapers, with the result that American women, who were experiencing a steep rise in the incidence of breast cancer—a malignancy that is histologically identical to breast cancer in men—had almost no idea of the potential link that had been discovered between the development of this disease and exposure to magnetic fields....

* * *

While the resolve of the Slater teachers to do something about the power lines was stiffening, the seventeen members of the E.P.A.'s Scientific Advisory Board subcommittee reviewing the E.P.A. draft report found themselves increasingly uneasy over its conclusion that power-line electromagnetic fields were a possible cause of cancer in human beings....

The epidemiology panel found that the authors of the E.P.A. draft had "achieved nearly complete coverage of pertinent work" but that their analysis of the epidemiological findings contained "too much unwarranted speculation about causal interpretation," which resulted in "giving emphasis to positive findings while de-emphasizing negative ones."...

* * *

Meanwhile, the teachers at the Slater school were growing impatient with the Fresno Unified School District officials for not having yet devised measures to protect them....

On May 14th, a hundred parents and children held a rally at the school.

After cordoning off the south side of the campus with yellow tape and hanging a huge sign that read "Danger, Electromagnetic Field" on the chain-link fence on Emerson Avenue, they marched up and down the sidewalk carrying signs that warned of the power-line health hazard and chanting "Safety for our kids!"...

The next meeting of the Fresno Board of Education, which was held on May 23rd, was attended by a standing-room-only audience that included nearly a hundred Slater parents. At the outset, Dr. Stallworth [of the county health department] said that he and his staff had confirmed seven cases of cancer among Slater teachers and one case of cancer in a Slater student, but that this number of cases did not constitute a cluster, which he defined as "an unusual occurrence of cancers." He went on to say that his conclusion was supported by Dr. Neutra, whom he described as "probably the most knowledgeable person in California on electromagnetic fields." Stallworth also said that there were no definitive data to suggest that power-line magnetic fields had a negative effect upon human health....

When someone in the audience asked Stallworth if he could explain why all the cancers that had been reported had occurred among women who worked on the side of the school nearest the power lines, there was prolonged applause, and it proved to be a question for which Stallworth had no answer. Shortly thereafter, Superintendent Abbott declared that because of the concerns of the Slater parents and the disruption of the educational program at the Slater school he believed it important to move students and teachers from the classrooms near the power lines until more definitive information was available. The members of the Board of Education then voted unanimously to adopt the resolutions proposed by the school district to accomplish this.

... [P]ublic concern had reached such a level that on January 15, 1991, the California Public Utilities Commission announced that it was opening an investigation "to explore the scientific evidence relating to possible health effects, if any, of utility employees' and consumers' exposure to electric and magnetic fields created by electric utility power systems," and to examine "the range of regulatory responses which might be appropriate." A press release that accompanied the announcement said that the Department of Health Services and the Public Utilities Commission were jointly conducting three research studies of the health risks associated with exposure to power-line magnetic fields....

* * *

... [T]he seventeen members of the Scientific Advisory Board subcommittee concluded that E.P.A. draft report on the potential carcinogenicity of electromagnetic fields had "serious deficiencies," and that there was "insufficient evidence from the human epidemiology data and from animal/cell experiments to establish unequivocal cause-and-effect relationships between low frequency electric and magnetic field exposure and human health effects and cancer." The fact is that the authors of the E.P.A. report had never claimed that power-line electromagnetic fields were an "unequivocal" cause of cancer but, rather, that they were only a "possible" cause of cancer, and the subcommittee had been asked not to determine whether the evidence of carcinogenicity was "unequivocal" but simply to review "the accuracy and completeness of the entire document and... whether the interpretation of the available information reflects current scientific opinion."

The subcommittee members also said that although some epidemiological studies reported an association between living close to power lines and "an increased incidence of some type of cancer," the E.P.A. report's conclusion that power-line magnetic fields were a possible cause of cancer was "currently inappropriate because of limited evidence of an exposure-response relationship and the lack of a clear understanding of biologic plausibility." At the same time, they covered all bets by warning that, because no factors other than electro-magnetic fields had been identified to explain the excess cancer risks found in the studies, the existing evidence that exposure to the fields was associated with the development of cancer "cannot be dismissed."

Curiously, the subcommittee members made no mention of the occupational studies in their review of the E.P.A. report, so the strong correlation between the findings of the childhood residential studies and the adult occupational investigations was totally ignored. As for animal studies, the subcommittee members pointed out (as the authors of the E.P.A. report had done) that no experiments had even been conducted to determine whether lifetime exposure to power-frequency magnetic fields could result in excess cancer in test animals. The fact that this should be the case twelve years after the publication of the first epidemiological survey showing a link between residential exposure to power-line magnetic fields and an excess risk of leukemia and other cancer in children reflected an appalling lapse on the part of the utility industry and EPRI [Electric

Power Research Institute], and also on the part of the E.P.A. and other governmental agencies....

A similarly dismissive attitude was displayed by officials of the Connecticut Department of Health Services, who had been asked to investigate a cancer cluster that had developed among the residents of Meadow Street, in Guilford, a town of some twenty thousand inhabitants that is on Long Island Sound, about fourteen miles east of New Haven. Between 1969 and 1989, seven tumors—among them two brain tumors, two cases of meningioma, and a malignant melanoma of the eye—were recorded among children and adults living on that street, which is only two hundred and fifty yards long and has only nine houses on it. Because all the tumors had developed in a handful of people who were either living or had lived for significant periods of time in four of six adjacent houses situated near an electric-power substation, and within a few feet of some main distribution lines carrying high current from the substation, it had been suggested that the unusual incidence of cancer and tumors among the residents of Meadow Street might be associated with their long-term exposure to the strong magnetic fields that are given off by such lines. This suggestion was reinforced by the many epidemiological studies showing that children and workers exposed to power-frequency magnetic fields were developing brain tumors at rates significantly higher than those observed in unexposed people, and by a British study showing the incidence of eye melanoma to be "notably high" among electrical and electronics workers, who are exposed to relatively strong magnetic fields.

At a meeting held at the Guilford Public Library on August 20, 1990, David R. Brown, chief of the Connecticut Department of Health Services' Division of Environmental Epidemiology and Occupational Health, told a group of a hundred or so Guilford residents that there was no cancer cluster on Meadow Street. To support this contention, one of Brown's associates displayed a map showing the location of ten meningiomas and nineteen other brain and central-nervous-system tumors listed by the Connecticut Tumor Registry as having occurred in Guilford between 1968 and 1988, and, pointing to the fact that the tumors appeared to be scattered throughout the town, said that this proved there was "absolutely no clustering" in Guilford. Two days later, Brown displayed the map at a Rotary Club meeting in Guilford, and told the Rotarians that he saw no need for the Department of Health Services to make any further inquiry into the incidence of cancer on Meadow Street....

By the end of the year, the Department of Health Services' handling of the situation in Guilford had prompted leading members of the Connecticut State Senate to call upon the Connecticut Academy of Science and Engineering—a nonprofit corporation that had been formed by the legislature "to promote the application of science and engineering to human health and welfare"—to conduct an independent review of the power-line problem. At the time, doubts about the academy's impartiality were raised when it was revealed that the academy had received financial contributions from Northeast Utilities—parent of the Connecticut Light & Power Company, which owns and operates the Meadow Street substation and the high-current wires leading from it—and that a high-ranking Northeast official was sitting on the academy's board of directors and another Northeast official was chairman of its nominating committee.

... The accuracy of the academy report was called into further question when it was learned that a member of the ad-hoc committee had written to [committee chairman Jan A. J.] Stolwijk several months before the final report was issued to remind him that committee members had been told that magnetic-field levels in the houses on Meadow Street had probably been "relatively high." None of this appeared to disconcert Stolwijk, who submitted a proposal to the Department of Health Services in September asking for $374,889 to investigate the association between the development of cancer in Connecticut children and how close they lived to power lines....

Meanwhile, officials of Northeast Utilities and Connecticut Light & Power, together with other utility officials across the nation, had been insisting for months that there was no proof that power-line magnetic fields could cause cancer, and no need for preventive measures or regulations to reduce exposure....

* * *

... [I]n the United States, where the cost of reducing such emissions will... be enormous, the question is whether government health officials and the utility officials will... acknowledge the existence of the power-line hazard, or whether they will persist in their efforts to deny it. Acknowledging the hazard would require that government and industry undertake to identify where the hazard exists in its most serious and concentrated form—a good place to start might be hundreds of schools and day-care centers that have been built perilously close to high-voltage or high-current power lines—and then set about

to remedy the hazard by rerouting such lines, or burying them in a manner that will drastically reduce their magnetic-field emissions. (The technology for doing so was developed and tested by the utility industry some time ago.) Given the record of the government and the industry in dealing with the power-line problem thus far, however, no one should expect that any of this will occur soon, if at all, unless a concerned and determined citizenry forces action.

As it happens, determined and prescient citizens have been confronting the power-line health issue across the nation. In 1990, opposition mounted by Residents Against Giant Electric (RAGE), a group of citizens in Monmouth County, New Jersey, who were concerned about the cancer hazard posed by power-line emissions, forced the Jersey Central Power & Light Company to abandon its plan to construct a pair of two-hundred-and-thirty-thousand-volt transmission lines through the town of Red Bank, Middletown, Holmdel, Hazlet, and Aberdeen. That same year, the efforts of a group called Rhode Islanders for Safe Power persuaded the town council of East Greenwich, Rhode Island, to enact a three-year moratorium on the construction of power lines carrying more than sixty thousand volts in that town. During 1990 and 1991, residents of the historic Old Town section of Alexandria, Virginia, who had discovered that high-current distribution wires carrying power to the city's business district were creating magnetic fields of more than forty milligauss in many homes, persuaded city officials to negotiate a franchise-and-operating agreement with the Virginia Electric Power Company, calling for the city and the utility to share the cost of burying the offending lines, and of redesigning power distribution in a thirty-six-block downtown area....

As might be expected, significant devaluation of residential property situated close to high-voltage and high-current lines has already occurred in various sections of the nation where the power-frequency hazard has become known, and even greater devaluation appears to be in the offing as word of the latest Swedish findings and other information about the problem is disseminated. Together with the health hazard itself, the devaluation is resulting in widespread concern and litigation....

[C]auses of potential litigation are the magnetic fields given off by faulty household wiring; by high-current conductors concealed in the walls, ceilings, and floors of commercial office buildings and other large structures; and by high-voltage transformers that can be found in almost any large building. Magnetic fields of well over a hundred milligauss were recently discovered, for example, in a state office building in Madison, Wisconsin, and in a back office in Manhattan. In both instances, the fields were found to be coming from transformers on the floor below, and were detected only because they caused serious malfunctioning in video-display terminals [VDTs] on the floor above.

As for the VDTs, of which some fifty million are estimated to be in use in the United States, they operate by generating extra-low-frequency magnetic fields, and thus provide an important additional source of long-term, chronic exposure. Pulsed magnetic fields of between one and five milligauss can be measured routinely at a distance of twelve inches from the screens of many VDTs, and fields two to three times as strong can be measured at the same distance from their sides, backs, and tops.

In spite of several studies showing that women who work with VDTs have a higher rate of miscarriage than other women, and other studies showing that VDT emissions can damage the fetuses of test animals, government health officials in the United States have failed to limit the magnetic fields that these devices are allowed to give off. Early this year, however, researchers at the Institute of Occupational Health, in Helsinki, found that women working with VDTs that exposed them to magnetic fields averaging about three milligauss suffered miscarriages at a rate close to three and a half times that of women using VDTs that exposed them to fields that averaged about one milligauss. The fact that this dose relationship is similar to the one established by the recent Swedish studies for exposure to power-line magnetic fields and the development of leukemia is serious cause for concern. Additionally worrisome is a recent study conducted by researchers at the University of Adelaide's Department of Community Medicine, who found that women working with computer monitors are developing primary brain tumors at nearly five times the expected rate. Considering the elevated rates of breast cancer in men with occupational exposure to electromagnetic fields, the sharp increase in recent years in the incidence of breast cancer among women, and the fact that women make up a majority of the work force using VDTs, it seems reasonable to wonder why no government agency has undertaken an epidemiological study to determine whether women who work with VDTs are developing breast cancer more readily that other women.

The fact that more studies will be needed to define the full dimensions of the magnetic-field hazard should not, however, be used by the nation's public-health officials as an excuse for further delaying measures to reduce exposure to power-line emissions. The public should understand that by extending the presumption of benignity to power-frequency magnetic fields in the absence of absolute proof of their carcinogenicity, public-health officials have already helped to perpetuate a situation in which thousands of people are at risk of developing malignant disease that could have been avoided. Indeed, in testimony submitted to the California Public Utilities Commission..., Neutra himself declared that "if the epidemiological results with regard to childhood cancer and occupational cancer were to be confirmed as real we would be talking about hundreds of preventable cases of cancer in the state each year."

A month or so after making this statement, Neutra finished a thirty-two-page draft of a report entitled "Exposures at the Slater School," ...

In the final question of the report, Neutra asked whether the magnetic-field-exposure conditions at Slater could have caused a cancer cluster. He began and ended a discursive four-and-a-half page reply by saying that he could not give definitive answer, but he went to some length to suggest that there was probably no association between the fields given off by the transmission lines on Emerson Avenue and the cancers that had developed among the teachers and staff members who had worked on that side of the school.

Berryman was disappointed to find that in the report there was neither confirmation nor denial of her suspicion that emissions from the power lines on Emerson Avenue might be connected with the cancers that had occurred among her colleagues. On November 5th, this suspicion was reinforced by the distressing news that still another of her fellow-teachers had developed cancer. The latest victim—the fourteenth, by her count—was a fourth-grade teacher in her early fifties, who had worked in Pod B for at least two years, and had just been operated on for a malignant tumor of the colon.

On the next day,... Berryman [received] some additional material from Neutra with a cover letter urging that it... be marked with comments. Among the new documents was a thirteen-page report on the cancer cases at Slater which had been written by Neutra and [Department of Health Services epidemiologist Eva] Glazer, who said that they had now confirmed eleven cases among past and present teachers and employees. The eleven confirmed cases were three breast cancers, two uterine cancers, two ovarian cancers, two melanomas, the brain cancer that had killed Katie Alexander, and the colon cancer that had killed Curtis Hurd. However, the list was incomplete, because it did not include two cases of cancer in employees who had declined to participate in the study, or the colon cancer that had been diagnosed in the Pod B teacher who had just undergone surgery. The difference between eleven and fourteen cases was extremely important, because after estimating once again that a thousand out of California's eight thousand schools might be situated next to power lines, Neutra and Glazer went on to declare that eleven cases of cancer could be expected to occur by chance alone among the teachers and staff members of no fewer than fifty-six of these thousand schools. However, according to a Poisson-distribution graph that the two health officials had attached to their report, only five and a half of the thousand schools could be expected to have fourteen cases of cancer, and less than one school out of the thousand could be expected to have sixteen cases.

The fact that only two more cancer cases would place Slater Elementary in a unique category among California schools was not lost on Berryman, who had suspected since January that the incidence of cancer among her colleagues was being underreported. At that time, she and Doris Buffo had telephoned fifteen or twenty former Slater teachers in the Fresno area, and learned that none of them had been approached by the Department of Health Services; this indicated that Neutra and Glazer, instead of going out and conducting a thorough survey of the cancer rate among Slater teachers and staff members, including the

eight-five or so who no longer worked at the school, had merely compiled a list of the cancer cases that had been reported to them. In a margin on the first page of their report, Berryman wrote the following sentence: "The credibility of your findings is seriously weakened by your failure to determine whether the teachers, teachers' aides, and other staff members who no longer work at Slater have developed cancer, and whether there has been any increased incidence of cancer among the students who have attended the school." She went on to note the colon cancer that had just been reported in the Pod B teacher. She also noted that the number of cancer cases had doubled since the two health officials had begun their investigation, a year and a half ago—all the cancers having occurred among people working on the side of the school nearest the power lines. Then she posed this question: "How many more cancers will it take?"

NO

Gary Taubes

FIELDS OF FEAR

The proposition that electromagnetic fields may be hazardous to your health began with Nancy Wertheimer, a Harvard-educated experimental psychologist who now works with the Department of Preventive Medicine at the University of Colorado. In the spring of 1974 and for much of the next two years, Wertheimer drove the streets of greater Denver searching for possible causative agents of childhood cancer.

What Wertheimer found was that the homes of children who developed cancer were, with suspicious regularity, located near high-current electric power lines. Wertheimer spent two more years with Ed Leeper, a friend with an education in physics, analyzing her data and checking her methods. "We stayed as quiet as we could," she told me recently. "We didn't want people getting anxious." ...

The scientific community paid little attention to Wertheimer's research until a decade later, when the *New Yorker* writer Paul Brodeur immortalized Wertheimer in a three-part "Annals of Radiation" series in June of 1989. A year later Brodeur's articles appeared in a book titled, with little ambiguity, *Currents of Death: Power Lines, Computer Terminals, and the Attempt to Cover Up Their Threat to Your Health.* Brodeur and *The New Yorker* returned to the subject in 1990 and 1992, in articles that were republished last year in a book titled *The Great Power-Line Cover-up: How the Utilities and the Government Are Trying to Hide the Cancer Hazard Posed by Electromagnetic Fields.*

Unlike Wertheimer's research, Brodeur's annals had almost immediate impact. In the years since the first series appeared, half a dozen government agencies have entered the business of assessing the health hazards of electromagnetic fields (known as EMF)—in particular, the magnetic fields emitted by both high-voltage power lines and "feeder" power lines, which go from house to house; appliances; home wiring; computer terminals; and anything else that plugs into a wall socket or carries electricity into a home or across the countryside. Congress has mandated that the Department of Energy organize a $65 million five-year research program, and the National Cancer Institute [NCI] is conducting a $5 million five-year study to assess whether exposure to EMF can cause or promote childhood leukemia, the most common form of childhood cancer. The motivation for the NCI study, says Martha Linet, an NCI epidemiologist, is less any evidence than the fact that "the public is very concerned and we, of course, are concerned as well."

The cost to society of public anxiety about EMF now exceeds $1 billion annually, according to a July, 1992, article in the journal *Science*, written by H. Keith Florig, of Resources for the Future, an environmental-research institute in Washington, D. C. Florig's estimate takes into account everything from the decrease in prices of real estate near high-voltage lines to the cancellation of or moratoria on new power-transmission projects to the cost of active efforts to reduce EMF exposure. Florig suggests that an appropriate budget for government research on the health effects of EMF could be "as large as [our] combined economic and health costs." Consider the huge savings to society, the argument goes, should further research lead either to a consensus that exposure to EMF is a significant health hazard or to proof beyond reasonable doubt that it is harmless.

The latter possibility is, surprisingly, the one that most scientists say is far more likely. Two recent studies, one by Britain's National Radiological Protection Board and one by the Oak Ridge Associated Universities (ORAU), conducted at the behest of the White House Office of Science and Technology and the Department of Labor, have reviewed the huge body of scientific literature on EMF and concluded that it is long on alarm and short on meaningful science.

The Oak Ridge committee reviewed some fifteen years' worth of literature on the biological effects of EMF and concluded that "epidemiologic findings of an association between electric and magnetic fields and childhood leukemia or other childhood or adult cancers are inconsistent and inconclusive," and that there is no compelling evidence "that these fields initiate cancer, promote cancer, or influence tumor progression."...

The British study was chaired by Sir Richard Doll, an Oxford University epidemiologist famous for his pioneering studies linking cigarette smoking to lung cancer. Doll called the evidence on EMF "much too weak to justify the conclusion" that EMF can cause childhood or adult cancer. He did add, however, that the weak evidence makes it all the more "urgent" to carry out high-quality, large-scale studies to lay the matter to rest.

The controversy over electromagnetic fields has set the institutionalized skepticism of science—the demand that extraordinary claims be supported by extraordinary evidence—against the alarmist attitude of citizens'-action groups and the press, which advocate a guilty-until-proved-innocent approach to environmental concerns. Whether the public has come out wiser rather than simply nervous remains to be seen.

* * *

Virtually all the existing evidence linking EMF to cancer comes from the science of epidemiology, which is the study of the incidence of diseases in populations and the factors that might cause or influence disease. Nancy Wertheimer, for instance, concluded that children who lived in homes near thick and presumably high-current electrical wires contracted cancer at two to three times the rate of children who lived in homes near thin and presumably low-current wires. Her study had serious flaws, as she readily admits, but over the years several other studies have made similar claims.

A second Denver study, nine years later, by David Savitz, who is now at the University of North Carolina, also reported a twofold increase in the risk of cancer for children living near high-current electrical wires. A Los Angeles study followed in 1991, reporting that the risk of contracting leukemia was doubled among children living near high-current lines. And finally, in late 1992, a Swedish study appeared that was hailed by the press as definitive. The Swedish researchers, Anders Ahlbom and Maria Feychting, of the Karolinska Institute, reported not only that magnetic fields seemed to increase a child's risk of contracting leukemia but also that the risk increased as exposure to magnetic fields increased—a phenomenon known in epidemiology as a dose response.

To those researchers inclined to believe that EMF can be harmful, these studies represent a consistent and reliable body of experimental data. Savitz, for instance, calls them "four reasonably well-done studies all pointing in reasonably the same directions."

Those researchers inclined toward skepticism challenge such assertions. Doll, for instance, told me when I spoke to him not long ago that although the Swedish study and a subsequent Danish study were carried out competently, the number of cases of childhood cancer identified is "perishingly small, really much too weak to justify the conclusion that you have got a cause-and-effect relationship." The Swedish study was based on what Ahlbom himself called "a handful of cases." the Danish study on even fewer.

None of the studies linked leukemia or other cancers to the actual magnetic fields measured in the homes. Instead the researchers could link cancer only to what are called proxy measures: in the Denver and Los Angeles studies the connection was with configurations of lines carrying electricity into homes which the researchers thought were likely to be carrying high currents. In Sweden it was the EMF calculated from historical records of power usage. Because the studies involve cases of childhood cancer that occurred many years in the past, epidemiologists in the field argue at length over whether these proxy measures might indeed best reflect EMF exposure at the crucial time. Even so, says Dimitrios Trichpoulos, the head of the epidemiology department at the Harvard School of Public Health, the need to rely on proxies to establish a cause-and- effect relationship makes the EMF-cancer link that much less convincing.

Another suspicious aspect of the studies is that they associate a various and shifting array of cancers with EMF. When the Swedish study came out, Savitz was quoted in *Time* as saying that up to that point the evidence had been stronger for brain tumors. The Swedish study, however, implicated EMF in leukemia and suggested that EMF had no effect on brain tumors. Last October the Danish study and a new Finnish study were published simultaneously in the *British Medical Journal*. The Danes reported a slight association between EMF and all childhood cancers grouped together, and none with leukemia alone. The Finns reported no positive association with any cancers. "They're all conflicting," Doll says.

One likely explanation is that the epidemiologists have fallen victim to what is known in science as a multiple-comparison problem, also known as "data dredging." In other words, re-searchers set out to compare the incidence of several types of cancer with several different measures of EMF strength, and find that some show a small positive association and some show a small negative association. The researchers report the positive ones, ignore the negative ones, and claim that they have confirmed the hypothesis that EMF can cause cancer.

The Swedish researchers, for instance, found no link between magnetic fields measured in the homes and any cancers, no link between distance from power lines and any cancers other than leukemia, and none between the fields calculated from historical records of electricity usage and either brain tumors or all childhood cancers together. They did find a link between calculated historical fields and childhood leukemia. "The results," the researchers concluded, "provide support for the hypothesis that exposure to magnetic fields increases the risk of cancer. This is most evident in childhood leukemia." This conclusion ignores the results regarding measured magnetic fields alone, which suggest the opposite hypothesis: that electromagnetic fields substantially protect against childhood leukemia. Taken as a whole, in fact, the data could equally be said to support the hypothesis that exposure to magnetic fields does not increase the risk of cancer. . . .

At the heart of the problem is that epidemiology is by most scientific standards a crude science. It has historically been capable of identifying causative agents of disease when the association is strong. One of the first major studies of cigarette smoking and lung cancer, for instance, published in the early 1950s by Doll and the late Sir Austin Bradford Hill, found that the risk of contracting lung cancer was at least ten times as high for cigarette smokers as for nonsmokers.

The published studies linking EMF to cancer, however, suggest that the risk of cancer is at most doubled by prolonged exposure to a strong electromagnetic field. This level of increased risk, says Ken Rothman, the editor of the journal *Epidemiology*, is "pushing the edge of what can be done with epidemiology." Epidemiologists and policymakers have worked under the guiding principle that the stronger the association between agent and disease, the less necessary is a credible biological mechanism explaining how that agent might cause the disease. As the epidemiological evidence gets weaker, the need for a plausible biological mechanism and for biomedical evidence—for instance, reproducible experiments in which the agent in question induces the disease in animals—grows stronger.

What's rarely mentioned in public discussions of electromagnetic fields is that the evidence against their having a biological effect of any consequence is strong. Doll says that the "solid weight of biological research" is against the EMF-cancer hypothesis, although he adds that "no hypothesis is too bizarre for someone to think of a reason to justify it." To begin with, cancer rates in America (with the notable exception of lung-cancer rates in women, attributable to smoking) have remained relatively unchanged in the past fifty years, while electrification of the country has increased enormously. . . .

* * *

The magnetic fields under discussion are 100 to 500 times less intense than the earth's magnetic field. Because they arise from alternating currents, however, they reverse direction sixty times a second, which the earth's magnetic field does not.

Citing as his source a retired chairman of the pharmacology department at Baylor University, Paul Brodeur has described the magnetic fields from alternating currents as ticking back and forth like a "metronome" and causing every molecule in the "brain and body in a child or adult standing next to a major power line" to vibrate back and forth in sixty-hertz time. "Anybody with a grain of sense," Brodeur says, "knows that day in and day out, week in and week out, that can't be very good for you."

Understanding the physical effects of these fields, however, requires a course in electromagnetism along the lines of freshman college physics, as well as common sense. Electromagnetic fields simply exert forces on charged particles —they push or pull. They do so in two ways: a static magnetic field, like the earth's, will exert a force on electrically charged particles that are moving; a changing magnetic field, like that of an alternating current, will exert a force on all charged particles, moving or not. The forces generated inside the human body by external sixty-hertz alternating currents when, for example, a person is standing directly under high-tension power lines are thousands of times less intense than the forces generated by the changing electric fields of the heart, brain, and muscles. They are also thousands of times less intense than the electrical forces, or "noise," produced by the natural random motion of ions and molecules in the body. (This random jiggling is known as thermal motion, because it manifests itself as heat.) And the forces generated inside the body by external alternating currents are thousands of times too weak to move a DNA or an RNA molecule in a cell, and trillions of times weaker than those

required to break the chemical bonds in such molecules or cause a mutation—the first steps in the initiation of cancer....

To explain how forces generated inside the body of EMF could have an effect a thousand, a million, or a trillion times greater than what seems physically possible, EMF researchers have proposed theories evoking esoteric phenomena from far-ranging fields of physics—soliton dynamics, Bose-Einstein condensation, electromagnetically induced pressure waves, and magnetic resonance. One theory, for example, proposed by Abe Liboff, a physicist at Oakland University, in Michigan, suggests that EMF can entrap ions in the brain and the body in "cyclotron resonance" and thus spin them at high speeds inside the brain and body like the particles in a particle accelerator. As the Oak Ridge report points out, Liboff ignores, among other aspects of physics, that ions in an accelerator are flung around in a vacuum by extremely strong magnetic fields designed to do just that, whereas ions in the body exist not in a vacuum but in a viscous medium (the brain, for instance) and are under the influence of negligible magnetic fields.

Liboff and his colleagues in EMF theory argue that the scientific community rejects their work because they are proposing a new paradigm and scientists who have grown up with the old paradigm are incapable of accepting such new concepts. Skeptics counter that the theories are, rather, poorly understood and misguided applications of known and accepted science. "People are very paranoid in this field," says William Happer, a physicist at Princeton University. "They think that nobody takes them seriously. They use the same jargon as other scientists; they write down differential equations and solve them. It's just that when you look at what goes into the equation, none of it makes sense."

* * *

The copious body of literature on EMF —at least 13,000 journal articles are being reviewed by an ongoing National Research Council committee on EMF— supports the conclusions of elementary physics and the proposal that electromagnetic fields are biologically harmless. The Oak Ridge report says, "Evidence is lacking to demonstrate that electric or magnetic fields act as cancer initiators by altering structural properties of DNA, function as cancer promoters by inducing or accelerating cell growth, or influence tumor progression." Researchers using EMF have been similarly unable to induce or promote cancer in animals in experiments that can be reproduced.

Although there are scattered reports of physiological changes generated by exposure to EMF, these changes are either irreproducible or show no particular relevance to the question of EMF and cancer. "The bottom line," says Gary Boorman, a scientist at the National Institute of Environmental Health Sciences, "is that all of the findings in the field so far are marginal, and most of them have not been replicated."

This scarcity of reproducible experiments has sparked the notion among EMF researchers that cancer can be induced or promoted only by a distinct, albeit unknown, combination of EMF variables. "This explanation is used," the Oak Ridge reports says, "to explain why so many studies, both *in vivo* and *in vitro*, are negative."

This theory also serves to obviate the usual requirement that a dose-response curve be identified before an agent is conclusively labeled a carcinogen. For ex- ample, if an exposure of two milligauss (a measure of magnetic-field strength) doubles your chance of contracting cancer, the usual expectation would be for four milligauss to triple or quadruple it. However, according to some EMF researchers, two milligauss might provoke cancer and four milligauss might not. Further complicating the matter, researchers have suggested that the EMF recipe that results in cancer might include some particular fluctuation of the earth's ambient magnetic field, which can differ from city to city and even from room to room. "Is it some combination of geomagnetic fields and sixty-hertz fields?" asks Raymond Neutra, the acting chief of the environmental-health-investigations branch of the California Department of Health Services. "Is it sudden spikes? Is is polarization?"

If your local electromagnetic fields are too strong or too weak, the logic goes, or not tuned to precisely the right wave function, they will have no effect. What seems to cause cancer in Buffalo might not in Sheboygan. Thus when Scientist B fails to replicate the experiment of Scientist A, the reason is not that Scientist A's experiment was poorly executed or interpreted incorrectly but that Scientist B did not use precisely the same cell line, or type of DNA or RNA, and did not expose the cells to precisely the same combination of geomagnetic field and EMF frequency, amplitude, and wave shape.

* * *

The big catch is that if electromagnetic fields have no detrimental biological effect, the absence of an effect will be impossible to prove. Outside mathematics it is simply impossible scientifically to prove the nonexistence of something. The best that science can do is to say that the existence of the phenomenon in question is highly unlikely and that the evidence in its favor is poor—which is what is being said today about EMF.

The public, the press, and even many scientists often fail to understand that the nonexistence of a phenomenon does not mean that every experiment will result in confirmation of its nonexistence. Experimental science is not nearly so clean. The history of science is littered with examples of what Irving Langmuir, the 1932 Nobel Prize winner in chemistry, called "pathological science," or "the science of things that aren't so"—of which the latest to hit the press was cold fusion. In these cases researchers publish hundreds of papers claiming to support the existence of an illusory effect, all of which are wrong....

Contributing to the pathology is the fact that once researchers publish a result confirming the existence of the phenomenon, they often cease to do the careful critical evaluation of their research that is a requisite of good science. "If you're an investigator working in EMF," says Gary Boorman, "and you can prove conclusively that there's nothing there, what you've done is create the demise of your field. Economics becomes very, very important here. Everything from lab space and post-docs to support and funding is tied to having an effect."

Langmuir suggested a half dozen characteristic symptoms of pathological science—among them that "the effect is of a magnitude that remains close to the limit of detectability" and that "the magnitude of the effect is substantially independent of the intensity of the cause" —all of which have been exhibited by the epidemiological research on EMF and cancer. The question becomes, How can scientists, policymakers, and the public tell the difference between a phenomenon that does not exist and never will and a phenomenon that may exist but will be confirmed only with more research? Langmuir suggested that real scientific discoveries, no matter how marginal the early data, blossom as more people and money enter the field—not the case with pathological science, which just goes "on and on."

So how do we tell about the presumed link between EMF and cancer? "What I would expect if it doesn't exist," Nancy Wertheimer says, "which I don't think I'm seeing but others think they are, is more and more studies that come up totally iffy, including the laboratory work and the epidemiology. Slowly you get this accumulation of more of the same, and it doesn't amount to anything."

Controversy alone, Charles Poole points out, will keep a field alive whether the phenomenon under examination is real or not. But rather than a series of studies' leading to a compelling scientific judgment, he says, "a highly plausible outcome for all this work is the eventual petering out of research interest." It can take decades of inconclusive and conflicting studies, though, before the research community decides to move on.

* * *

The public concern engendered by Paul Brodeur's exposés has ensured a steady flow of funding for further research. Brodeur's work presents a picture different from that of the scientific data, one arrived at by a technique that Wertheimer, who continues to believe that EMF may be hazardous, describes as leaving out evidence not in accord with Brodeur's own interpretation. "Brodeur served an important function of journalists," she says. "He got people excited. It's not a scientific approach, because he left out most of the negative evidence."

David Savitz, whose studies have supported an association between EMF and cancer, agrees, saying that Brodeur "interprets the evidence differently than I do and most other scientists I know." He adds that Brodeur's later articles, which became *The Great Power-Line Cover-up*, have "less and less scientific merit and are more and more misleading." Savitz, like Wertheimer, believes that Brodeur played an important role by generating public interest in the issue. "I would rather the public be motivated by hard evidence," he says, "but that may not be the realistic world of setting research priorities."

Brodeur presents studies as incontrovertible when most scientists consider them inconclusive and inconsistent, and portrays scientists as petty and self-interested if they have had the temerity to suggest that the studies are less than incontrovertible. Brodeur also presents a smattering of research results—those reporting biological effects from EMF—as if they represent the bulk of the literature and a consistent body of research....

At a meeting last November of the National EMR Alliance, a coalition of more than 300 citizens' groups fighting to reduce what they believe are hazardous exposures to EMF, Brodeur explained in a speech that consensus scientific opinion differs from his own because those scientists who disagree with his position have sold out. Those doing the buying, he said, are the Electric Power Research Institute, known as EPRI, which is the research arm of the utility industry, and the lawyers for the utility industry.

"A lot of the scientific community is being bought on this issue," Brodeur continued. "I'm not saying most of it. The problem isn't the ones that are being bought;

the problem, as it always is, is the eighty-five or ninety percent of honest scientists who have been approached but aren't saying anything. The silence of the community [is] because scientists and medical doctors hate to criticize one another. You know they've got to go to meetings, they have to drink and nibble a canapé with these guys. You don't want to come out and attack a guy for taking money."

Brodeur also explained to his audience that the utility companies are likely to win any court cases on EMF, "because even now they have got almost all the expert witnesses lined up." Brodeur and lawyers for the alliance suggest that citizens' groups sue utility companies for property damage, claiming that power lines have drastically reduced nearby real-estate values. To win such cases in many states, according to John Ward, a Baltimore attorney, "requires only proof of public fear of [EMF] from power lines and proof that such fear diminishes the market value of the property. The reasonableness of the public's fear is deemed either established or irrelevant." As Ward told the alliance during the meeting last fall, "When the voice of sweet reason doesn't work, property-damage cases are the club."

Brodeur suggested at the meeting that newspapers are reluctant to report the harmful reality of EMF, because they, too, must pay tribute to interested parties: "Seventy-five percent of almost any newspaper's revenue," he explained to the credulous audience, "between fifty and seventy-five percent comes from real-estate advertisement, and this problem is having a major effect on real-estate advertisement."

Many of the major players in EMF research have similar explanations for why the scientific community has rejected their research. "Most people who say this is impossible come from the engineering side of things," says Abe Liboff, the progenitor of the cyclotron-resonance theory. "Scientists are different." Louise Young, one of the authors of *Power Over People*, a 1973 exposé of the alleged environmental hazards of high-voltage transmission lines, says that because the electric utilities, through EPRI, are the major source of research funds in the field, money goes only to researchers who will report evidence that living near EMF is safe—an assertion that is documentably wrong....

These arguments have a certain persuasiveness, even if they are at best highly debatable. For whatever reason —perhaps the influence of Hollywood— Americans have a marked willingness to distrust any scientist who professes to know better than the lay experts. The best place to go for scientific expertise, however, is often the scientific experts. What makes Brodeur's conspiratorial interpretation all the harder to understand is the level of alarm raised compared with the maximum possible level of the threat. Scientists on both sides of the issue say that they are dealing at the very most with rare diseases and an increased risk that is almost infinitesimal—especially compared with all the other risks of everyday life, from driving and smoking to choice of diet. As Savitz puts it, the possibilties are "the absence of effect and a fairly subtle and modest one."

Anders Ahlbom, the co-author of the Swedish study, says that if his results do turn out to be incontrovertible, and "if you make a very simplified assumption —say, living close to a power line doubles your risk of leukemia—then you still have to put this into a public-health perspective." Seventy cases of childhood leukemia are diagnosed each year in Sweden, out of which one might be attributed to living near high-power transmission lines. Suppose you have a day-care center around your power lines," Ahlbom says, "which is fairly common" in Sweden. "Suppose you move your child to a day-care center that requires driving several more miles. You may actually increase your risk" of harming your child, in a car accident.

As epidemiologists await the results of the National Cancer Institute's EMF study, due in 1995, and of a similar large study in Britain, members of the public will have to make their own decisions. Doing so will involve weighing the unknown and at most extremely small risks of EMF against the known risks of everyday life. In California, the epidemiologist Charles Poole observes, parents have suggested that the authorities close down schools near power lines and bus the children to other schools. Poole, who refers to himself as an "agnostic" on the EMF issue, says "You know, the buses don't have seat belts and kids die every year in bus crashes. We don't know there's any risk at all in electromagnetic fields from power lines. But people have a fear of the unknown; they have a fear of these invisible rays. This could all easily turn out to be a false alarm."

POSTSCRIPT

Does Exposure to Electromagnetic Fields Cause Cancer?

Seven people (both adults and children) living on the same street in Guilford, Connecticut, a street with only nine houses on it, developed cancer over a relatively short period of time. In Montecito, California, children attending the local elementary school have developed lymphoma and leukemia at more than 15 times the expected rate. And in Fresno, California, 15 teachers and staff members at an elementary school have developed cancer in recent years. The factor common to all three groups is living or going to school near high-voltage power lines giving off high levels of magnetic fields. While the Department of Health in each area refutes the claim that the power lines play any role, some researchers believe that there could be some relationship. Currently, there is no definitive answer to why the high rates of cancer occurred among these residents and students. Readings that discuss possible links between electromagnetic fields (EMFs) and cancer include "Electric Link," *New Scientist* (June 18, 1994); *The Great Power-Line Coverup* (Little, Brown, 1993); "Shocking Charges," *American Health* (May 1993); *Currents of Death: Power Lines, Computer Terminals, and the Attempt to Cover Up Their Threat to Your Health* (Little, Brown, 1990); and "Annals of Radiation," *The New Yorker* (June 1989).

Proving that exposure to high levels of electromagnetic fields is a risk is extremely difficult. Many scientists claim that the elevated cancer rates in Guilford, Montecito, and Fresno are simply flukes. Also, most of the studies showing a relationship between EMFs and cancer have not been able to be duplicated by other scientists, which also indicates a statistical fluke. What is certain is that many people are fearful of EMFs: In several states anxious citizens have delayed plans by electric companies to expand high-voltage transmission lines. Houses next to power lines sell more slowly and for less money. Parents of children attending schools near power lines are demanding that either the schools move or the lines move. And cancer victims are suing utility companies for millions of dollars.

Clearly, more research is needed to determine if there is a genuine risk and, if so, what the best way is to reduce exposure. For further reading on the subject, see "Electromagnetic Fields," *Consumer Reports* (May 1994); "Is Electricity Endangering Your Family?" *McCall's* (November 1993); "Electrical Emissions: Dangerous or Not?" *The New York Times* (June 22, 1993); "Shocking Charges," *American Health* (May 1993); "Do Cellular Phones Cause Cancer?" *Fortune* (March 8, 1993); and "Electromagnetic Fields: In Search of the Truth," *Popular Science* (December 1991).

PART 7

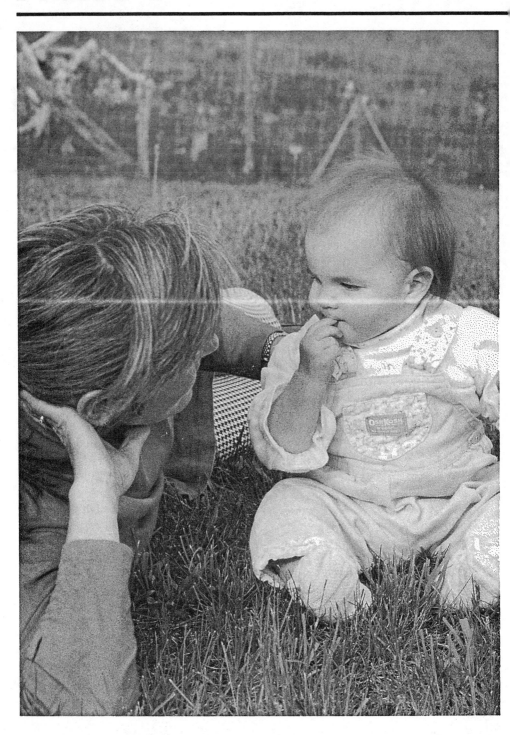

Making Choices for the Health Care Consumer

A shift is occurring in medical care toward informed self-care: People are starting to reclaim their autonomy, and the relationship between doctor and patient is changing. Many patients are asking more questions of their doctors, considering a wider range of medical options, and becoming more educated about what determines their health. Some individuals are rejecting traditional medicine altogether and seeking alternative health providers, while others are rejecting only some aspects of traditional medicine, such as immunizations. This section debates some of the choices consumers may make regarding their health care.

- Should All Children Be Immunized Against Childhood Diseases?

- Are Chiropractors Legitimate Health Providers?

ISSUE 19

Should All Children Be Immunized Against Childhood Diseases?

YES: Royce Flippin, from "The Vaccine Debate: Kids at Risk?" *American Health: Fitness of Body and Mind* (July/August 1990)

NO: Richard Leviton, from "Who Calls the Shots?" *East West: The Journal of Natural Health and Living* (November 1988)

ISSUE SUMMARY

YES: Health writer Royce Flippin argues that since measles and some other potentially dangerous childhood diseases are making a comeback, all children should be immunized against them.

NO: Health journalist Richard Leviton maintains that many vaccines are neither safe nor effective and that parents should have a say in whether or not their children receive them.

A number of infectious diseases are almost completely preventable through routine childhood immunizations. These diseases include diphtheria, meningitis, pertussis (whooping cough), tetanus, polio, measles, mumps, and rubella (German measles). Largely as a result of widespread vaccination, these once-common diseases have become relatively rare. Before the introduction of the polio vaccine in 1955, epidemics of the paralyzing disease occurred each year. In 1952 a record 20,000 cases were diagnosed, as compared to the last outbreak in 1979, when only 10 paralytic cases were identified.

Measles, which can cause serious complications and death, has also declined considerably since the measles vaccine became available. In 1962 there were close to 500,000 cases in the United States, as compared to under 4,000 cases in late 1980. Measles still kills some children and causes permanent damage to others who have not been immunized. In some parts of the country, particularly in urban areas, measles epidemics rage among nonimmunized children of all ages, who pass the disease along to each other.

Unfortunately, measles is not the only disease making a comeback. In 1983 an outbreak of whooping cough in Oklahoma affected over 300 people. By 1988 nearly 3,000 cases nationwide had been diagnosed. Whooping cough is a serious and sometimes fatal disease, especially among young infants. Although the risks of whooping cough and other childhood diseases are serious, many children remain unimmunized because their parents either cannot afford vaccination, are unaware of the dangers of childhood diseases, or believe that the risks of vaccination outweigh the benefits—the last of these is the basis for this debate.

The whooping cough vaccine has been the subject of more concern than any other immunization. While almost all of the 18 million doses administered each year cause little or no reaction, about 50 to 75 children who receive the vaccine suffer serious neurological injury, a few of which lead to death. Although some consider this risk to be too high, before the vaccine was available, nearly 8,000 children died annually from whooping cough. Still, many parents who are concerned about the dangers of the vaccine have chosen not to have their children vaccinated.

In the following selections, Royce Flippin argues that vaccines are much safer than the diseases they prevent and that parents must continue to have their children immunized. Richard Leviton asserts that many vaccines, particularly whooping cough, are not safe or effective and that parents must have a say in whether or not their children receive them.

YES   Royce Flippin

THE VACCINE DEBATE: KIDS AT RISK?

Measles outbreaks swept through the nation last year, leaving more than 16,000 children and young adults feverish and dotted with red itchy spots—up from 3,400 cases in 1988. The numbers are expected to be even higher this year. In 1989, the fretful "whooping" cough of pertussis—the deadly scourge of the '30s and '40s—struck more than 3,700 American children, a rate more than double that of the early '80s. And the number of reported cases is only a small fraction of the actual caseload, health officials fear.

Though these childhood diseases are almost entirely preventable by vaccines, immunization rates in the U.S. have dropped significantly in the past 10 years. Incredibly, more than one in five American two-year-olds now go unprotected against either polio, measles, rubella or mumps. One in seven have never received a full series of shots against diphtheria, tetanus and pertussis (the DTP shot—formerly called DPT). Those are national estimates; in some urban centers as few as 40% of tots are fully immunized. Many of the unprotected children are impoverished. Their parents often can't afford the $80 to $150 per child (plus office fees) for a complete set of shots.

But beyond cost or oversight, there's also genuine concern about the safety of some vaccines—measles, mumps, polio and especially the pertussis shot for whooping cough. Critics especially fault pediatricians for failing to single out children at high risk of being injured by these shots. Now comes news that a vaccine against the varicella virus that causes chicken pox might become available as soon as next year, pending FDA approval. Published studies indicate it's a safe and effective vaccine for normal kids, says the CDC's Dr. Laura Fehrs.

While public health officials push for more immunizations, some parents' groups are charging that many vaccines themselves are unsafe, and that the public hasn't been fully informed about the danger of adverse side effects. Many parents whose children have had severe, sometimes lasting complications from vaccines have joined grassroots organizations such as Dissatisfied Parents Together. This group was formed in 1982 to spread the word about the risks of pertussis and other vaccines and lobby for better record-keeping and safer vaccines, as well as compensation for those who suffer vaccine injuries.

Medical researchers, caught in the middle of the debate, have struggled to determine the true risk to kids, while scientists race to produce a new generation of safer vaccines.

A SHOT IN THE DARK

By far the vaccine that has inspired the most fear is the whole-cell pertussis shot (so called because it's made of entire dead bacteria). Linked with complications ranging from fever to seizures, the vaccine is even accused of causing brain damage and death.

Other vaccines have come under scrutiny as well: Measles and mumps vaccines, given as part of the MMR shot (measles, mumps, rubella), can cause fever, rashes and swollen glands in children. (Rubella, the other part of the shot, has been suspected of sometimes causing rheumatoid arthritis when given to adults.) The oral polio vaccine can in extremely rare instances actually cause the disease.

The pertussis vaccine, however—usually given in a series beginning at two months of age—is the subject of worldwide controversy. In the mid '70s fear of adverse vaccine reactions in Great Britain drove immunization rates down to near 30% for pertussis. Several years later, as the "herd immunity" effect of group vaccination wore off, whooping cough cases began to climb. The English reported 66,000 cases in 1978—compared with an annual rate between 2,000 and 17,500 for the years 1969 through 1977. As the disease spread, more and more people opted to get shots.

Today, 75% to 80% of the English are immunized and the case load dropped to 11,700 last year. In 1976, Japan's pertussis vaccination rate dropped to about 10% but now is back up to over 80% in part because of a new, purified form of the vaccine. Sweden, however, hasn't vaccinated against pertussis since 1979, and the disease is prevalent.

Today, some scientists are saying the worst fears about the vaccine simply aren't justified. Last March in the *Journal of the American Medical Association* (*JAMA*), investigators studying 38,000 Tennessee schoolchildren found no association between the pertussis vaccine and the incidence of serious neurological effects or brain damage (encephalopathy). An editorial in the same issue cited two other recent studies with similar findings and suggested there was no absolutely no doubt of the shot's safety. "It's time for the myth of pertussis vaccine encephalopathy to end," declared Dr. James Cherry, chief of infectious diseases at the UCLA Medical Center.

But Barbara Loe Fisher, executive vice president of Dissatisfied Parents Together, isn't convinced. Fisher believes adverse reactions are underreported: It was only after the passage of the National Childhood Vaccine Injury Act in 1986—an effort spearheaded by her group—that doctors were required to report all reactions.

In her book *A Shot in the Dark*, Fisher and her coauthor describe scores of horrifying accounts of complications among children within hours or days of receiving a DTP shot. Some children recovered, but others were left paralyzed, brain damaged—some even died. Fisher's own son collapsed in shock within hours of a DTP shot, she says, and was left with multiple learning disabilities. "If you look at these studies, they just don't hold up," she says. "My feeling is that because vaccine manufacturers are involved in the funding of most of them, you're not getting an unbi-

MEASLES REDUX

Think you're done with shots? It turns out the measles vaccine given to some baby boomers was less than perfect: Almost one-quarter of the victims in last year's outbreak were college-aged or older. Health authorities are now urging everyone vaccinated between 1963 and 1968 to consider being revaccinated with the more effective "live" vaccine now available. Those born before 1957 probably had the disease and are immune. However, adds George Seastrom, a public health advisor with the CDC, "People born before 1957 who have never had measles should also consider getting vaccinated."

Other preventable diseases pose even higher risks for adults. According to the National Foundation for Infectious Diseases, influenza and pneumonia account for up to 60,000 deaths a year in the U.S., and the 300,000 cases of hepatitis B reported annually cause 5,000 deaths each year. Also, 11 million women of child-bearing age go unprotected against rubella, which is known to cause birth defects, and the vast majority of tetanus and diphtheria cases from 1985 to 1987 occurred in people over 20 who lacked adequate immunization.

However, there is some good news. Confirmed cases of paralytic polio are now so rare in the Americas that international health officials predict they'll have chased the crippling disease from the Western Hemisphere by year's end. With an intensive global vaccination drive, they say polio could be eradicated from the globe—as was small pox in 1977—by the end of the decade.

ased opinion." As an example, she points out that Lederle-Praxis, a maker of pertussis and other vaccines, funds Cherry as an independent third-party investigator.

Cherry responds: "I was involved in a recent Denmark study, which found no cause-and-effect relationship between epilepsy and pertussis vaccine, and that was funded by an unrestricted grant from Lederle. This means they had no control over the study. The research was done and peer-reviewed, and published in a respectable journal [*The Journal of Pediatrics*]."

That aside, Dr. Marie Griffin, the Vanderbilt University epidemiologist who led the *JAMA* study, says she wouldn't go quite as far as Cherry's editorial. "Our study is reassuring," she says, "but it was not conclusive. Maybe if we'd looked at 3 *million* children we would have seen a difference. We don't know."

What her study does show, Griffin explains, is that serious complications from the vaccine aren't common. Her group found no cases of brain damage or serious neurological disease within four weeks of receiving DTP shots.

ASSESSING THE RISKS

The situation is complicated by the fact that vaccines are initially given in infancy,

THE DON'TS OF PERTUSSIS VACCINATION

Most kids who get the pertussis vaccine have no serious side effects. But in rare instances, major complications do arise. The CDC has now developed the following checklist to help identify high-risk kids who should *not* get the pertussis portion of the DTP vaccine.

- Anyone over age seven.
- Children with a fever-related illness.
- Those with a history of convulsions (with or without fever).
- Children undergoing immunosuppressive therapy.
- Children with an underlying neurological disorder, such as epilepsy or infantile spasms.

Children who've had one of the following reactions to a previous DTP shot *should not* receive any more pertussis shots: allergic hypersensitivity; fever of 105° or higher within 48 hours of the shot; a collapse or shock-like state within 48 hours; persistent crying for three or more hours, or unusually high-pitched crying within 48 hours; convulsions (with or without fever) within three days; impaired or reduced consciousness within a week.

The grassroots organization Dissatisfied Parents Together lists the following as high-risk factors *not* officially recognized by the CDC:

- Any illness, including runny nose, cough, ear infection or diarrhea, up to one month prior to a DTP shot.
- A family member who has reacted severely to DTP.
- A personal or family history of severe allergies.
- Premature delivery, low birth weight or birth complications.
- A family history of convulsions.

For other vaccines the CDC recommends: Measles, mumps, rubella and oral polio vaccines should not be given to women who are pregnant or considering becoming pregnant in the next three months. They also should not be given to anyone suffering immune-deficiency diseases, or taking medication that suppresses immunity. People with allergies to neomycin should consult a doctor before receiving measles, mumps, rubella or intramuscular polio vaccine. Those with egg allergies should also check with a doctor before getting measles, mumps and influenza vaccines. Tetanus and diphtheria vaccines should not be given if the patient has had a previous allergic or neurological reaction to the shots. At no time should a vaccine be administered to an adult or child suffering from an illness with high fever.

when pre-existing neurological illnesses first manifest themselves. For instance, Cherry suspects a form of epilepsy called infantile spasm may be truly to blame in some cases. The condition peaks at three to five months. "Vaccines bring it out, but the illness will happen anyway—or perhaps is already happening at the time of the vaccination."

Children are also prone to seizures in infancy. Dr. Gerald Fenichel, a pediatric neurologist at Vanderbilt, says that fever-induced convulsions occur in 4% of all children. "Several articles suggest that in genetically predisposed children seizures can be induced by the fever associated with pertussis vaccine—or measles vaccine, for that matter," he says. Doctors have identified which kids—at high risk for reactions—should not be immunized (see "The Don'ts of Pertussis Vaccination").

Griffin was surprised her study found few vaccine-related seizures. But Danish investigators recently did find a higher-than-normal rate of fever-induced seizures in children following their DTP shots; and two large studies reported a slight post-DTP fever in most children, a fever of 105° or more in one out of 330 shots, and convulsions or collapse in one out of 875 DTP vaccinations.

While such relatively common episodes aren't life-threatening, they're frightening, says Dr. Allen Mitchell, associate director of the Sloan epidemiology unit at the Boston University School of Medicine, who publishes a newsletter called *Pediatric Alert*. Mitchell says pediatricians have become sensitive to parental anxiety over the shots and their possible complications. "It appears more and more doctors are giving acetaminophen with the DTP shot to prevent high fever," Mitchell says. "This practice may lessen the chance of fever-induced seizures, and also reduce the discomfort that often follows the shot."

DETOXING THE PERTUSSIS SHOT

Meanwhile, scientists say they're closer than ever to a solution—a safer vaccine. In animal studies, a new genetically altered strain of "acellular" pertussis vaccine gave effective protection with no toxic side effects, according to a report in *Science*.

That was achieved by altering two key amino acids in the pertussis toxin, says coinvestigator Dr. Joseph Barbieri of the Medical College of Wisconsin.

Is this the vaccine of the future? "It depends on how it does in clinical trials," Barbieri says, adding that such trials have begun in Italy. A different form of acellular vaccine, which relies on chemical purification and detoxification, is already being used in Japan.

By most accounts it will be years before a totally nontoxic pertussis vaccine goes mainstream here. Meanwhile, the Department of Health and Human Services is looking into the issue of adverse reactions to pertussis and rubella vaccinations. HHS has asked the Institute of Medicine in Washington, DC, to examine the available evidence and present a report by next summer.

For the time being, people who choose not to get their kids immunized can be grateful for the generally high U.S. vaccination rate, which prevents diseases from reaching pandemic proportions. "It's like paying your taxes," says Dr. Charles Gordon, a New York pediatrician. "We can survive if a few people don't—but if no one pays, we're all in trouble."

NO

Richard Leviton

WHO CALLS THE SHOTS?

One day in 1980 Barbara Fisher held down her two-and-a-half-year-old son, Christian, so the doctor could give him his fourth DPT (diphtheria-pertussis-tetanus) shot. Neither Fisher nor the doctor knew that Christian, with respect to DPT vaccine, was a high-risk child. He had experienced a violent "local reaction" to his third injection, an experience a physician would diagnose, had one noticed it, as a contraindication against further vaccination.

Within hours of his fourth shot, Christian suffered what his mother now realizes was a classic collapse/shock reaction to pertussis. "I didn't report it to my doctor," says Fisher today. "I had not been informed of what a severe reaction was, and I didn't know I was witnessing one." She thought Christian might be undergoing a relapse of the flu. Fisher didn't want her doctor to regard her as "one of those hysterical mothers who calls up every time the child sneezes."

In the ensuing months it became obvious to Fisher that something had gone wrong with the DPT vaccination. Christian forgot his alphabet. He became hyperactive and emotionally fragile. He had staring spells, lost weight, and developed chronic diarrhea, upper respiratory infections, and allergies. Fisher still trusted her physician, who assured her that Christian was "just going through a stage." "But," says Fisher, "my whole family knew something drastic had happened to Christian, that he had become a totally different child overnight."

Today Barbara Fisher is a much wiser and infinitely better-informed mother. She knows that after his fourth DPT shot her "once precocious" Christian suffered a mild encephalopathy that left him with minimal brain damage, multiple learning disabilities, and an impaired immune system. Fisher, like many mothers, was left raging with many unanswered medical questions.

"Why was I so willing to suspend my common sense and deny reality in order to believe in the infallibility of medicine and my doctor? I believed vaccines were completely safe and effective because that is what I was led to believe by all I had read or heard in the media, by what I had been told by my pediatrician, and because I came from a family full of doctors and nurses and other health professionals who had dedicated their lives to medicine. I had absolutely no idea that a vaccination could result in brain damage or death."

Young Christian Fisher, however, was one of the lucky ones. He is not dead or mentally retarded or suffering from convulsions. There are 67,000 infants vaccinated with DPT every week in America but nobody—not medical professionals, the government, or mothers—has accurate casualty statistics. But that there have been significant vaccine-associated damages is meticulously documented in Fisher's provocative book, coauthored by Harris Coulter, *DPT: A Shot in the Dark* (Warner Books, 1985).

For Barbara Fisher, educating the public about the dangers of adverse reactions to DPT has become a paramount social responsibility. Christian's experience instantly politicized her. And she cites the familiar equation: Knowledge equals power.

"It is time we as parents begin to take back the right and responsibility for our children's health instead of taking the easy way out and leaving the decisions up to our doctors." Thus in 1982 Fisher founded Dissatisfied Parents Together (DPT) in Washington, D.C., to spearhead the drive for greater public awareness and to initiate legislative change. Fisher's DPT coalition, with chapters in many states, has a huge natural constituency. Each year another $3^1/_2$ million babies are born in America, who will be legally required to have some ten vaccinations by the age of six.

Barbara Fisher has become a major figure in the controversy over mandatory vaccination policies. On the other side of the controversy are some of the leading policymakers in American medicine —the American Academy of Pediatrics, the federal Centers for Disease Control, and the American Medical Association. They unilaterally endorse vaccination programs. "There is an ineluctable conflict between public health and individual rights and this is a regrettable fact," observes Stanley Plotkin, M.D., chairman of A.A.P.'s Committee on Infectious Diseases and director, Division of Infectious Diseases at Children's Hospital of Philadelphia.

"Public health makes the assumption that the health of a group of people is more important," he says. "When you're dealing with contagious diseases the action of a single individual may impact on others. We do not recognize the right of parents to put their children at risk of developing an infectious disease. We feel that a policy that protects children is superior."

Navigating the waters across which such volleys are fired requires today's parents to be both wary and well-informed.

AN ARSENAL OF VACCINES

The concept behind vaccination is to artificially produce immunity to an infectious disease by introducing a small amount of the disease virus or bacteria into the body. The immune system wages a mini-campaign against the foreign materials and develops antibodies tailored for that disease organism, for future reference, in case the child contacts the pathogens in the environment.

This is called active immunization and theoretically provides lasting, effective protection against specific diseases. "The goal is to mimic the natural infection by evoking an immunologic response which presents little or no risk to the recipient," informs the 1986 *Red Book*, the pediatrician's standard reference work on vaccinations, published by the A.A.P.

...Today's vaccines use either live or killed infectious agents, usually a virus or bacteria. They are typically injected; a type of polio vaccine is taken orally. The oral polio vaccine is cultured from the kidney cells of the African green monkey.

In addition to the active immunizing antigen, vaccines contain a suspending fluid (sterile water), trace amounts of preservatives (including formaldehyde and mercury-derivatives), stabilizers, antibiotics, and adjuvants (aluminum phosphate).

While there are no national vaccination laws, the fifty states are fairly uniform in their requirements for mandatory vaccinations as a prerequisite for school admission. Children must be vaccinated against the five traditional childhood diseases of mumps, measles, rubella, diphtheria, and pertussis, plus tetanus and polio.

Mumps is a routine, relatively innocuous viral disease that lasts one to two weeks and requires no medical treatment. Two-thirds of infected children develop a self-limiting illness with swollen salivary glands, fever, headache, and appetite loss, but afterwards they have lifetime immunity. A single vaccination of live virus is given at age fifteen months, usually as part of a triple injection called MMR (measles-mumps-rubella). The mumps component, however, is not required in sixteen states.

Measles is a contagious viral disease that lasts two weeks. Characteristic symptoms are a high fever and a rash of pink spots, but more serious complications include eye and ear inflammations, pneumonia, or, in rare instances, encephalitis. The live virus vaccine was introduced in America in 1963 although the measles mortality rate had already dropped radically from 13.3/100,000 cases to 0.3/100,000 by 1955.

Rubella (German measles) is often a benign disease with symptoms so mild they often escape detection. There is a three-day rash, fever, a slight cold, and sore throat. The principal danger is congenital rubella syndrome (CRS), whereby a pregnant woman can expose her fetus to injury if she contracts rubella in her first trimester. A children's mass immunization program for rubella began in 1969 after a CRS epidemic among 20,000 babies in 1964.

Diphtheria has nearly disappeared from America, where it was once greatly feared as a highly contagious bacterial disease with a mortality rate at 3–10 percent. Medical treatment with penicillin or erythromycin is usually indicated. Although mortality rates from diphtheria had dropped by 50 percent before a vaccine was developed, today three to five doses are required in all fifty states.

Pertussis, or whooping cough, is probably the most virulent of the traditional childhood diseases and it can be life-threatening. The infectious agent, *Bordetella pertussis*, was first isolated in France in 1906. Pertussis vaccination, using whole-cell killed virus, began in 1936 and became widespread by 1957. Pertussis symptoms, including a paroxysmal cough, usually afflict infants younger than two years. Today thirty-nine states require three to five injections, beginning at age two months.

Tetanus, technically not a childhood disease, is a potentially dangerous, sometimes fatal, random bacterial infection. Tetanus infection can produce severe neurologic symptoms and muscular spasms (the spasms in the jaw gave the disease the name of "lockjaw"), and worldwide it has a 30–50 percent mortality rate. It is especially prevalent in tropical countries. A regimen of one to five tetanus inoculations are required by forty-seven states, beginning at age two months.

Poliomyelitis infection actually produces no symptoms in 90 percent of its recipients and only 1–2 percent of children infected develop its classic, virally produced symptoms. Polio vaccine, required at three to four doses nationwide, comes in two forms: Salk killed-virus injection and Sabin live-virus oral vaccine.

BRAVE NEW VACCINES

... The A.A.P. is categorically opposed to any kind of optional vaccination approach, states G. Scott Giebink, M.D., professor of pediatrics at the University of Minnesota Medical School and a member of the A.A.P. infectious diseases committee. "This is because the virtual eradication of many of the vaccine-preventable diseases has been based on universal rather than optional, or partial, immunization. All of the programs have been incredibly effective—but not because only a few people had the vaccines."

Childhood diseases are still a significant public health threat, requiring prevention, Giebink stresses. "That's the primary reason for continuing a strong and universal immunization program as these diseases are rampant in the world. I'd place the public health benefits first."

Alan Nelson, M.D., president of the A.M.A., agrees. "The data that support the advantages of vaccinations in terms of neurologic injury or mortality to those unprotected are so clear-cut that our public policy still has to support mass immunization. There are few things in medicine that are totally risk-free. That's why we have to measure the benefits against the risks, but with vaccinations the benefits clearly outweigh the risks."

Nelson cites the example of Britain. "There the choice of parents was expressed and DPT vaccination rates have dropped, but the experience has been bad in terms of epidemics and outbreaks of pertussis ever since."

The primary issue at stake is the communicability of infectious diseases, says Walter Orenstein, M.D., director of the Division of Immunization at the CDC in Atlanta. "It's a community decision. When we have children vaccinated, we not only protect the children, we protect the community at large. Parents who decide not to have their children vaccinated not only are not protecting their children, but potentially their actions are leading to danger for other children in that community. If this happened on a large scale, that would put an entire community at risk." ...

CONTRAINDICATIONS

Not everyone shares this rosy prognosis for preventive vaccination for nearly all diseases. In the mid-1980s a combination of television documentaries, major newspaper stories, and several books—most prominently, Fisher and Coulter's *DPT* —raised public awareness to a shocked appreciation of problems with the mass vaccination approach. Major fissures in the otherwise solid medical edifice were suddenly revealed. The issues are complex and myriad, and often emotionally tinged.

The DPT shot, among all vaccinations in use, produces the most serious adverse reactions. Before 1985 parents were never adequately advised (if at all) of the potentially harmful side-effects of DPT, state Fisher and Coulter. Even today pediatricians still usually downplay the risks. Adverse reactions, which are medical contraindications against further injections, run the gamut from localized skin reactions to seizure, brain inflammation, and death. In 1988, more than forty years after the DPT vaccine was introduced, no accepted parameters have been developed for prescreening hypersensitive children who might be at major risk from DPT.

Prior to 1988 there was not a nationally mandated reporting system either, one which required physicians or health departments to file reports on adverse reactions. Thus accurate data on the prevalence of adverse reactions is lacking and estimates vary widely. Often pediatricians fail (or refuse) to make the connection between a DPT injection and adverse reactions, even when they occur within hours of each other. Coulter and Fisher did their own calculations, based on the best available published data, and came up with some staggering damage estimates.

They calculated that, based on an infant population of 3.3 million per year eligible for DPT shots, 4,248 children have either post-injection convulsions or collapse, 10,377 have high-pitched screaming within forty-eight hours, and 18,873 infants have some form of significant neurological reaction within two days. Possibly as many as 943 deaths and 11,666 cases of long-term damage are attributable to DPT.

There is also considerable disagreement over the level of efficacy of the DPT vaccine, state Fisher and Coulter. Estimates range from 63 to 94 percent. DPT was never adequately tested for safety, its artificially induced immunity lasts only two to five years, and it is regarded as "one of the crudest vaccines on the market." American medical authorities are inexplicably reluctant to adopt the newer and apparently safer Japanese acellular pertussis vaccine.

Given these conditions, Fisher's DPT coalition is understandably strongly in favor of making vaccinations a voluntary act. Fisher would like the DPT vaccine to function freely in the marketplace, like other consumer goods. "Then you will have the good, safe, effective vaccines used, and the poor ones will be dropped. That will give an incentive to the drug companies and government to come up with the most effective and the safest vaccines possible."

Most European nations now allow optional vaccinations for DPT. Voluntary programs are actually generating "control group" data for natural infection rates in countries without mass vaccination. Communist countries such as the Soviet Union, Poland, and East Germany still require vaccinations.

The examples of Britain, West Germany, and Sweden are often cited on both sides of the DPT debate. In these countries, when vaccination rates plummeted in the 1970s and incidence of pertussis infection climbed, a corresponding higher incidence of infantile complication or death did not occur, as many had predicted it would. In 1984, researchers at London's Epidemiological Research Laboratory concluded, in contrasting twenty-five deaths at an 80 percent vaccination rate in 1974 with twenty-three deaths at a 30 percent vaccination rate in 1977, that "since the decline in pertussis immunization, hospital admission and death rates from whooping cough have fallen unexpectedly."

The A.M.A., however, is not convinced that the European model of optional pertussis vaccination is medically worthy of importation to America.

"The incidence of pertussis is cyclic and the severity could also run in cycles," observes A.M.A.'s Nelson. "It's still a very bad disease, a terrible, tragic disease. The burden is on those who say the disease is not still an extraordinarily bad illness to prove that. I don't think you will find very many physicians willing to say we don't have to worry about pertussis anymore, that its severity has lessened."

Medical authorities contend that the kind of documentation Fisher and Coulter present, culled from interviews with over 100 mothers of presumed vaccine-damaged children, are "anecdotal" and not scientifically admissible.

"Most of the pertussis controversy revolves around observations that are anecdotal and unconfirmed," states Plotkin of the A.A.P. "The value of such anecdotes is very limited. On the basis of the information available, I would think there are only rare reactions to pertussis vaccine."

Extensive studies in the U.S. and Britain, explains Giebink, have shown "quite conclusively that some of the most serious of these nervous system disorders are in fact not caused by the vaccine but are only temporally related with it. We've looked at some of the particular diseases using scientific methods and we have not been able to show a cause-and-effect relationship."

CDC's Orenstein concurs. "These adverse events are so rare that we can't detect them. A lot of the responsibility falls on the parent who has to make the connection and file a report. Some of them may forget in their crisis. Suppose we do get all the adverse events reported?

It doesn't mean that any of these events are *caused* by the vaccination."

It is precisely statements like these that have infuriated mothers whose babies have suffered damages "temporally" following DPT injections, whatever the true causality might be. Many mothers say their physicians don't listen to them, caution them against hysteria or making trouble, are complacent or patronizing. Other women contend their doctors lied to them and betrayed their trust. Barbara Fisher excoriates this "cavalier disregard for vaccine toxicity and human life."

"We are so conditioned to the idea that our doctor's word is to be trusted without question," said one mother whose infant died thirty-three hours after a DPT shot. "I am a nurse. I watched my son die that day, and I didn't even know what was happening until it was all over."

Mother-activists like Fisher find something immoral lurking within the risk-benefit equations of medical science, especially in light of the lack of exemption options for parents in many states.

"The epidemiologists look at mass vaccination the way a military general studies a battle. A general knows he must sacrifice men to take a hill. This is how government health officials see mass vaccination. They start getting into the idea that some children are expendable. I cannot think of any other instance in our society where we say it's okay to kill children, to have them brain-damaged, because it's for the greater welfare of society."

As Fisher tersely puts it, "When it happens to your child, the risks are 100 percent."

HOLISTIC IMMUNOLOGY

There might be more reasons than symptomatic contraindications arguing the case against mandatory vaccination. According to a variety of holistic practitioners, including M.D.'s, homeopaths, and naturopaths, the general practice of vaccination may have long-term damaging effects on the vitality of the immune system. One such bold M.D. was the late "People's Doctor," Robert Mendelsohn.

Mendelsohn had very impressive credentials to support his strident criticism of vaccinations. He was a practicing pediatrician for twenty-five years, professor at the University of Illinois Medical School, Chairman of the Medical Licensure Committee for Illinois, author of three popular medical guidebooks, and publisher of a medical newsletter for consumers.

For Mendelsohn, vaccinations were a "medical time bomb," the "most threatening" of which was DPT. "The greatest threat of childhood diseases lies in the dangerous and ineffectual efforts made to prevent them through mass immunization," he said. "Although I administered them myself during my early years of practice, I have become a steadfast opponent of mass inoculation because of the myriad hazards they present."

Vaccinations, said Mendelsohn, are one of the harmful sacraments of the modern religion of medicine. "In the total absence of controlled studies, all vaccines today remain, scientifically speaking, unproven remedies—the polite term for medical quackery. The only proven characteristic of vaccines is their devastating adverse effects." Mendelsohn also suggested there might be a causal link between degenerative diseases and immunizations.

Richard Moskowitz is an M.D., homeopath, and former president of the National Center for Homeopathy, now practicing at The Turning Point clinic in Watertown, Mass. He is one of many holistic practitioners who have corroborated Mendelsohn's early indications. In Moskowitz's view *all* vaccinations may be injurious to the functioning and integrity of the immune system.

Moskowitz argues that vaccination may produce a form of immunosuppression and chronic immune failure. The injected virus, because it has been artificially weakened before injection, no longer initiates "a generalized, acute inflammatory response." Instead, it tricks the body into an antibody response—"an isolated technical feat" and only an aspect of the overall immune ability. Worse, the virus may persist in the blood for prolonged periods, perhaps permanently.

"Far from producing a genuine immunity, vaccines may actually interfere with or suppress the natural immune response," says Moskowitz. "By making it difficult or impossible to mount a vigorous, acute response to infection, artificial immunization substitutes a much weaker *chronic* response with little or no tendency for the body to heal itself spontaneously."

Evidence indicates that the individual vaccinations may each have unique deleterious consequences on the immune system. Tetanus may interfere with the immune reaction. It has been linked with peripheral neuropathy, allergic reactions, and laryngeal paralysis. Rubella has been tentatively associated with arthralgia (joint pain) and arthritis. A 1980 report in *Mutation Research* indicated that children who underwent repeated smallpox vaccinations in Czechoslovakia showed chromosomal aberrations in their white blood cells, indicating a mutagenic effect.

The British journal *Medical Hypothesis* reported in 1988 in a study of 200 patients with chronic Epstein-Barr virus syndrome that the disease was attributable to the live rubella virus found in the vaccine. In 1987 a consultant for the World Health Organization announced in the London *Times* that the prevalence of smallpox vaccinations over a thirteen-year period in seven African nations actually triggered the AIDS virus outbreak in those countries. In 1985 a scientist at Harvard's School of Public Health revealed that STLV-3, an AIDS-type virus, had been found in the green monkey *(Cercopithecus)* whose kidney cells were routinely used to culture oral polio vaccine.

Other anomalous long-term medical trends implicating vaccinations have recently been brought to light. Widespread measles vaccinations seem to be shifting the incidence of the disease into older age groups; 80 percent of cases are now occurring in people aged ten to nineteen and with atypical, often untreatable symptoms. Vaccination immunity is clearly less than complete, as 1988 CDC figures showed that of 795 reported cases of pertussis in infants aged three to six months, 49 percent of them had been fully vaccinated.

While holistic health providers are finding alarming grounds for connecting today's auto-immune anomalies and a weakened immune response with vaccines, Giebink of the A.A.P. states unequivocally, "Those are all groundless speculations." ...

IN SEARCH OF WILLING DOCTORS

All fifty states allow a medical exemption for high-risk children. Generally what is required is a written statement by a licensed M.D. indicating that the proposed vaccination is medically contraindicated, based on a previous adverse reaction, a family history of reactions, or a personal history of convulsions, neurological disorders, severe allergies, prematurity, or recent severe, chronic illness.

While individual state regulations vary slightly in terminology, essentially the intention remains uniform, as this excerpt from the New York state regulation makes clear: "If any physician licensed to practice medicine in this state certifies that such immunization may be detrimental to a student's health, the requirements of this section shall be inapplicable until such immunization is no longer found to be detrimental."

Philip Incao, M.D., is a licensed New York state physician with offices in Harlemville, New York, near Albany. Incao has been signing medical exemptions for most of the fifteen years of his family practice. But Incao, who practices anthroposophic medicine (see "The Promise of Anthroposophical Medicine," July 1988 *EW),* as developed by the Austrian philosopher Rudolf Steiner (1861-1925), makes a broader interpretation of "detrimental."

Anthroposophical medicine states that the struggle with childhood infectious diseases is salutary for the child's personal and spiritual development and they should not be suppressed; homeopathic medicines may be used to ameliorate the process, however. In this model the illness is seen as an acute, inflammatory event which mobilizes the immune system. It enables the child's "Ego" (the Higher Self, in other vocabularies) to remodel the inherited body according to its own blueprint.

None of Incao's medical exemptions have been refused. Beginning in 1986, however, his unconventional practice may have provoked New York state health officials to begin what has been a smoldering form of harassment and informal investigation of his anthroposophical procedures. While the medical exemption is nationally available, it shouldn't be surprising to find that most doctors are reluctant to grant it, even in conditions of obvious contraindications —because it bucks too much against the orthodoxy. *DPT: A Shot in the Dark* is full of harrowing examples of distraught families scouring an entire state in search of a sympathetic M.D. to sign their medical exemption.

On the positive side, Washington state recently licensed naturopaths to give vaccinations, which means they can also grant exemptions. In some states, including Florida, chiropractors are allowed to write medical exemptions. The cracks in the orthodoxy may be gradually widening to allow parents more latitude.

BROADENING RELIGIOUS BELIEFS

An exemption from vaccinations based on religious beliefs is permitted in all states except West Virginia and Mississippi. Recent favorable litigation in New York has expanded the legal interpretation of religious beliefs, thereby granting parents further options.

The New York statute defines the parameters for religious exemptions by stating that mandatory vaccination requirements "Shall not apply to children whose parents are bona fide members of a recognized religious organization whose teachings are contrary to the practices herein required." This exemption works fine if a parent in fact belongs to a recognized religion. But what happens if a family has sincere beliefs but is outside

the folds of any church? In 1984 a family in Clinton, New York, found out. They refused to have their two daughters vaccinated and took the issue to court. And they won.

Robert and Kit Allanson had initially secured a medical exemption for their daughters Naomi and Marika, but the school rejected it. The girls were expelled from school, their return pending on vaccination. Allanson secured the legal services of Attorney James Filenbaum and they immediately filed a suit in federal court, suing the school district, superintendent, and principal for $2 million. They also demanded a religious exemption for their girls.

The only weakness in the Allanson strategy was that they didn't belong to any church and the nearest recognizable label they had for their convictions was macrobiotics. The prosecutor had a field day with this.

At the trial, however, Filenbaum brought in a minister and the chairman of the religious department at nearby Hamilton College to testify on behalf of the religious authenticity of the Allansons' beliefs, however much those beliefs might lack an institutional context. After five-and-a-half months of testimony, charges of child neglect, and, Robert Allanson says, "hand-to-hand combat with the government," the Allansons prevailed as the U.S. district judge ruled in their favor.

The Allanson case was a valuable precedent for everyone, even outside of New York. Since the 1984 ruling, Filenbaum has argued another dozen religious exemption cases (in addition to advising hundreds of other clients) and has won nearly all of them. . . .

PERSONAL BELIEFS

Probably the best compromise all around is now legally available in twenty-two states. This is a harassment- and red-tape-free exemption on the grounds of personal or philosophical belief.

Vermont is a "triple-exemption" state which approved the personal belief exemption in 1981. According to Bob O'Grady, administrator of the Epidemiology Division in the Vermont State Health Department in Burlington, of Vermont's 98,600 students enrolled in public and private schools (kindergarten through twelfth grade), .5 percent (493 children) take the personal belief/religious exemption and .2 percent (197 students) take the medical exemption. Clearly 690 exempt and unvaccinated students representing about .7 percent of the school population is not viewed as a threat to public health.

All that is required to obtain the joint religious/philosophical exemption in Vermont, says O'Grady, is a written statement from the parent indicating that she has "a religious or moral conviction opposed to vaccination." The exemption is automatically granted. One needn't even specify the nature or details of the beliefs. Since Vermont has one of the highest vaccination rates (at 98.9 percent) in the country, the option of offering medical, religious, and philosophical exemptions for a tiny minority is a satisfactory compromise among conflicting demands, says O'Grady. "I would have to judge that most people in Vermont feel it is, too."

California also has the personal belief exemption, mandated in 1961 when polio vaccinations were made legally necessary for school admissions. Here a parent must file a letter with the school stating that vaccination is contrary to his or her beliefs, explains Lauren Dales, M.D., chief of the Immunization Unit, California State Department of Health Services in Berkeley.

However, the health officer has the option to "temporarily exclude" a child from school "during the incubation period" if the child is believed to have been exposed to an infectious disease and is still at risk for developing symptoms. Other than that, the California statute "doesn't leave any grounds for a parent's application not to be accepted," says Dales. In his ten years with the department, he's never heard of a complaint from parents.

In California, of 475,000 new pupils each year, about 3,000 take the philosophical/religious exemption and about 1,000 take the medical. "We don't have a problem with these exemptions," says Dales. "We obviously don't want to see disease outbreaks, but when the exemptions are coming in at the low level they are, we don't think they are epidemiologically critical." ...

WHO DECIDES?

The right of freedom of choice in vaccinations is clearly a difficult one to wrest from the hands of the medical establishment, as Barbara Fisher realizes after six years of strenuous effort.

"We haven't gotten anywhere near as far as we had wanted to. We have tried to be as credible as possible. We did our homework before we went out and criticized vaccines. We're dealing with a very powerful and wealthy pharmaceutical industry, with the government, health agencies, and organized medicine. That's a formidable force we're up against."

The exact nature of this "formidable force" may actually lie below the skin of the vaccination controversy and, as Fisher maintains, it may well touch at the "very heart of what is wrong with American medicine today."

The controversy really comes down to two diametrically opposite medical views. Plotkin of the A.A.P., for instance, does not recognize the right of a parent to subject a child to infectious disease. Anthroposophical physician Incao recognizes the necessity for a child to undergo the maturing struggles of early childhood infectious illnesses whereby "the higher self remodels the body in accordance with spiritual ideals."

This stark contrast raises important questions. Do we have the right to be sick anymore? Have we become overly afraid of being sick? Can illness be legislated out of existence, as something aberrant and unnatural?

The fundamental issue could also be seen as a question of one's rights: Does an individual have the right to oversee his/her own immune system (and his or her children's) and its interaction with the environment and the rest of society?

"We're so afraid of nature," says Incao. "What is the purpose of our life? If this purpose is to allow our individuality to unfold and express itself to the fullest, then this happens through the process of the immune system unfolding and reacting as self meets nonself. We become susceptible to infectious disease when we open ourselves to the world. Then we can become full human beings."

And for that voyage of discovery, concludes Incao, vaccinations are contraindicated.

RESOURCES

DPT (Dissatisfied Parents Together)
128 Branch Road
Vienna; VA 22180
(708) 938-DPT3

DPT: A Shot In the Dark, by Harris L. Coulter and Barbara Loe Fisher, Warner Books, 1985.

Dangers of Compulsory Immunization: How to Avoid Them Legally, by Tom Finn, Family Fitness Press (P.O. Box 1658, New Port Richey, FL 34291-1658), 1987.

Immunization: The Reality Behind the Myth, by Walene James.

POSTSCRIPT

Should All Children Be Immunized Against Childhood Diseases?

Currently, all 50 states require children to be vaccinated before enrolling in school. However, the safety of various vaccines, particularly the whooping cough (DPT) vaccine, continues to be the subject of debate. Although both the American Academy of Pediatrics and the U.S. Public Health Service continue to endorse the whooping cough vaccine, many parents and health providers feel that the risks are too high. Steven Black, codirector of the Kaiser-Permanente Pediatric Vaccine Study Center in Oakland, California, feels that the DPT vaccine is far from ideal. Newer vaccines, he believes, reduce the risks of injury by a significant percentage (see "The Perils of Pertussis," *American Health,* June 1991). Unlike the current DPT vaccine, which uses whole, killed bacteria cells to trigger the formation of antibodies, the new immunizations contain materials that produce immunity without as many side effects. The new vaccines, currently available in Japan but not yet in the United States, cause a significantly lower percentage of some side effects such as high fever and swelling, but whether or not they will reduce the incidence of brain damage is unclear.

Parents of young children are facing two crises relating to immunizations: First, widespread publicity about the genuine but extremely rare adverse effects of the whooping cough vaccine; and second, drug manufacturers' concerns about producing vaccines without protection from expensive lawsuits brought by parents of injured children. As a result, fewer companies are willing to produce vaccines. This, in turn, will lead to vaccine shortages and higher costs (which will be passed on to the consumer).

Vaccines other than the DPT vaccine are also thought to be harmful. A 1980 article in *Mutation Research* indicated that children who had smallpox vaccinations in Czechoslovakia showed harmful changes in their white blood cells. Also, in 1988 the British medical journal *Medical Hypothesis* reported a study of 200 patients with a chronic viral disease, Epstein-Barr syndrome. The article claimed that the disease was caused by a live rubella (German measles) virus that was found in a vaccine that was given to the patients.

The controversies surrounding vaccination continue. The medical community's endorsement of vaccination is evident in the following: "Declining Childhood Immunization Rates Becoming Cause for Concern," by J. W. Zylke, *Journal of the American Medical Association* (September 11, 1991); "Why Aren't We Protecting Our Children?" by A. Jurgrau, *RN* (November 1990); and

"Complying With Vaccine Law Will Help Prevent Errors," by M. R. Cohen, *Nursing* (August 1990). In *Immunization: The Reality Behind the Myth* (Bergin & Garvey, 1988), Walene James claims that immunization is not the answer to disease control. Barbara Fisher and Harris Coulter echo James in their book *DPT: A Shot in the Dark* (Warner Books, 1985).

ISSUE 20

Are Chiropractors Legitimate Health Providers?

YES: Rick Weiss, from "Bones of Contention," *Health* (July/August 1993)

NO: Editors of *Harvard Medical School Health Letter,* from "Low Back Pain: What About Chiropractors?" *Harvard Medical School Health Letter* (January 1988)

ISSUE SUMMARY

YES: Rick Weiss, a staff writer for *Health* magazine, reports on the benefits of chiropractic care and contends that patients with back pain who are treated by chiropractors are generally more satisfied with their treatment than those treated by medical doctors.

NO: The editors of the *Harvard Medical School Health Letter* argue that although some people may be helped by chiropractic treatment, many chiropractors adhere to a philosophy that is unproven at best and harmful at worst.

After nearly a century on the fringes of health care, chiropractic is seeking respectability; in some ways, it is gaining it. Chiropractic now ranks behind medicine and dentistry as the third largest primary health care profession in the Western world. Americans spend over $2 billion on chiropractic care each year, and over 30 hospitals in the United States have chiropractors on staff. And spinal manipulation, the primary therapy practiced by chiropractors, has achieved some recognition as a valid treatment for back pain.

The field of chiropractic was begun in 1895 by D. D. Palmer, a "magnetic healer" and tradesman living in Davenport, Iowa. Palmer allegedly cured a janitor's deafness by pressing on one of the man's spinal vertebrae. Palmer believed that misalignment of the spine, which he called "subluxations," could cause virtually all human diseases. He theorized that when these subluxations irritate the spinal nerves—which exit the spinal cord through openings between the vertebrae and branch off to the body's limbs and organs—diseases and pain would develop. According to Palmer, pressure from nerve irritation could be relieved, and health could be restored, by manipulating the appropriate vertebrae. This manipulation is the basic spinal adjustment practiced by all chiropractors.

Today, few chiropractors—who must attend at least two years of undergraduate school and four years of chiropractic college before they can be licensed by national and state boards—still believe in Palmer's view that subluxations cause nearly all health problems. However, most acknowledge that disease is caused by both infectious agents, such as bacteria and viruses, and health behaviors, such as sedentary lifestyles and smoking. Despite these modern beliefs and in accord with Palmer's original theory, chiropractic has remained preoccupied with the spine as the primary factor in health and disease. Chiropractors still subscribe to the theory that misaligned vertebrae impair the nervous system, causing a lowering of the body's defenses and resulting in disease. Good health, they believe, requires that vertebrae be kept in proper alignment, which is achieved only through spinal manipulation.

Spinal manipulation has been used for thousands of years to treat back pain, but there are conflicting opinions on whether or not it really works. Scientists who have evaluated the effects of chiropractic have concluded that spinal manipulation is probably helpful for some patients with back pain, specifically when the pain has been present for three weeks or less and so long as there are no tumors, fractures, or other abnormalities. For other types of back pain, medical experts are divided.

Because of the lack of definitive scientific evidence, and because chiropractic is strongly identified with spinal manipulation, traditional medicine has, overall, been suspicious of chiropractic and has not considered it to be a legitimate medical treatment. Until 1980 the American Medical Association (AMA) considered it to be unethical for a doctor to refer a patient to a chiropractor; any doctor who did so risked losing his or her membership in the AMA. Although the AMA dropped this position in 1980, many doctors still refuse to refer patients to chiropractors.

Nevertheless, chiropractors are licensed to practice in the United States, and their services are covered by workers' compensation in all 50 states. Most states also cover chiropractic care under Medicaid and partially under Medicare, although private insurance coverage varies by state. Some chiropractors have also been recruited by some health maintenance organizations (HMOs), while others have gained admitting privileges at about 100 hospitals around the country. But overall, chiropractors have remained separate from traditional medical practices.

In the following selections, journalist Rick Weiss argues that there is a benefit to chiropractic care and that it is a cost-effective, beneficial therapy for certain back pain sufferers. The editors of the *Harvard Medical School Health Letter*, representing traditional medicine, acknowledge that some people may be helped by chiropractic treatment, but they maintain that many chiropractors adhere to a philosophy that could be harmful.

YES   Rick Weiss

BONES OF CONTENTION

Sid Williams is a big man, a former Georgia Tech defensive end, who looks appropriately messianic for someone claiming to know the supreme secret to good health. His brilliant white hair sweeps back in electrifying waves, dark eyes peer out from beneath a thick, bony brow, and he rails with the passion of a Southern preacher. "I'll tell you one thing," he booms in a thick Georgia accent, sitting barefoot on the porch of his vacation home on Florida's Gulf coast. "You're not talking to a quack-charlatan-cultist."

He bristles, because he's been called all these things, and much worse, during his 40-year career as a chiropractor. Then he shrugs and laughs, intoxicated with the knowledge that the tide of public opinion has begun to turn in his favor.

As president and founder of Life College in Marietta, Georgia—the country's largest chiropractic college—and chairman of the 6,000-member International Chiropractors Association, Williams has suffered the slings of mockery and criticism through many of his profession's most difficult years. "It got to the point where if nobody was giving us a hard time, we'd start to think something was wrong," he says. But lately he and his 50,000 colleagues have begun to savor the pleasures of respect from an ever widening circle of supporters.

Chiropractors today make up this country's third largest medical profession (after physicians and dentists) and are licensed to practice without supervision or referral from medical doctors in every state. Hospitals are increasingly adding chiropractors to their medical staffs, and their spine-crunching services are widely reimbursed by Medicare, Medicaid, workers' compensation, and private insurance.

Most important, chiropractors have attracted a huge following of dedicated patients. Some 15 to 20 million Americans visited a chiropractor last year, the majority of them for treatment of low-back pain. Many return for treatments week after week, seemingly addicted to the trademark laying on of hands known as a chiropractic adjustment.

At first glance it seems that they've made a smart choice. Several studies in the past two decades have hinted that chiropractors have something important to offer, especially when it comes to low-back pain. The largest and most impressive single study, published in 1990, found that patients with chronic low-back pain treated at chiropractic clinics ended up with less pain and more mobility than those treated in hospitals. Chiropractors also point to another big study, published in 1991, which concluded that people with acute low-back pain not caused by neurological complications could significantly boost their odds of recovering within three weeks by getting spinal manipulation.

Chiropractors are apparently economical, too. Workers' compensation costs for a back-pain patient seeing a chiropractor are about one-tenth those for a patient treated by a medical doctor. That's no small matter, given how common backaches are. Seventy to 80 percent of adults are affected by back pain at some point in their lives, and it is second only to childbirth as the most common reason for hospitalization in the United States. And although nearly 90 percent of backaches disappear on their own within six weeks, the human and monetary costs are enormous. Back pain causes millions of missed workdays every year, at a cost of billions of dollars in compensation claims and lost productivity.

"The insurance companies love chiropractors because for occupational injuries and low-back pain they get their patients back to work sooner," says Norman Gevitz, a medical historian at the University of Illinois at Chicago.

But despite chiropractors' growing popularity with patients and insurers, there are reasons to think twice before surrendering your body to a chiropractor's care. For one thing, astonishingly little is known about what a chiropractic adjustment really is, what effects it has on the body, and what ailments it might exacerbate or cure. Even the seemingly

positive findings from the big back-pain studies in 1990 and 1991 are less compelling than some chiropractors care to admit. In fact, neither study clearly differentiated between the techniques used by chiropractors and those used by other specialists, like physical therapists, leaving unresolved the question of whether chiropractors have anything truly unique to offer.

For ailments other than back pain, there is even less documentation for the benefits of chiropractic. (The word *chiropractic* may sound odd by itself, but that's the correct term.) Chiropractors are bursting with anecdotal reports of cures for asthma, headaches, hair loss, even blindness. But their reliance on individual testimonials rather than controlled clinical trials leaves chiropractors vulnerable to the criticism that these patients could just as easily have recovered on their own.

Perhaps most disturbing, no research has ever substantiated the chiropractic theory of disease, which belittles the importance of infectious agents and posits instead that a vaguely defined spinal defect, called a subluxation, underlies virtually every medical disorder from diabetes to cancer.

Chiropractors describe subluxations as kinks in the spine that pinch one or more nerves, interfering with the body's ability to stay well. Intuitively, the idea makes some sense. Nerves do, after all, serve as conduits throughout the body. And their ability to transmit messages can indeed be affected by injuries to the spine, causing nerve and muscle symptoms like shooting pains, numbness, or paralysis.

But there is absolutely no proof that subluxations can cause organ failure or immune dysfunction, as chiropractors traditionally claim. Or that common back pain can be caused by a subluxation.

Indeed, there is no proof that subluxations exist at all, much less that their "adjustment," whatever that might be, improves nerve transmission and enhances health. Subluxations don't show up on X rays, for instance. Yet chiropractors persist in making widespread use of X rays in a futile search for these phantom flaws, despite increasing concern about the cancer-causing potential of radiation.

"The big question is, What is the scientific evidence for chiropractic?" says Gevitz. "Research is increasing, but there is still very little evidence to support any of what they do."

* * *

Criticisms like these only inflame Williams, known to colleagues as Dr. Sid. In his winter home on St. Armands Key, an exclusive island reached by a causeway from Sarasota, Dr. Sid talks of having cured not only countless injured backs but all manner of maladies from diabetes to baldness.

"I've had people come in and get adjusted, and later they found they could see better than before," he declares, waving a hand through the humid Florida air. "They ask, 'Doctor, did you do anything to my eyes?' And I say, 'Of course I did. I turned the power on in your *whole body,* and aren't your eyes part of your body?'"

He shakes his head as if in disbelief that anybody could fail to see the significance of what he's saying. "What are medical doctors doing? Giving chiropractors their cricks, backaches, and strains. We do something for everything," he says. "Rigor mortis is the only thing that we can't help!"

But Dr. Sid ought to know why medical doctors have been wary of chiropractors' extravagant claims and why his pro-

fession is still vulnerable to charges of cultism. He more than anyone in the field has dedicated his life to preserving chiropractic's unorthodox past. He's even turned the house next door into a colorful shrine—a sort of Graceland of Chiropractic—in memory of Bartlett Joshua (B.J.) Palmer, the man responsible for developing chiropractic into the widely recognized specialty it is today.

Palmer, whose father founded chiropractic almost a century ago, spent his winters in that one-story beach house until his death in 1961. Life College and Dr. Sid bought the house in 1979 and filled it with precious artifacts from B.J.'s life. Here is preserved B.J.'s original chiropractic adjustment table, with the telltale hole cut into the maroon padded headrest to accommodate a patient's nose and mouth while lying face down. Here on walls painted red, orange, blue, yellow, and green hang photographs of B.J. standing with his close friend John Ringling, who overwintered his famous circus in Sarasota and persuaded B.J. to buy property there. And here are some racy pieces of buxom female statuary, suggesting that the chiropractic guru's interest in anatomy wasn't entirely dorsal.

B.J. was a teenager living in Davenport, Iowa, when his father, a bearded fishmonger and self-taught healer named D. D. Palmer, performed what seemed like a medical miracle. The patient was a janitor named Harvey Lillard, and he had been deaf since injuring his back 17 years earlier. On September 18, 1895, acting on a hunch, the elder Palmer delivered a sharp blow to Lillard's back, instantly restoring the man's hearing.

From Lillard's recovery Palmer hypothesized that the brain is essentially a dynamo, or battery, that distributes a healing energy to organs via the nerves

in the spine. He called that energy Innate Intelligence and reckoned that when
nerves become pinched by a misalignment of the spine—what he called a subluxation—then the organs fed by those
nerves lose their vigor. He speculated that
subluxations might arise at the moment
of birth from the harrowing trip down the
birth canal, from childhood injuries, or
from work-related postural stresses later
in life. Whatever their cause, the result
would be illness or, as Palmer put it, "disease."

Palmer termed his newfound specialty
"chiropractic" (from the Greek *cheir*,
"hand," and *praxis*, "practice"), and soon
his son B.J. took to spreading the bone-
jarring gospel that virtually every ailment is but a subluxation in need of adjustment. A natural-born salesman, B.J.
gave dramatic lectures about the benefits of chiropractic and started a network of chiropractic colleges. During the
1930s he frequently sang the praises of
chiropractic on his Davenport radio station, WOC ("Wonders of Chiropractic"),
in the evenings after a sportscaster named
Ronald Reagan gave the latest scores.

B.J. enjoyed his role as a medical
heretic. An incorrigible punster, he would
quip to physicians: "My analysis is better
than urinalysis." He summarized the difference between doctors of chiropractic
(D.C.s) and medical doctors (M.D.s) with
the equations "D.C. equals disease con-
quered; M.D. equals more dope—more
death."

The American Medical Association
[AMA] was not amused. It told physicians in the 1960s that it was unethical
to associate professionally with the "cult
of chiropractic." And in 1963 it formed a
Committee on Quackery, whose primary
goal was to drive chiropractors out of
business.

Chiropractors fought back. In 1976 they
filed an antitrust suit against the AMA,
charging it with conspiracy to monop-
olize medicine. And in September 1987,
almost 92 years to the day after Harvey
Lillard got his back popped, chiropractors won a stunning victory: Although
limited to practicing only their own form
of medicine-spinal manipulation without
drugs or surgery-they gained the legal
right to work alongside physicians in hospitals and to practice without referrals
from M.D.s.

B.J. didn't live to see that beachhead
reached. Neither did he live to hear
the skeptics maintain that today's cash-
strapped hospitals appreciate chiropractors primarily for their ability to attract
new patients. Or that doctors' growing
acceptance of chiropractors boils down
to relief that somebody else is willing to
take their back-pain patients, with whom
they've never had much success.

But if B.J. missed his chance to spar
with these skeptics, he's been well
represented by Dr. Sid, who keeps B.J.'s
spirit alive with a peculiar passion. Dr.
Sid talks, dresses, and wears his hair like
B.J. did. He drives a white and yellow
Cadillac like B.J. did. He even engraved
his initials in the driveway of his home as
B.J. did in the driveway next door.

Recently Dr. Sid went so far as to
surround the Palmer house and his own
with a stately wrought iron fence set in
white concrete stanchions. With its 60-
foot flagpole, the two-home site looks
like a diplomatic complex. "I call it the
B.J. Palmer–Sid E. Williams Chiropractic
Embassy Compound," he says. "The
chiropractic language is spoken here."

But as Dr. Sid well knows, chiropractors are hardly unified under a single
flag or even a single language. Rather,
chiropractors have for decades been em-

broiled in a civil war. On one side are Dr. Sid and his fellow "straight" chiropractors, who see themselves as the pure conscience of chiropractic tradition. Firmly believing that most illnesses can be traced to subluxations, they reject most drugs and surgery in favor of spinal manipulation. Although straights account for only about 15 percent of all chiropractors, straight chiropractic colleges graduate hundreds more every year, and they promise to remain a potent political force within the profession.

On the other side are so-called "mixers," who favor blending the principles of chiropractic with those of other healing arts, ranging from herbalism to modern medicine, with the goal of using what works best. These chiropractors tend to focus on the treatment of musculoskeletal disorders, such as back and neck problems. They advocate less reliance on chiropractic tradition and more on peer-reviewed clinical trials, arguing that chiropractors must get themselves onto firmer scientific footing or risk losing the modicum of credibility they have garnered so far.

Standing tall beneath the ceiling fans of his living room, Dr. Sid expresses little patience for those chiropractors who would, in his terms, sell out to mainstream medicine. "Why don't these guys just become medical doctors?" he asks.

Of course, he adds, medical doctors will be sorry come the chiropractic Armageddon. "Let's suppose the world realizes that subluxations are really the problem," Dr. Sid says. "The first thing you notice, you need fewer drugs, less surgery, fewer hospitals. This must really frighten medical doctors, but they're going to have to swallow their cud on this one. Who would have thought the Berlin wall would come down? Or that communism would end?" he asks, pacing between overstuffed chairs. "Well, medicine will be recognized as a failed theory, too. These medical doctors think they're supermen, jumping off tall buildings. But they're going to hit the cement. Hard."

A warm glow rises in his cheeks, and for a moment he looks almost beatific. "I'm in love with chiropractic," he says. "You fix somebody with an adjustment and see them walk away so happy. What's the explanation? A preacher says, 'It's an act of God!' A medical doctor says, 'It's a physiological impossibility!' But the chiropractor says, 'Hell, it's an everyday occurrence.'"

* * *

A couple of thousand miles north of Sarasota, it's a bitter winter day in Lombard, Illinois, home of the National Chiropractic College. In a room furnished only with an adjustment table and a chair, Carol DeFranca asks her chiropractor for relief.

DeFranca has a bad cold. Her head is congested. Her limbs ache. The muscles of her diaphragm and neck are sore from days of coughing and sneezing.

Scott Chapman, a handsome young chiropractor wearing a sharply pressed white shirt and silk tie, stands behind his patient while she sits on the padded table. His right hand steadies her forehead while the left gently massages the back of her neck. His voice is confident and soothing. "These muscles are working overtime," he says.

Chapman has DeFranca lie face down on the padded table, opens the back of her hospital gown, and with strong fingers familiarizes himself with the subtle terrain of her back and neck. He pounds with his fist on the back of his own hand as it rests on her backbone, and works her ribs like flexible levers to manipulate her spine. The idea, he says, is to discover spinal misalignments or strained joints, then apply just the right amount of force in the right spot to put the body back in balance.

In a decisive moment, he cups his hands together, rests them precisely on a couple of vertebrae in the middle of her back, leans precipitously over her, and with a short, sharp pump—and a resounding crunch—performs the first of several "high-velocity thrust" adjustments. "Mmmmmph," DeFranca says, with apparent relief.

"Am I attacking the virus directly?" Chapman asks rhetorically while positioning himself for the next maneuver. "No," he answers himself, clearing a few errant tresses from DeFranca's shoulder. "Am boosting her immune system? Maybe. There have been some preliminary studies suggesting that adjustments may actually influence immune function. But my main goal is to relieve the musculoskeletal components of her illness, those aches and pains that are secondary to having a cold or flu."

The remaining adjustments follow in short order. Using one hand to stabilize DeFranca's head, Chapman reaches around to the side of her neck, pauses, and lets loose with a powerful but apparently precise shove. The telltale crunch reverberates throughout the room. After another adjustment DeFranca sits upright, her face flushed and vibrant, and says she's still congested but feels a lot better.

Having stood by silently throughout this treatment, John Triano, director of National College's ergonomic and joint laboratory, now speaks up from one side of the room. As a chiropractor with a master's degree in neurophysiology, Triano is a leader in the nascent effort to get chiropractic free of its fundamentalist past and into the scientific fold. In his view, people like Dr. Sid do the profession more harm than good.

"Some chiropractors are so insecure in what they do, even the notion of doing research frightens them," Triano says. "These people revere heritage so much that they confuse it with truth."

Triano takes nothing for granted. He's among a new breed of chiropractors who commit the ultimate blasphemy of suggesting that subluxations may not exist. He has looked at thousands of spinal X rays and knows how good they are at revealing all kinds of damage. Has he ever seen a subluxation? He pauses. "With my eyes closed," he replies with a smile.

Looking casually professorial, with his neatly trimmed beard, brown suede jacket, and cowboy boots telling of his years of training in Colorado, Triano makes his way down a corridor in the clinic and reflects on DeFranca's adjustment. "The thing that sets chiropractic apart from physical therapy and massage is the high-velocity thrust you've just seen," he says. "And until a few years ago there was zero information on what that thrust really is; what forces are involved and how they affect the spine."

Recently, Triano says, he took it upon himself to gather that information. In the ergonomics laboratory at National College, Triano constructed what looks like the Adjustment Table From Hell. The table is wired with more than $100,000 worth of high-tech apparatus: force detectors that measure the amount of pressure being applied in any direction; high-resolution infrared cameras to track how much a person's body moves when it absorbs a chiropractic thrust; and a device that measures electrical activity and contractions in a patient's muscles before, during, and after an adjustment.

"The day we first tested the system, it took us four and a half hours to measure something that lasted only zero point one two five seconds," Triano says. "That's how long the thrust lasts. One hundred and twenty-five thousandths of a second, then it's over."

Triano found that a typical chiropractic thrust peaks at about 200 pounds of force or the equivalent of having a baby elephant sitting (very briefly) on your spine. Neck adjustments are in the range of ten to 30 pounds. The infrared cameras revealed, among other things, that the head moves more during a neck adjustment than had been suspected, suggesting that chiropractors ought to hold it more firmly to add precision to this common maneuver.

Experiments like these are time consuming and expensive, but Triano is convinced that chiropractors have little hope of proving the efficacy of what they do without defining how an adjustment actually affects the spine. He hopes that by coming to understand the precise nature of an adjustment, chiropractors may be able to work backward and figure out exactly what it is in their patients' backs that they are actually fixing.

To resolve that question would be no mean feat. The human spine is an extraordinarily complex structure composed of 33 individual bony units, or vertebrae, stacked upon one another like a column of lined up napkin rings, most of them separated from each other by disks of shock-absorbing cartilage and a lubricating joint fluid. (Nobody knows for sure what causes the popping noise of-

ten heard during an adjustment, but some researchers propose that it may be the sound of tiny gas bubbles exploding as the fluid-filled joint space suddenly expands, much the way a champagne bottle pops when its cork is pulled out.)

Encased within this hollow stack of vertebrae are hundreds of nerve fibers that transmit information between the brain and various organs and limbs. They exit in pairs at regular intervals through tiny openings between vertebrae, wending their way through the many muscles and ligaments that help support the spine.

There are hundreds of things that can go wrong with all these moving parts: The muscles supporting the spine can become strained; the ligaments that bind muscle to bone can get stretched or torn; the joints of the vertebrae can wear away; and the cushiony disks between vertebrae can dry out, ooze fluid, and even rupture, pressing against nerves and causing pain.

Most people, however, won't ever find out what's causing their back pain—even if they visit an orthopedist, a physician trained in musculoskeletal disorders. That's because spines vary from person to person, and even if an X ray or other test detects an abnormality in a spine or disk, there's no guarantee that the apparent anomaly is what's causing the pain.

Given such vagaries, perhaps it's not surprising that millions of people seem unbothered by chiropractors' inability to explain exactly why or how their treatments work. But it does bother Triano, and he believes that it's only a matter of time before answers emerge.

"The state of chiropractic today is comparable to our understanding of diabetes in the 1930s," Triano says. "Back then we knew there was a disease called diabetes, and that people who have it sweat a lot, urinate a lot, and have to make changes in their diet or they might die. But we didn't know what was wrong with them. That's where we're at with chiropractic. We know what patients look like, we know they benefit from adjustments, but we still don't have a good grasp of what's really going on.

"The difference between people like Sid Williams and myself is in our willingness to accept that we don't know what is going on," Triano says. "People like Sid Williams believe they have the answer, that subluxations are the root of all evil. But there's no evidence that their belief system is true. In fact, there *is* evidence that the main tenets of chiropractic are *not* true. But so what? This is how science works. I'm convinced that some of what I do is helpful for my patients, and I am convinced that with more research I'll be able to help even more."

* * *

Triano is not the only one who's convinced. Surveys indicate that back-pain patients who go to chiropractors are more satisfied with their care than are those who go to medical doctors. But might these patients benefit just as much from a physical therapist or an inexpert massage from a friend? If chiropractors really have something unique to offer, why have they had such a difficult time gathering the kind of scientific proof that might persuade the unconverted?

Convincing studies *are* hard to design. Even the best single study to date—the one that compared back-pain patients who went to chiropractic clinics to those who went to hospitals—didn't look at how the treatments performed by chiropractors differed from those performed by hospital personnel.

In that study, patients who went to the hospital were treated mostly by physical therapists, who typically use less force than chiropractors do, pushing on the spine and limbs to stretch and strengthen muscles and increase range of motion. But some physical therapists also use high-velocity techniques that resemble chiropractic maneuvers, and some of what chiropractors do resembles physical therapy. So it's possible factors other than manipulative technique contributed to the quicker recoveries in chiropractic patients.

"This is an important distinction," says Paul Shekelle, a physician and expert in chiropractic at RAND, a research organization in Santa Monica, California. Chiropractic does seem to help a lot of people with back pain, he says, but lots of things might be influencing their rate of recovery. "Maybe chiropractors are better psychiatrists or offer better positive reinforcement."

This is a disturbing concept for chiropractors, who have worked hard to usher their profession to the gates of scientific validation and who see themselves primarily as skillful manipulators of the body, not ministers of the psyche. But it's worth considering whether the key to chiropractic's popular success might indeed be something outside the purview of standard scientific research.

"Chiropractic's paradigm is different from that used by medicine, and in some ways harder to study," says Walter Wardwell, a professor emeritus in sociology at the University of Connecticut who has made a lifelong study of the profession. "Chiropractic isn't interested so much in the germs in the environment as in the body's ability to cure itself." And nobody,

Wardwell says, not even the best medical doctor, really understands the nature of healing.

The questions are timeless: How does the body pull itself together after injury? Can the mind help or hinder that process? What is the role of a healer? And most relevant, what are the health benefits of physical contact—of plain and simple touch?

"An M.D. will give a pill, a prescription, but no tactile contact," medical historian Gevitz says. "Chiropractors feel around. They have a nice tactile sense, and patients feel relieved. Sometimes you hear this pop, and that can be a wonderful placebo."

He uses the word without apparent judgment. Because the funny thing about placebos, inactive as they supposedly are, is that they work. People get better, even if nobody understands why.

Besides, Shekelle adds, even standard medicine isn't as scientific as many would believe. He notes that U.S. surgeons have in the past 30 years performed hundreds of thousands of carotid endarterectomies—surgical procedures that ream out people's clogged carotid arteries—in the untested belief that the procedure might help prevent strokes. "There's a lot going on in medicine that is just as unproven as chiropractic," Shekelle says.

Add to that chiropractic's excellent safety record (only a handful of serious injuries have ever been reported out of many millions of adjustments), and the question of whether chiropractors have enough science on their side starts to take on a somewhat hollow ring. After all, people don't need a scientist to tell them when they feel better. And for most of life's various aches and pains—especially those that have no apparent cause and

that medical doctors admit they can do little about—isn't relief all anybody really cares about?

* * *

Back on St. Armands Key, Dr. Sid relaxes on his porch to the sound of palm fronds clicking overhead. In calm moments like these, it's easy to be lulled by his unfailing self-confidence and by his pointed critiques of standard medical care. Anybody who has been to a medical doctor, especially for back pain, knows how unsatisfactory such a visit can be. By contrast, imagine a half hour on the table under Dr. Sid's big, strong hands. Who wouldn't feel better?

Well, lots of people. People with infections. People with tumors. And probably a lot of people with back problems, who might benefit more from anti-inflammatory drugs, muscle relaxants, or exercise regimens. The problem is that many everyday ailments, including most backaches, vary so much from person to person that it's difficult to know what kind of therapy will work best. For garden variety back pain, chiropractors do seem to have as good a shot as anyone at speeding recovery. But for many ailments chiropractic will be of no benefit at all, and in some cases it may even exacerbate the problem. The bottom line: Find a chiropractor who is willing to call it quits when adjustments aren't helping and has the wisdom to refer patients to a physician when appropriate.

Many chiropractors are working toward codifying that kind of assurance. At a ground-breaking conference held in California last year, 35 chiropractors from all over the country drafted preliminary guidelines that would define, for the first time, those ailments for which chiropractic is probably useful and those for which medical attention may be preferable. The conference marked the culmination of three years of discussions within the profession, and most of the nation's chiropractors have welcomed the resulting document—especially since the federal government may soon require similar assessments of efficacy before approving reimbursement through Medicaid and Medicare.

But Dr. Sid and his followers are vehement in their opposition to those guidelines, claiming the rules will only get in the way of their simple, 100-year-old mission: to find the hidden glitch in each patient's spine and fix it.

"Don't say I'm against research," Dr. Sid says. "But a damned fish peddler figured this out! That's the problem: This thing is so simple, but everybody tries to make it so complicated."

NO

Editors of *Harvard Medical
School Health Letter*

LOW BACK PAIN: WHAT ABOUT CHIROPRACTORS?

About one out of every five backs that pass you on the street is causing its owner some distress. Sooner or later almost everybody becomes acquainted with low back pain. Fortunately, painful backs tend to get better by themselves. About two-thirds of cases of low back pain improve within 30 days —regardless of the treatment they do or don't receive. That may seem too long, though, to someone who has to work or wants to play. Rather than wait it out, many people go in search of help. The specialists they turn to most often are orthopedic surgeons; next most commonly they go to chiropractors. Lots of other practitioners are available to treat back pain: internists, neurologists, family physicians, physiatrists, osteopaths, acupuncturists, physical therapists, massage therapists. Why is it that chiropractors get so much of the "back business"?

Two reasons come to mind. The first, which everyone would agree on, is that nobody else is all that effective with low back pain. The second, which is less certain, is that chiropractors have something special to offer their patients.

FACTIONS AND PHILOSOPHY

The field of chiropractic was invented in 1895 by an Iowa grocer, D. D. Palmer. Palmer's notion was that the central nervous system controls all the body's functions—principally through the nerves that come out of the spinal cord. Each of these nerves must pass through a small aperture between two vertebrae. If two vertebrae were improperly aligned, Palmer reasoned, a nerve could become pinched. The nerve would then tend to misfire, and the part of the body served by it would not function well. If this situation persisted, or became severe, illness would result. Palmer wasn't much impressed by the idea that germs, for example, cause illness. He preferred to think that all symptoms were expressions, one way or another, of malfunctioning nerves. Nerves could be made to work better if they were relieved of pressure caused by slight dislocations of vertebrae (termed "subluxations"). Thus, in his view, adjusting the spine was the best possible treatment for all kinds of illness.

Some of the principles underlying chiropractic practice are philosophical or spiritual—not the sort of statements that can be proved or disproved by scientific methods. The basic ideas about subluxations and pinched nerves can be scientifically studied, though. And there's every reason to believe that this body of chiropractic lore is simply wrong. It has been shown that many organs of the body work well enough even if their nerve supply is cut off completely. And subluxations are not abnormal; every spine has slight "misalignments." Nerves are rarely pinched or damaged as a result of these variations of normal anatomy, and specific physical symptoms are not usually associated with irregularities in a particular area of the spine.

One group of chiropractors—known as the "straights"—has continued in the tradition established by Palmer. Identified with the International Chiropractors' Association, this faction continues to see pinched nerves as a cause of dizziness, eye and ear problems, high blood pressure, glandular troubles, skin disorders, hay fever, congestion, low blood pressure, rheumatism, impotence, knee pains, bed wetting, hemorrhoids, and ankle swelling—to name but a few of the conditions that they imply will be relieved by spinal adjustment. (State and federal laws limit how explicit chiropractors can be in stating such claims.)

The majority of chiropractors in the United States, however, are "mixers" and are more likely to be members of the American Chiropractors' Association. They share a general philosophy derived from Palmer: that illness results from a kind of disharmony in the body, a failure of the natural drive to health. But mixers don't make spinal manipulation the end-all and be-all of their practice. Mixers may attempt to treat their patients by modifying diet, giving vitamin supplements, or offering counseling and education. However, by law and as an aspect of their philosophy, chiropractors do not use medical treatments, such as prescription drugs or surgery. Virtually all chiropractors do take x-rays (occasionally a great many x-rays) to examine the spine.

Finally, there is the National Association for Chiropractic Medicine, which is a minority voice in the field. According to its president, the NACM is "an organization that was formed specifically to reject and renounce the untenable historical chiropractic theory." Chiropractors associated with the NACM limit their practice to treating joint conditions that may be relieved by mobilization or manipulation, and they advocate basing chiropractic practice on research that meets accepted scientific standards. This group is seeking to become more closely allied with regular medicine in a cooperative relationship.

MANIPULATION AND BACK PAIN

If you ask whether chiropractic treatment of low back pain works for some people some of the time, the answer is yes. So do all types of therapy, including placebo treatments against which potentially more effective treatments are often tested. Nevertheless, studies suggest that chiropractic adjustments provide more immediate reduction of pain than placebo treatments, and they often appear to produce speedier improvement than standard medical approaches.

Few well-conducted trials have compared chiropractic to other forms of therapy. But, although neither plentiful nor perfect, some studies of chiropractic approaches to low back pain have been carried out. Manipulation is the best studied.

Manipulation is a hands-on therapy that is not well standardized. The term may be applied differently in different settings. Chiropractors often use the term "spinal adjustment" for their procedure. In any case, the patient with low back pain is often placed on his or her side while the practitioner grasps the uppermost shoulder and a hip or bent knee for leverage. The shoulder and pelvis are then pressed in opposite directions, so as to rotate the torso. This maneuver sometimes produces a cracking sound that seems to emanate from the spine. This sound has been attributed to the sudden release of gases dissolved in the joint fluid; it may signal what is probably a temporary change in the relative positions of some vertebrae. Skilled practitioners seem able to apply pressure to, and "crack," a single intervertebral joint.

Trials conducted under varying conditions and using practitioners with various kinds of background have demonstrated that manipulation is indeed better than nothing at relieving back pain for a short while. An acute episode of back pain in someone who does not have a long history of the problem seems most responsive to this form of treatment. After a few weeks, though, manipulated backs appear to be no better or worse off than backs that have been left to their own devices. It is, thus, unlikely that chiropractic treatment is making some fundamental or "curative" change in the spine. There is less support for the use of manipulation to treat established, chronic low back pain, although some sufferers do experience transient relief from manipulation.

One quite well-designed study of manipulation used massage as the control therapy in order to test the possibility that personal touch is more important than the specific technique. The therapists in this study were both chiropractors and physicians trained in manipulation or massage. The subjects, who had never before undergone manipulation, were unable to guess accurately which treatment they had been given, and thus their prejudices presumably did not affect their perception of relief obtained by one treatment or the other. The efficacy of therapy was evaluated both by asking patients whether they felt better and by testing to see whether they had gained flexibility. By both criteria, manipulation reduced pain immediately after treatment more effectively than massage. Six to seven weeks later, however, neither group was significantly more free of pain than the other.

The outcome of this study is, on the whole, typical. When compared with other nonsurgical treatments, such as anti-inflammatory drugs, pain killers, heat treatments, and so forth, manipulation often appears to have a short-term advantage but loses its edge in the long run. None of the trials has been perfect, so there is plenty of opportunity for debate and difference of opinion (and for taking refuge in claims of "clinical experience").

WHY THE CONFUSION?

Studies of manipulation for back pain are not very satisfactory, but neither are studies of many other treatments. The hurdles to designing and executing good

NO Editors of *Harvard Medical School Health Letter* / 363

research on pain of any kind are many and large.

To take just one example, it can be very difficult to test alternative treatments on comparable groups of subjects. British researchers sought to compare patients reporting to a chiropractic clinic with others who went to a hospital clinic. Half of each group was to be referred to the other treatment center, but over a third of the chiropractic patients refused to enter the study for fear that they would be sent to a hospital for conventional treatment, whereas only 6 percent of the hospital patients refused to have chiropractic manipulation. Likewise, keeping subjects "blind" to the therapy they are receiving (as was achieved in the study of manipulation versus massage) often is not feasible.

A real possibility, suggested by the trials of manipulation, is that the treatment works well for some people with low back pain and poorly for others. The problem is to know in advance which will be which.

PROS AND CONS OF CHIROPRACTORS

Manipulation is not the exclusive "property" of chiropractors. Doctors of osteopathy, who have training quite similar to that of medical doctors, apply a form of manipulation, as well as prescribing drugs and performing surgery. Some other health professionals outside chiropractic are also trained in manipulation. But the majority of experienced practitioners are chiropractors. New York Chiropractic College, to give an example, allots 15% of its students' classroom time to courses in technique, including manipulation. The curriculum, which continues for 10 trimesters, also includes courses in

anatomy, physiology, biochemistry, microbiology, and pathology. Practical experience in internships consumes another 20% of the students' time. Manipulation then becomes a significant component of the chiropractor's daily work.

Chiropractors emphasize that their approach to treating disease is "drugless" and "natural." These may or may not be virtues, depending on the condition that is being treated. But a consequence is that chiropractors spend a lot of time in developing a relationship with their patients and often see their patients with considerable frequency. If a warm and supportive association is developed, a sense of well-being may be promoted in nonspecific but nonetheless important ways.

In treating back pain, chiropractors often stress education about the back and its care. This may appeal to patients and, if well done, is very helpful. On the other hand, many chiropractors adhere to a philosophy of disease and treatment that at best is unproven and at worst is wrong. To the extent that a chiropractor encourages patients to avoid effective treatment, he or she is doing them a disservice. But chiropractic and regular medicine do not appear, in practice, to be mutually exclusive. A Canadian survey found that 97% of chiropractors refer patients to physicians for care and that 84% also had patients referred from physicians. It appears that patients generally use chiropractic care in addition to, not instead of, regular medical care. Chiropractors are licensed to practice in most states, though state licensing laws vary in the scope they grant to chiropractors.

Whatever the realities of referral back and forth between chiropractors and physicians, the American Medical Association has called chiropractors "unscientific cultists," has resisted licensing of chiropractors, and has opposed any professional interaction between them and physicians. As of last August, however, this policy was found by a Federal district judge to violate antitrust legislation.

In 1968 the Department of Health, Education, and Welfare recommended that chiropractic not be included in the Medicare program. A law passed 4 years later allowed some chiropractic services to be covered. The policies of private insurance companies may extend coverage to chiropractic treatment, but there is considerable variability, and most seem to be quite restrictive with respect to the conditions they cover.

A patient need not accept Palmer's views of disease and health to accept manipulation as a potential avenue to relatively rapid relief of low back pain. On the other hand, anyone willing to wait it out is likely to find that there is no need to seek intervention at all.

As a rule of thumb, it seems fair to say that if manipulation is going to help, the benefit should be evident after no more than half a dozen treatments. Repeated manipulations over a prolonged period without significant improvement are seldom worthwhile. Spinal disorders are not the only causes of back pain. Manipulation therapy without a proper diagnostic work-up (not just x-rays) is ill-advised and may even be disastrous for patients whose back pain is due to abdominal disease, osteoporosis, cancer, or other metabolic diseases.

POSTSCRIPT

Are Chiropractors Legitimate Health Providers?

Currently, 1 in 20 Americans visit a chiropractor each year. These visits, generally speaking, are not enthusiastically endorsed by traditional physicians. Chiropractic has not yet become mainstream despite the large number of people who use this service. The reasons, chiropractors claim, is that spinal manipulation is more an art than a science.

Gerald Leisman, a neurologist (not a chiropractor), claims that the process of subluxations is deductive, not scientific, as are most methods of determining an unknown cause of pain. Leisman believes that for most back pain sufferers, there *is* no scientific way to establish a specific diagnosis, since back pain often does not show up on an X ray or produce abnormal blood or fluid values. This lack of scientific evidence in chiropractic, he maintains, does not negate the benefits of spinal manipulation.

Scientific research into the benefits of chiropractic care is still limited. The National Institutes of Health and the National Science Foundation, both primary funding sources for research in medicine and science, have yet to fund chiropractic research. Chiropractors, thus far, have had limited access to funding and research facilities, which would allow them to scientifically evaluate the effectiveness of chiropractic treatment.

The evaluation of chiropractic treatment is also difficult because of the diversity of chiropractic practices. Different chiropractors believe in a variety of ideologies and practice in many different ways. Some chiropractors feel that spinal manipulation should be used only for back pain, while others believe that it can benefit certain illnesses, such as high blood pressure and the common cold. Most chiropractors, however, treat only muscle and bone disorders, headaches, and back pain. Also, the majority of reputable chiropractors do not attempt to treat infectious diseases or other illnesses and are trained to spot these conditions and refer patients to a physician.

As medical costs continue to rise in the United States, chiropractic care may claim a valid place in the health care system. This cost factor is discussed in "A Low Cost Cure for Back Pain?" *Kiplinger's Personal Finance* (February 1992) and in "Does Anything Work for Back Pain?" *Consumer's Reports on Health* (February 1992). For additional reading on chiropractic and other alternative health care, see "Chiropractors," *Consumer Reports* (June 1994); "Promising New Ways to Solve Medical Problems," *New Choices* (November 1993); "Homeopathy: Too Much Ado About Nothing," *Skeptical Briefs* (December 1993); and "Unconventional Medicine in the United States," *The New England Journal of Medicine* (January 12, 1993).

CONTRIBUTORS
TO THIS VOLUME

EDITOR

EILEEN L. DANIEL, a registered dietitian, is an associate professor in the Department of Health Science at the State University of New York College at Brockport. She received a B.S. in nutrition and dietetics from the Rochester Institute of Technology in 1977, an M.S. in community health education from SUNY College at Brockport in 1978, and a Ph.D. in health education from the University of Oregon in 1986. A member of the Eta Sigma Gamma National Health Honor Society, the American Dietetics Association, the New York State Dietetics Society, and other professional and community organizations, she has authored or coauthored over 30 articles on issues of health, nutrition, and health education in such professional journals as the *Journal of Nutrition Education*, the *Journal of School Health*, and the *Journal of Health Education*.

STAFF

Mimi Egan   Publisher
Brenda S. Filley   Production Manager
Libra Ann Cusack   Typesetting Supervisor
Juliana Arbo   Typesetter
Lara Johnson   Graphics
Diane Barker   Proofreader
David Brackley   Copy Editor
David Dean   Administrative Editor
Richard Tietjen   Systems Manager

AUTHORS

BRUCE AMES, a genetic toxicologist, is a professor of biochemistry and molecular biology and the director of the National Institute of Environmental Health Sciences Center at the University of California, Berkeley, where he has been teaching since 1968. He has authored or coauthored over 300 publications, and he has received the General Motors Cancer Research Foundation Prize, the Tyler Prize for his work in environmental science, and the Gold Medal Award of the American Institute of Chemists.

MARC BARASCH is a journalist and a former editor of *New Age Journal*.

FRANCES M. BERG is a nutritionist and the founder, publisher, and editor of *Healthy Weight Journal*. She is also an adjunct professor in the Department of Community Medicine and Rural Health of the School of Medicine at the University of North Dakota in Grand Forks, North Dakota. She is the author of eight books, and she writes a weekly "Healthy Living" column, which is syndicated in over 50 newspapers.

DENNIS BERNSTEIN is an associate editor for *Pacific News Service* and a coproducer of KPFA's *Flashpoints* radio show.

ROBERTA BLOTNER is the director of the Institute on Alcohol and Drug Abuse at the City University of New York's John Jay College of Criminal Justice.

PAUL BRODEUR is an author and a staff writer for the *New Yorker*. He has published a number of books on asbestos, ozone depletion, and the link between electromagnetic fields and cancer, including *Currents of Death: Power Lines, Computer Terminals, and the Attempt to Cover Up Their Threat to Your Health* (Simon & Schuster, 1989) and *The Great Powerline Coverup: How the Utilities and the Government Are Trying to Hide the Cancer Hazard Posed by Electromagnetic Fields* (Little, Brown, 1993).

DANIEL CALLAHAN, a philosopher who specializes in biomedical ethics, is a cofounder and the president of the Hastings Center in Briarcliff Manor, New York. He received a Ph.D. in philosophy from Harvard University, and he is the author or editor of over 30 publications, including *The Troubled Dream of Life: Living With Mortality* (Simon & Schuster, 1993).

RICHARD A. COOPER, a physician, is the dean of the Medical College of Wisconsin and the director of its Health Policy Institute.

JASON DePARLE is a former editor of the *Washington Monthly*.

EZEKIEL J. EMANUEL is an assistant professor of medicine, social medicine, and clinical epidemiology at Harvard Medical School and a practicing oncologist at the Dana-Farber Cancer Institute, both in Boston, Massachusetts. He has published widely on advance directives and end-of-life care issues, euthanasia, the ethics of managed care, and the physician-patient relationship. He has received numerous awards, including the American Medical Association's Burroughs Wellcome Leadership Award and a Fulbright Scholarship.

LINDA L. EMANUEL is a physician and a researcher with the Division of Medical Ethics at Harvard Medical School in Boston, Massachusetts.

FAITH T. FITZGERALD is an internist and a professor of medicine at the University of California, Davis. She has written on a wide variety of topics in medicine, including protean disease states, medical education, physical diagnosis, and bioethics. She is a master of the American College of Physicians and sees patients in both hospital and clinical settings.

ROYCE FLIPPIN is a freelance health and science writer living in New York City. He writes on a variety of health issues, including physical psychology (how the body affects the mind) and exercise and fitness. He is also a former senior editor of *American Health: Fitness of Body and Mind*.

MICHAEL FUMENTO, a former AIDS analyst and attorney for the U.S. Commission on Civil Rights, is the science and economics reporter for *Investor's Business Daily*. He has written two books, *The Myth of Heterosexual AIDS* (New Republic Books, 1990) and *Science Under Siege* (William Morrow, 1993), and he is the author of numerous articles on AIDS, which have appeared in publications worldwide.

MARY GORDON is a novelist and a short story writer. She is the author of *Men and Angels* (Ballantine Books, 1986) and *The Other Side* (Viking Penguin, 1989).

HERBERT HENDIN is the executive director of the American Suicide Foundation in New York City and a professor of psychiatry at New York Medical College. He is a graduate of the Columbia University Psychoanalytic Center, where he also taught for 15 years. He recently completed a study of assisted suicide and euthansia in the United States and the Netherlands.

VICTOR HERBERT, a physician and an attorney, is the chair of the Committee to Strengthen Nutrition at the City University of New York's Mount Sinai School of Medicine. He is also the chief of the Hematology and Nutrition Research Service for the Bronx Veterans Affairs Medical Center in New York City.

KEVIN R. HOPKINS is an adjunct senior fellow of the Hudson Institute in Indianapolis, Indiana, a nonprofit research organization founded in 1961 to analyze and make recommendations about public policy for business and government executives as well as for the public at large.

MICHAEL F. JACOBSON is a microbiologist and the director of the Center for Science in the Public Interest, a health and nutrition consumer advocate group.

WILLIAM B. JOHNSTON is the vice president and a senior research fellow of the Hudson Institute, a nonprofit research organization founded in 1961 to analyze and make recommendations about public policy for business and government executives as well as for the public at large.

ANDREW G. KADAR is an attending physician at Cedars-Sinai Medical Center in Los Angeles, California, and a clinical instructor in the School of Medicine at the University of California, Los Angeles.

JOSEPH P. KANE, a Catholic priest, has served as chaplain at Rikers Island Jail for over 20 years. He has helped develop a curriculum on criminal justice issues for Jesuit high schools and a training manual for correctional chaplains. Father Kane is a coeditor of a collection of original articles about the criminal justice system entitled *Who Is the Prisoner?*

JEROME P. KASSIRER is a physician.

THEA KELLEY is a freelance journalist based in San Francisco.

GERALD KLERMAN (d. 1992) was a professor of psychiatry at Cornell Medical College. He also taught at Harvard University and Yale University, and he was the administrator for the Alcohol, Drug Abuse, and Mental Health Administration under President Jimmy Carter.

LESLIE LAURENCE is a health and medical reporter.

RICHARD LEVITON, a health journalist, is a senior writer for the *Yoga Journal*, published in Berkeley, California, and a regular contributor to *The Quest*. He has written over 150 feature articles, many of which have been reprinted in Canada, Germany, Australia, and many other countries throughout the world.

PATRICIA LONG is a journalist specializing in health issues.

GERALD W. LYNCH is the president of the John Jay College of Criminal Justice, a unit of the City University of New York.

NANCY F. McKENZIE is an author and the executive director of Health/PAC.

LAWRIE MOTT is a senior scientist with the Natural Resources Defense Council. Active on a variety of pesticide issues at both the state and national levels, she is a member of the advisory board for Americans for Safe Food, the board of directors of the Pesticide Education Center, and the advisory board of the Environmental Media Association. She was also appointed to the EPA administrator's Pesticide Advisory Committee and the University of California's Advisory Committee for Public Education on Food Safety.

NATIONAL TASK FORCE ON THE PREVENTION AND TREATMENT OF OBESITY of the National Institutes of Health in Bethesda, Maryland, was composed of nine scientific members from universities throughout the United States. Among their goals was to address concerns about the effects of weight cycling and to provide guidance on the risk-to-benefit ratio of attempts at weight loss, given current scientific knowledge.

JAMES NOLAN, a physician and a professor of medicine, is the chair of the Department of Medicine at the State University of New York College at Buffalo and the president of the Association of Professors of Medicine.

TIMOTHY E. QUILL is an associate professor of medicine and psychiatry at the University of Rochester in Rochester, New York, and the chair of the university's Program for Biopsychosocial Studies. He is the author of numerous publications on physician-patient communication and end-of-life decision making, including *Death and Dignity: Making Choices and Taking Charge* (W. W. Norton, 1993).

JOANN ELLISON RODGERS is a journalist.

J. NEIL SCHULMAN is a novelist, a screenwriter, and a journalist living in Los Angeles, California. He has taught a graduate course for the New School for Social Research, and he has lectured at Northwood University. He is the author of two award-winning novels, and his *Los Angeles Times* article "If Gun Laws Work, Why Are We Afraid?" won the James Madison Award. His latest book is *Stopping Power: Why 70 Million Americans Own Guns* (Synapse-Centurion, 1994).

KAREN SNYDER is a pesticide researcher in the San Francisco office of the Natural Resources Defense Council, which addresses almost every major environmental issue facing the United States, including air and water pollution, energy use and development, wilderness preservation, nuclear armament, and control of toxic substances.

IRWIN M. STELZER studies economic and regulatory policy issues as the director of Regulatory Policy Studies at the American Enterprise Institute in Washington, D.C., a privately funded public policy research organization. The U.S. economic and political columnist for London's *Sunday Times*, the *Boston Herald*, and Australia's *Courier Mail*, he has written and lectured on economic and policy developments in the United States and Britain, particularly as they relate to privatization and competition policy.

JACOB SULLUM is the managing editor of *Reason* magazine.

ELLEN SWITZER is a freelance writer who specializes in medicine, psychology, and law.

GARY TAUBES is a freelance journalist in New York City. He is also a contributing editor for *Discover* and a correspondent for *Science*. He is the winner of the 1995 American Institute of Physics' Science Writing Award.

GEORGE E. VAILLANT is the director of adult development at Harvard University. He received an M.D. from Harvard Medical School in 1955, and he has taught at Tufts University, Harvard Medical School, and Dartmouth Medical School. A recipient of the Jellinck Prize for alcoholism research, he is also the author of *The Wisdom of the Ego* (Harvard University Press, 1993).

BETH WEINHOUSE is a health and medical reporter.

RICK WEISS is a staff writer for *Health* magazine.

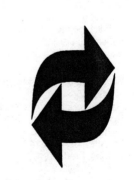

INDEX